This book presents a new, "triarchic" theory of human intelligence that goes beyond IQ in its conceptualization and implications for assessment. The theory has three parts. The first deals with the relations between intelligence and experience. It describes the role that intelligence plays at various points in our continuum of experience with tasks and situations, from the time we first encounter them to the time they have become thoroughly familiar. The second deals with the relations between intelligence and the external world. It describes the interplay between intelligence and the contexts in which it is exercised and, indeed, defined. The third deals with the relations between intelligence and the internal world of the individual. It describes the mental mechanisms that underlie what we consider to be "intelligent performance."

Robert J. Sternberg begins by sketching the history of intelligence research. He then outlines the three parts of the theory and adduces supporting evidence, including evidence from studies of "practical" as well as "academic" intelligence. He considers the issues raised by exceptional intelligence and by intelligence testing.

His conclusions will be of interest to all those concerned with intelligence, its development and its measurement.

Beyond IQ

Beyond IQ

A triarchic theory of human intelligence

ROBERT J. STERNBERG

Yale University

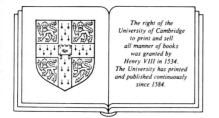

The right of the
University of Cambridge
to print and sell
all manner of books
was granted by
Henry VIII in 1534.
The University has printed
and published continuously
since 1584.

CAMBRIDGE UNIVERSITY PRESS

Cambridge

New York   New Rochelle   Melbourne   Sydney

Published by the Press Syndicate of the University of Cambridge
The Pitt Building, Trumpington Street, Cambridge CB2 1RP
32 East 57th Street, New York, NY 10022, USA
10 Stamford Road, Oakleigh, Melbourne 3166, Australia

© Cambridge University Press 1985

First published 1985
Reprinted 1985, 1986, 1987

Printed in the United States of America

Library of Congress Cataloging in Publication Data
Sternberg, Robert J.
Beyond IQ.
Includes bibliographical references and indexes.
1. Intellect.   2. Intelligence tests.   I. Title.
II. Title: Beyond I.Q.
BF431.S7378   1985   153.9   84-11322
ISBN 0 521 26254 2 hard covers
ISBN 0 521 27891 0 paperback

This book is dedicated to that triarchy of mentors and role models who have been most influential in shaping my professional values, standards, and ways of thinking over the years:

GORDON BOWER   WENDELL GARNER   ENDEL TULVING

Contents

Preface

The general goal of this book is to present a new, "triarchic" theory of human intelligence. I believe the theory goes beyond many previous theories in its scope and answers a broader array of questions about intelligence than has been answered in the past by most single theories, including my own former componential theory. Indeed, the theory is to some extent an outgrowth of the componential theory: That theory is now one of three subtheories that comprise the triarchic theory.

The first subtheory, a contextual subtheory, specifies how intelligent behavior is defined in large part by the sociocultural context in which this behavior takes place. Contextually intelligent behavior is specified to involve (a) adaptation to a present environment, (b) selection of a more nearly optimal environment than the one the individual presently inhabits, or (c) shaping of the present environment so as to render it a better fit to one's skills, interests, or values. The normal course of intelligent functioning in the everyday world entails adaptation to the environment; when the environment does not fit one's values, aptitudes, or interests, one may attempt to shape the environment so as to achieve a better person–environment fit; when shaping fails, an attempt may be made to select a new environment that provides a better fit. Alternatively, one may attempt to shape the old environment when selection fails. What is involved in adaptation, selection, and shaping can be determined, to some extent, by examining people's conceptions of intelligence within a given sociocultural milieu. The "implicit" theories of persons thus derived can then serve as a framework for explicit theorizing about intelligence. Contextual theories, in general, and this one, in particular, do not place sufficient constraints upon behavior in order fully to characterize what constitutes intelligent behavior. Hence, a contextual theory can serve only as a subtheory of a full theory of intelligence.

The second subtheory, an experiential subtheory, posits that for a given task or situation, contextually appropriate behavior is not equally "intelligent" at all points along the continuum of experience with that behavior or class of behaviors. Rather, one's intelligence is best demonstrated when one is (a) confronted with a relatively (but not totally) novel task or situation or is (b) in the process of automatizing performance on a given task or in a given situation. These two facets interact to some extent: Efficacious automatization of processing allows allocation of additional resources to the processing of novelty in the environment; conversely, efficacious adaptation to novelty allows automatization to occur earlier in one's experience with new tasks and situations. Thus, one cannot simply classify a task as either requiring intelligence or not requiring intelligence. The extent to which it requires intelligence depends upon the point in an individual's experiential continuum at which the task is encountered. The same holds true for situations. Although this subtheory constrains the contextual subtheory in stating at what points along the experiential continuum contextually appropriate behavior is more and less intelligent, it does not specify the mental structures or mechanisms involved in intelligent behavior.

The third subtheory, a componential subtheory, specifies the structures and mechanisms that underlie intelligent behavior. Contextually appropriate behavior emitted at the relevant points in the experiential continuum is intelligent as a function of the extent to which it involves certain kinds of mental processes: Metacomponents control one's information processing and enable one to monitor and later evaluate it; performance components execute the plans constructed by the metacomponents; knowledge-acquisition components selectively encode and combine new information and selectively compare new information to old information, so as to allow learning of new information to take place. This subtheory thus specifies the cognitive processes involved in adaptation to, selection of, and shaping of environments. The componential subtheory completes the triarchy of specifications that defines the extent to which a given behavior is *intelligent*.

In sum, the contextual subtheory relates intelligence to the external world of the individual; it addresses the questions of *what* behaviors are intelligent for whom and of *where* these behaviors are intelligent. The subtheory specifies the potential set of *contents* for behaviors that can be characterized as intelligent. The experiential subtheory relates intelligence to both the internal and external worlds of the individual; it answers the question of *when* behavior is intelligent. This subtheory specifies the relation between intelligence as exhibited on a task or in a situation, on the one hand, and *amount of experience* with the task or situation, on the other. The componential subtheory relates intelligence to the internal world of the individual; it answers the question of *how* intelligent behavior is generated. In particular, the subtheory specifies the potential set of *mental mechanisms* that underlie intelligent behavior, regardless of the particular behavioral contents. The three subtheories, taken together, can be used to understand individual differences, or *who* is intelligent. I hope that I will provide in the course of the explication of the subtheories sufficient evidence to establish *why* it is that certain behavior can be considered, on a theoretical basis, to be more intelligent than other behavior.

The first, contextual subtheory, is "relativistic" with respect to both individuals and the sociocultural settings in which they live. What constitutes an intelligent act may differ from one person to another. The second, experiential subtheory, is relativistic only with respect to the points at which novelty and automatization are relevant for a given individual. But the relevance of the two facets to intelligence is claimed to be universal. The third subtheory is universal: Although individuals may differ in what mental mechanisms they apply to a given task or situation, the potential set of mental mechanisms underlying intelligence is viewed to be the same across all individuals and sociocultural settings. Thus, the vehicles by which one might wish to measure intelligence (test contents, modes of presentation, formats for test items, etc.) will probably need to differ across sociocultural groups and possibly even within such groups; but the underlying mechanisms to be measured and their functions in dealing with novelty and in becoming automatized do not differ across individuals or groups.

The book has three specific goals as well as the general goal noted at the beginning.

First, it presents the first full statement of the triarchic theory. Prior to this book, the componential subtheory was all I had to offer by way of a theory of human intelligence. But as the years have gone by, I have become increasingly aware of the incompleteness of this subtheory as an account of human intelligence. The present theory remedies some (I hope, many) of the incompletenesses of the componential account.

Second, the book serves to update the presentation of my theorizing since the publication of my 1977 book, *Intelligence, Information Processing, and Analogical Reasoning: The Componential Analysis of Human Abilities.* This earlier book is now out of date: My subsequent theory and empirical research have been presented in a series of articles and book contributions that have followed the earlier book. The present book pulls together and integrates under the rubric of the triarchic theory the material that until now has been presented only in scattered fashion.

Third, the book is intended to serve as a metatheoretical statement of the form theories of intelligence might take in the future, as well as an initial statement of a theory that takes this form. I believe that previous theories, such as the componential one, have tended to address only very limited aspects of human intelligence. For whatever value they may have had as theories of *cognition*, they have been of lesser value, because of their incompleteness, as full-scale theories of *intelligence*. I believe the present theory goes beyond many past theories in both the breadth of questions addressed and the depth of the answers proposed.

The book is divided into five parts comprising twelve chapters, which in combination give a thorough presentation of the triarchic theory and existing tests of it.

Part I consists of just Chapter 1, "Conceptions of intelligence." This introductory chapter discusses the history of theory and research on intelligence and places the triarchic theory in a historical context of theories of human intelligence.

Part II, on subtheories of the triarchic theory, consists of three chapters. Chapter 2, "The context of intelligence," presents my contextual subtheory and describes why intelligence should be understood in part in terms of the individual's attempt to adapt to, select, and shape real-world environments. Chapter 3, "Experience and intelligence," presents an experiential subtheory that places certain constraints upon the contextual subtheory. The subtheory holds that two facets of contextually appropriate behavior, response to novelty and automatization of information processing, are part of what makes such behavior "intelligent." Chapter 4, "Components of intelligence," presents my componential subtheory, which specifies the mental structures and mechanisms involved in intelligent behavior. It thus completes the set of constraints that needs to be applied to the contextual subtheory, as well as to the experiential subtheory, in order to have a reasonably complete theory of intelligence.

Part III, presenting tests of the triarchic theory, describes the theories of cognitive functioning nested under the triarchic theory, especially the componential subtheory, and presents the results of numerous tests of these theories of cognitive functioning. This part of the book is divided into five chapters. The organization of these chapters into sets of chapters dealing with fluid, crystallized, and practical aspects of intelligence derives from the contextually derived implicit theory of intelligence presented in the preceding part of the book. Chapters 5 and 6 deal with "fluid" aspects of intelligent functioning. Chapter 5, "Fluid abilities: inductive reasoning," presents a componential theory of inductive reasoning and tests of this theory. Chapter 6, "Fluid abilities: deductive reasoning," presents a componential theory of deductive reasoning and tests of this theory. Chapters 7 and 8 deal with "crystallized" aspects of intelligent functioning, but also with the question of how fluid abilities give rise to crystallized ones. Chapter 7, "Crystallized intelligence: acquisition of verbal comprehension," describes a theory of acquisition of verbal information (and particularly vocabulary) from context and relates acquisition processes to present levels of knowledge. Chapter 8, "Crystallized intelligence: theory of information processing in real-time verbal comprehension," describes a theory of how verbal information, and especially vocabulary, is processed in real time. Chapter 9, "Social and practical intelligence," extends the triarchic theory to more worldly domains. It presents limited theories of adaptive functioning and tests of the theories as they apply to social and practical adaptation in the world.

Part IV, discussing some implications of the triarchic theory, contains two chapters. Chapter 10, "Exceptional intelligence," deals with the implications of the theory for understanding intellectual giftedness and retardation. Chapter 11, "Implications of the triarchic theory for intelligence testing," views current intelligence tests from the perspective of the triarchic theory, and suggests how such tests might be changed.

Part V, the concluding remarks, consists just of Chapter 12, "Integration and implications," which discusses some general issues regarding intelligence that arise out of the theory and the tests of the theory that have been conducted.

In sum, I present in this book a new triarchic theory of human intelligence and the evidence that supports the theory. Although this theory, like every other theory of intelligence or any other psychological construct, will have only a limited half-life, I hope that the theory helps us better understand the nature of intelligence and is useful in guiding research on intelligence in productive directions.

Many people have contributed immeasurably to the development of the ideas presented in this book. In particular, I must thank the present and past members of my research group at Yale both for their valuable collaborations in the research described here and for their continuous influence on, contributions to, and critiques of my thinking. Because of their tremendous contributions, over the eight years I have been at Yale, to the work presented in this book, I would be doing them a great disservice not to mention them individually by name: Cindy Berg, Liz Charles, Barbara Conway, Janet Davidson, Cathryn Downing, Mike Gardner, Bob Greene, Marty Guyote, Danny Kaye, Jerry Ketron, Maria Lasaga, Diana Marr, Tim McNamara, Georgia Nigro, Jan Powell, Bathsheva Rifkin, Brian Ross, Bill Salter, Miriam Schustack, Louise Spear, Judi Suben, Sheldon Tetewsky, Roger Tourangeau, Meg Turner, Rick Wagner, Evelyn Weil. Janet Davidson and Bob Greene had the kindness and patience to read through and comment upon the entire book manuscript, for which I am especially grateful. My students and staff have in no way been "junior componential analysts" or "junior triarchic theorists." To the contrary, they have worked highly independently, bear major responsibility for many of the ideas in our joint research, and have disagreed with me at least as often as they have agreed. I owe them a tremendous debt.

I also owe an equally great debt to my family and friends, who have supported and put up with me over the years, and to the agencies that have supported my research: the National Science Foundation, the Office of Naval Research, the Army Research Institute, the Spencer Foundation, and the Ministry for the Development of Intelligence of the Government of Venezuela. I am particularly indebted to the Office of Naval Research, which has provided by far the "lion's share" of support, and to Marshall Farr, who has been my primary contract monitor for this organization. Finally, I am grateful to my faculty colleagues at Yale, for their contribution to the congenial atmosphere in which I have worked, and to my teachers and advisers, who have over the years helped shape me as a professional psychologist. This book is dedicated to three of these teachers who have been particularly important in my professional development.

R. J. S.

Part I

Introduction

Part I contains just a single chapter, "Conceptions of intelligence," presenting a review of past and present ideas about the nature of human intelligence. The chapter discusses two kinds of theories of intelligence: explicit and implicit. Explicit theories are the formal accounts of intelligence that are formulated by psychologists; implicit theories are the informal notions about intelligence that we carry around with us. Whereas explicit theories form the basis for most empirical research, implicit theories form the basis for our daily actions based upon our beliefs regarding the nature of intelligence. Because implicit theories, in a sense, give rise to explicit theories, it is important to understand both kinds of theories, how they are interrelated, and how they evolve. All of these issues are discussed in the introductory chapter.

1 Conceptions of intelligence

Intelligence is among the most elusive of concepts. Certainly, there are few other concepts that have been conceptualized in as many different ways. The various conceptions of intelligence that have been proposed have usually sounded related to each other; unfortunately, the nature and extent of the interrelations remain fuzzy. In this chapter, I discuss some of the alternative conceptions of intelligence that have been proposed in the past and attempt to clarify the nature of their interrelations.

Accounts of intelligence are of two basic kinds: explicit theories and implicit theories. Each of these kinds of theories will now be considered in turn.

Explicit theories of intelligence

Explicit theories of intelligence are based, or at least tested, on data collected from people performing tasks presumed to measure intelligent functioning. For example, a battery of mental ability tests might be administered to a large group of people and the data from these tests analyzed in order to isolate the proposed sources of intelligent behavior in test performance. Although investigators proposing explicit theories might disagree as to the nature of these sources of intelligence – which might be proposed to be factors, components, schemata, or some other kind of psychological construct – they would agree that the data base from which the proposed constructs should be isolated ought to consist (directly or indirectly) of performance on tasks requiring intelligent functioning.

Explicit theories of intelligence come in a variety of forms. I will discuss here the two forms of theorizing that have been the most influential in the psychology of human intelligence – differential theorizing and cognitive theorizing. Although these two views have probably been the most influential ones in North American and British conceptions of the nature of intelligence, they are not the only views that have been advanced (see, e.g., Hebb, 1949, and Hendrickson, 1982, for physiological views and Piaget, 1972, for a

3

genetic – epistemological view). These other views are not discussed here, but descriptions of these and other views can be found elsewhere (see, e.g., Dockrell, 1970; Eysenck, 1982; Resnick, 1976; Sternberg, 1982c).

Differential theories of the nature of human intelligence

Differential (or psychometric) theories of intelligence, so called because of their bases in the study of individual differences among people, have in common (with rare exceptions) their attempt to understand intelligence in terms of a set of underlying abilities – for example, verbal ability, reasoning ability, and the like. These underlying abilities are identified through a mathematical technique called factor analysis. This technique starts with a matrix of intercorrelations (or covariances) for a set of tests and identifies "latent" sources of underlying variation in test scores that are theorized to give rise to the observable variation in test scores. These latent sources of individual differences are called factors. Thus, it is proposed that individual differences in performance on intelligence tests can be decomposed into individual differences in these factors, each of which is posited to represent a distinct human ability.

Given that the large majority of differential theories have in common the use of factors as a basis for understanding intelligence, one might wonder how the differential theories differ from one another. The primary differences are in terms of (a) the number of factors posited by the theory and (b) the geometrical arrangement of the factors with respect to one another. Consider how number and geometrical arrangement can form the bases for alternative theories of intelligence.

Variation in number of factors. Differential theorists vary greatly in the number of factors they purport to be important for understanding intelligent behavior. Indeed, the range in numbers of factors for major theories is from 1 to 150.

At the lower end, Spearman (1927) proposed that intelligence comprises two kinds of factors, a general factor and specific factors. The ability represented by the general factor permeates performance on all intellectual tasks; each of the abilities represented by the specific factors permeates only a single task, and hence these abilities are not of much psychological interest. Thus, there is just one factor of major psychological interest, the general factor, or g, as it has often been called. Spearman made two (not necessarily mutually exclusive) famous proposals regarding the nature of g. One proposal was that individual differences in g might be understood in terms of differences in the levels of mental energy individuals could bring to intellectual task performance. The other proposal was that individual differences in g could be understood in terms of differences in people's abilities to utilize three "qualitative principles of cognition" (Spearman, 1923): apprehension of experience, eduction of relations, and eduction of correlates. In order to understand what each of these three principles represents, consider an analogy of the form A : B :: C : ?, for example, LAWYER : CLIENT :: DOCTOR : ?. Apprehension of experience refers to encoding (perceiving and understanding) each of the given terms of the analogy. Eduction of relations refers to inference of the relation between the first two analogy terms, here, LAWYER and CLIENT. Eduction of correlates refers to application of the inferred principle to a new domain, here, applying the rule inferred from LAWYER to CLIENT so as to produce a completion for DOCTOR : ?. The best answer to this analogy would presumably be PATIENT. Given that analogies directly embody these principles, it is not surprising that Spearman (1923, 1927) and many others subsequently have found analogies such as the one above to be among the best available measures of *g*. (See Sternberg, 1977b, for a review of relevant literature.)

In a more "middle-of-the-road" position, one finds Thurstone (1938), who proposed that intelligence comprises roughly seven "primary mental abilities." Consider the identity of each of these abilities and how it is commonly measured:

1. *Verbal comprehension.* This ability is typically measured by tests of vocabulary (including both synonyms and antonyms) and by tests of reading comprehension skills.

2. *Verbal fluency.* This ability is typically measured by tests that require rapid production of words. For example, the individual might be asked to generate as quickly as possible, and within a limited period of time, as many words as he or she can think of that begin with the letter *d*.

3. *Number.* This ability is typically measured by arithmetic word problems where there is some emphasis upon both computation and reasoning, but relatively little emphasis upon extent of prior knowledge.

4. *Spatial visualization.* This ability is typically measured by tests requiring mental manipulation of symbols or geometric designs. For example, the individual might be shown a picture of a geometric design in some degree of angular rotation, followed by a set of pictures in various orientations that are either identical (except for degree of rotation) to the original object or else are mirror images of the original objects. The individual would have to indicate whether each item is the same as the target or instead is a mirror image.

5. *Memory.* This ability is typically measured by a test of recall-memory for words or sentences or by paired-associates recall of names with pictures of people. A typical paired-associates test would present people with a set of pictures paired with the names of the people they depict. The people would be given some fixed amount of time to study the set of pictures and names.

After time was called, the people would be presented with the pictures and be asked to provide the name corresponding to each picture.

6. *Reasoning.* This ability is typically measured by tests such as analogies (e.g., LAWYER : CLIENT :: DOCTOR : ?) and series completions (e.g., 2, 4, 7, 11, ?).

7. *Perceptual speed.* This ability is typically measured by tests requiring rapid recognition of symbols – for example, rapid crossing-out of *l*'s that are embedded in a string of letters.

At the upper extreme in terms of number of proposed factors is Guilford (1967; Guilford & Hoepfner, 1971), who at one time proposed that intelligence comprises 120 distinct factors and has more recently increased this number to 150 (Guilford, 1982). According to Guilford, every mental task involves three ingredients: an operation, a content, and a product. There are five kinds of operations: cognition, memory, divergent production, convergent production, and evaluation. There are five kinds of contents: visual, auditory, symbolic, semantic, and behavioral. And there are six kinds of products: units, classes, relations, systems, transformations, and implications. Since the subcategories are independently defined, they are multiplicative, so that there are $5 \times 5 \times 6 = 150$ different mental abilities.

Guilford and his associates have devised tests that measure many of the factors posited by the model. As of 1982, Guilford claims to have demonstrated the existence of 105 of the 150 possible factors. Guilford (1982) has also made clear that, although the 150 factors are logically independent, they can be psychologically dependent in the sense of being intercorrelated. Consider how just a few of these abilities are measured. Cognition of visual relations (called cognition of figural relations in the 1967 version of the model) is measured by tests such as figure analogies or matrices. Memory for semantic relations is measured by presenting to examinees a series of relationships, such as "Gold is more valuable than iron," and then testing retention in a multiple-choice format. Evaluation of symbolic units is measured by same–different tests, in which subjects are presented with pairs of numbers or letters that are identical or different in minor details. Subjects are then asked to mark each pair as "same" or "different."

Variation in geometric structure of factors. As noted earlier, two models positing the same number of factors – and even the same contents for factors – might still differ because of their positing of different geometric arrangements of these factors. The four best-known structures are an unordered arrangement, a cubic arrangement, a hierarchical arrangement, and a radex arrangement.

Unordered arrangements consist of lists of factors all of which are asserted to be equal in importance to each other. Thurstone's (1938) primary mental abilities might be seen as a good example of this kind of arrangement. Thurstone suggested simply that intelligence could be understood in terms of seven factors. They are not ordered in any particular way: Any permutation of the list is as valid as any other.

The best-known "cubic" theorist is Guilford. Guilford (1982) has represented the structure of intellect as a large cube composed of 150 smaller cubes. Each dimension of the cube corresponds to one of the three categories (operation, content, product), and each of the 150 possible combinations of the three categories forms one of the smaller cubes.

Hierarchical arrangements are probably most popular in the contemporary differential literature on intelligence. According to this kind of view, abilities are not of equal importance. Rather, certain abilities are more global, and hence more important, than others. Spearman's (1927) factorial model, with a general factor and less important specific factors, might be seen as the original hierarchical model, although it is not clear that Spearman thought of his theory primarily in this way. Holzinger (1938) elaborated upon Spearman's point of view by suggesting that there exist group factors intermediate in generality between the general factor and the specific factors. These group factors permeate performance on some class of tasks (and in any case, more than one task), but are not involved in performance of all mental tasks in a given test battery. Burt (1940) proposed a five-level hierarchical model, with the "human mind" at the top, the "relations level" right below it, associations below that, perceptions below associations, and sensation at the bottom of the hierarchy. Vernon (1971) proposed a more sophisticated hierarchical model, suggesting that g could be decomposed into two broad group factors, verbal–educational ability and practical–mechanical ability. He further proposed that these broad group factors could be further decomposed into narrower group factors, although this further decomposition is of less interest in his theory.

Finally, Guttman (1965) has proposed a radex structure for intelligence. A radex can be thought of as a circle. Each test found on intelligence test batteries can be placed somewhere in the circle. Tests nearer the center of the circle measure abilities more "central" to intelligence. Thus, the purest measures of intelligence would be at the center of the circle, and the least pure measures would be at the periphery of the circle. Arrayed around the interior of the circle are differing kinds of task contents and required processes – for example, verbal tasks, numerical tasks, and geometric–pictorial tasks.

Critique. In sum, differential or psychometric theories of intelligence differ primarily in terms of the numbers of factors they posit and in terms of the geometric arrangements of these factors. On their face, the theories seem quite different. It is not clear that at a deeper level these differences are as consequential as they initially would seem. Indeed, the amount of agreement among these theories could be seen as substantially greater than the amount of disagreement.

First, the theories share common metatheoretical assumptions. All assume that intelligence can be understood in terms of latent sources of individual differences or "factors." These factors are believed to provide, in some sense, a "map" of the mind. Because the factors are identified on the basis of observed individual differences in mental-test performance, all of the theories assume that the primary basis for identifying the dimensions of intelligence ought to be observed individual differences. Also, the kinds of tests that have served as the bases for measuring these individual differences have been quite similar. All are in the tradition of Binet and Simon (1905, 1908), although they differ in the details of exactly what skills they measure.

Second, the alternative theories are, in many cases, mathematically nearly equivalent. One might wonder how such different factor structures could result from essentially the same mathematical technique, factor analysis, being applied to roughly comparable sets of subjects taking roughly comparable sets of tests. The answer lies largely in the placement of axes in a "factor space." Factors can be represented in a space, where each factor is a dimension in the space. When a factor analysis is performed, the locations of points (tests) in the factor space are fixed, but the locations of the factor axes are not. In other words, it is possible to have many – indeed, infinite – orientations of factor axes. It turns out that many of the theories differ from one another primarily in terms of orientation of the factor axes in the factor space and hence are (roughly) equivalent mathematically. From this point of view, the different theories say the same things in different ways. Recent cognitive – experimental research suggests that the various factorial theories can all be mapped into a common set of information-processing components of task performance (Sternberg, 1980c, 1980f). In other words, no matter what factor structure one uses, the basic processes contributing to the factors are the same. This point of view will be elaborated later in the book.

Third and finally, some of the differences among theories appear, on closer examination, to be ones of emphasis rather than of substance. For example, Spearman's and Thurstone's theories appear to be radically different. But by the end of his career, Spearman was forced to concede the existence of group factors; indeed, he even collaborated with Holzinger on the development of a theory that encompassed group factors as well as the general and specific ones. Similarly, Thurstone was forced, by the end of his career, to acknowledge that a higher-order general factor existed that in some sense incorporated the primary mental abilities. The primary evidence for such a higher-order factor is that the primary mental abilities are not statistically independent, but rather are intercorrelated with each other: People who tend to be high in one ability tend to be high in others as well, and people who tend to be low in one ability tend to be low in others as well. When one factors these factors, one obtains a general, higher-order factor. The main difference between Spearman and Thurstone may thus have been in the emphases they placed on higher- versus lower-order factors. Spearman emphasized the former, Thurstone the latter. Humphreys (1962) and Jensen (1970) have provided excellent accounts of how hierarchical models can be formed that incorporate the ideas of factors both at the level of Spearman's general factor and at the level of Thurstone's primary mental abilities.

There have been what at times have seemed like unending debates over the merits of factor analysis as a means for uncovering the nature of intelligence. (See, e.g., Burt, 1940; Eysenck, 1953, 1967; Humphreys, 1962; Royce, 1963, 1979; Sternberg, 1977b, 1979b.) I have come to view these debates as misconceived, in large part because it really does not make sense to evaluate a methodology independent of its use. To the extent one's goal is to isolate rather global, structural constellations of individual differences in test performance, factor analysis certainly can be useful. As so often happens with multivariate methods, this method has been subjected at times to fairly serious misuse (cf. Guilford, 1952; McNemar, 1951; Sternberg, 1977b, for discussions of some of these misuses). When a method is subjected to misuse, it is tempting to blame some intrinsic property of the method rather than to blame the misusers. To the extent that there has been a generalized and serious misrepresentation, it is perhaps in claiming too much for what factor analysis has told us about intelligence. More attention should have been paid to a careful accounting of just what questions about intelligence factor analysis can and cannot answer (see Sternberg, 1980f). But the same could be said for many other methods as well. When a method is first applied to the study of a problem, it is quite natural for overly strong claims to be made: The limitations of the method simply have not yet become clear. But over the years, these limitations do become more clear, and it is necessary to pay attention to both strengths and weaknesses of the method as applied to various kinds of problems. In the case of factor analysis, it was certainly useful in providing initial structural models, and recent uses of confirmatory factor analysis (e.g., Frederiksen, 1982; Geiselman, Woodward, & Beatty, 1982) demonstrate that factor analysis will continue to play an important role in understanding the nature of intelligence. We even have, at this time, some fairly clear notions as to what this role is likely to be, but a full discussion of this topic is beyond the scope of this book.

Cognitive theories of the nature of human intelligence

Cognitive (or information-processing) theories of intelligence have in common their attempts to understand human intelligence in terms of the mental

processes that contribute to cognitive task performance. A primary difference among views is in the level of cognitive functioning that they emphasize
in attempting to seek this understanding. At one extreme, there exist investigators who have proposed to understand intelligence in terms of sheer speed
of information processing and who have used the most simple tasks they
could devise in order to measure pure speed uncontaminated by other variables. At the other extreme, there exist investigators who have studied very
complex forms of problem solving and who have deemphasized or dis-
counted speed of functioning in mental processing. In general, greater emphasis upon speed of processing has been associated with investigators studying the simpler forms of information processing, whereas greater emphasis
upon accuracy of and strategies in information processing has been associated with investigators studying the more complex forms of processing.
Consider a sampling of the range of levels of processing that have been
studied. Again, no claim is made for the completeness of this survey, although it does seem to be fairly representative of the kinds of work that have
been done.

Pure speed. Proponents of the notion that individual differences in intelligence can be traced back to differences in sheer speed of information processing have tended to use simple reaction time and related tasks in order to
make their point. In a simple-reaction-time paradigm, the subject is required
simply to make a single overt response as quickly as possible following
presentation of a stimulus. This paradigm has been widely used, ever since
the days of Galton, as a measure of intelligence (Berger, 1982). Although
Galton (1883) and Cattell (1890) were strong supporters of the importance of
sheer speed in intellectual functioning, the levels of correlation obtained
between measures of simple reaction time and various standard measures of
intelligence, none of which are perfect in themselves (e.g., IQ test scores,
school grades, and the like), have been rather weak. Wissler (1901) obtained
correlations close to zero, as did Lemmon (1927). Lunneborg (1977) obtained correlations with eight psychometric measures of intelligence ranging
from -.17 to -.42, with a median of -.38. (Negative correlations would be
expected because longer reaction times are presumed to be associated with
lower levels of intelligent performance.) In my view, some of the most
trustworthy results are those attributable to Jensen (1980, 1982), who has
reported correlations for two samples: One of the correlations was in the
middle -.20s, the other around .10. Clearly, if there is any relationship at all
between measures of pure speed and of psychometrically measured intelligence, the relationship is a weak one.

Choice speed. A complication of the above view is that intelligence derives
not from simple speed of processing, but rather from speed in making

choices or decisions to simple stimuli. In a typical "choice-reaction-time" paradigm, the subject is presented with one of two or more possible stimuli, each requiring a different overt response. The subject has to choose the correct response as rapidly as possible following stimulus presentation. Correlations with psychometric measures of intelligence have been somewhat higher than those obtained for simple reaction time (Berger, 1982). Lemmon (1927) found a correlation of -.25 between choice reaction time and measured intelligence. Lunneborg (1977) found variable correlations. In one study, correlations ranged from -.28 to -.55, with a median of -.40. In a second study, however, correlations were trivial. Jensen (1982) reported a correlation of -.3 for one sample, but a correlation close to zero for another. Lally and Nettelbeck (1977) obtained a correlation of -.56, but in a sample with a very wide range of IQs (57 – 130); such samples tend to boost correlations.

An interesting finding in the research both of Jensen (1979, 1982) and of Lally and Nettelbeck (1977) is that the correlation between choice reaction time and IQ tends to increase with the number of stimulus – response choices involved in the task. In fact, these investigators found a roughly linear relation between the level of correlation obtained and the log to the base 2 of the number of choices (bits) in the task, at least through eight choices (three bits). But the correlations for typical ranges of subject ability nevertheless seem to peak at slightly over the -.4 level. Thus, increasing the number of choices in a choice-reaction-time task seems to increase correlation with IQ, but the task still is a long way off from providing what would seem to be a causal account of individual differences in psychometrically measured IQ.

Speed of lexical access. Hunt (1978, 1980) has proposed that individual differences in verbal intelligence may be understood largely in terms of differences among individuals in speed of access to lexical information in long-term memory. According to this view, individuals who can access information more quickly are able to profit more per unit time of presented information and hence to perform better on a variety of tasks, especially verbal ones. Hunt, Frost, and Lunneborg (1973) and Hunt, Lunneborg, and Lewis (1975) initiated a paradigm for testing this theory that makes use of the Posner and Mitchell (1967) letter-comparison task. Subjects are presented with pairs of letters - such as *AA, Aa,* or *Ab* - that may be the same or different either physically or in name. For example, *AA* contains two letters that are the same both physically and in name; *Aa* contains two letters that are the same in name only; and *Ab* contains two letters that are the same neither in name nor in physical appearance. The subject's task is to indicate as rapidly as possible whether the two letters are a match: In one condition, subjects indicate whether or not the letters are a physical match; in another condition, the same subjects indicate whether or not the letters are a name match. The measure of interest is each subject's average name-match time minus physical-match time. This measure is taken to be an index of the time it takes to access lexical information in long-term memory. Physical-match time is subtracted from name-match time in order to obtain a relatively pure measure of lexical access time that is uncontaminated by sheer speed of responding. Thus, whereas those who study simple reaction time are particularly interested in sheer speed of responding, Hunt and his colleagues do what they can to subtract out this element.

A number of investigators have used this paradigm as a basis for understanding individual differences in verbal intelligence (e.g., Hunt et al., 1975; Keating & Bobbitt, 1978; Jackson & McClelland, 1979). Unlike the simple- and choice-reaction-time tasks, the lexical-access task yields a remarkably consistent picture with respect to its relationship to measured intelligence: Correlations with scores on verbal IQ tests are typically about -.3. Thus, lexical-access time seems to be related at some level to intellectual performance. But again, it is obviously, at best, one contributor to individual differences in what is measured by standard psychometric IQ tests (which are themselves highly imperfect measures of intelligence, broadly defined): The correlation is too weak to make any strong statement regarding the direction of causality.

Speed of reasoning processes. A number of investigators have emphasized the kinds of higher-order processing involved in reasoning in their attempts to understand intelligence (e.g., Pellegrino & Glaser, 1980, 1982; Sternberg, 1977a, 1977b; Sternberg & Gardner, 1983; Whitely, 1980). Following in the tradition of Spearman's qualitative "principles of cognition," these investigators have sought to understand individual differences in intelligence in terms of individuals' differential processing of information in tasks such as analogies, series completions, syllogisms, and the like. There have been two main emphases in this work, namely, on performance processes and executive processes. This work will be summarized now, and more will be said about it later.

Investigators seeking to understand intelligence in terms of performance processes seek to discover the processes individuals use in problem solving from the time they first see a problem to the time they respond to the problem. Consider, for example, the widely studied analogy item. In a typical theory of analogical reasoning, performance on the analogy item is decomposed into component processes such as *inferring* the relation between the first two terms of the analogy, *mapping* the higher-order relation that connects the first half of the analogy to the second half, and *applying* the relation inferred in the first half of the analogy to the second half of the problem (Sternberg, 1977b). The motivating idea is that individuals' skills in solving these problems derive from their ability to execute these processes rapidly. Moreover, the processes involved in analogy solution have been shown to be quite general across various kinds of inductive-reasoning problems (Greeno, 1978; Pellegrino & Glaser, 1980; Sternberg & Gardner, 1983). Thus, the components are of interest because they are not task-specific, but rather are quite general across a variety of problem-solving tasks (see also Newell & Simon, 1972, for a similar logic applied to other kinds of complex problems).

How well does the performance-process approach work? For the three components noted above (inference, mapping, application), Sternberg (1977b) found a median correlation of -.16 for schematic-picture analogies and of -.34 for verbal analogies. In a geometric-analogies experiment, only application was reliably estimated for individual subjects, and it showed a median multiple correlation (taking into account error rates as well as latencies) with psychometric test performance of .34. Mulholland, Pellegrino, and Glaser (1980), also using geometric analogy problems but with a different breakdown of components, obtained results that were roughly comparable to these. Sternberg and Gardner (1983) obtained much more reliable estimates of the reasoning process parameters than had Sternberg (1977b). They administered to subjects three different tasks – analogies, series completions, and classifications – with three different contents – schematic-picture, verbal, and geometric. Correlations between a combined reasoning component (including inference, mapping, and application) and psychometrically measured intelligence were -.70 for analogies, -.50 for series completions, and -.64 for classifications, averaged over contents. Correlations were -.70 for schematic-picture items, -.61 for verbal items, and -.67 for geometric items, averaged over tasks. This approach seems capable of yielding rather high correlations and thus to hold some promise for understanding individual differences in psychometrically measured intelligence, although again, it seems highly unlikely that this approach provides anything close to a full account of intelligence.

Investigators seeking to understand intelligence in terms of executive processes seek to discover the processes by which individuals make decisions such as (a) what performance components to use in solving various kinds of problems, (b) how to combine the performance components into an overall strategy, (c) how to represent information, (d) how to trade off speed for accuracy, and so on (Brown, 1978; Flavell, 1981; Sternberg, 1980f). Sternberg (1980f) has proposed that these executive processes or "metacomponents" are highly general across tasks involving intelligent performance and that they are in large part responsible for the appearance of a general factor in mental ability tests. According to this view, what is "general" across the tests is the execution of the metacomponents of task performance. Because metacomponents are difficult to isolate from task performance, existing data regarding the relationship betwen these metacomponents and psychometrically measured intelligence are spotty, at best. Some relevant data are reported in Sternberg (1981d). Two metacomponents, global planning and local planning, were isolated from a complex-reasoning task. Global planning measures general strategic planning of solution strategy across a range of item types. Local planning measures specific strategic planning for an individual item. It was found that global planning scores correlated .43 with measured intelligence and that local planning scores correlated -.33 with measured intelligence. Thus, more intelligent individuals tended to spend relatively more time than others in global planning, but relatively less time than others in local planning (see also Chapter 8 for studies of metacomponential functioning in the domain of reading).

Critique. The cognitive theories differ in the "levels of processing" about which they theorize (see Craik & Lockhart, 1972; Sternberg & Salter, 1982) and in the kinds of tasks that serve as foci for information-processing analysis. But as was true in the case of the psychometric theories, the cognitive theories are more similar than they might at first appear to be.

First, all of the theories assume, at some level, that intelligence can be understood in terms of constituent information-processing components. The unit of analysis is a real-time operation upon a particular kind of mental representation. Thus, whereas the differential theories are based upon a static structural entity, the factor, the cognitive theories are based upon a dynamic process entity, the component. In the first flush of enthusiasm that accompanied the introduction of cognitive theorizing in the study of intelligence, cognitive researchers seemed to be claiming, either implictly or explicitly, that understanding processes was more important than understanding factors (see, e.g., Hunt et al., 1973; Sternberg, 1977b). This claim was misguided. The two kinds of entities address different questions – one about structure, the other about process – and ultimately they can be used to help understand each other (Sternberg, 1980c). Arguments about which kind of entity is more basic (e.g., Carroll, 1980) are, in my opinion, fruitless, because there exists no empirical means for answering this question, nor is it even clear what the question means at a substantive level.

Second, there is a common emphasis in cognitive theories upon speed of processing. This emphasis, too, contrasts with the emphasis in psychometric theorizing and testing upon accuracy. Not all cognitive theorists, of course, emphasize speed in their theorizing (see, e.g., Baron, 1982; Newell & Simon, 1972; Simon, 1976). But this emphasis has been predominant in cognitive research. On the one hand, this emphasis may reflect genuine beliefs about the psychology of human intelligence. On the other hand, it may reflect the heavy use by cognitive researchers of reaction-time methodologies, in which case methods may be dictating theory (at least in part) rather than the other way around. Even attempts to understand both speed and accuracy of processing simultaneously (e.g, Mulholland et al., 1980; Sternberg, 1977b, 1980d) have been based upon tasks with relatively low error rates in which speed rather than accuracy has been the dominant dependent variable under consideration. To the extent that there is a problem in the use of reaction time, it is not with reaction time per se, but rather with its use when it may not be wholly appropriate.

Third and finally, the theories draw their empirical support from performance on tasks that are easily prepared, one might even say "canned," for use in the laboratory. The difference between a simple reaction-time task and an analogies task can be seen as quite large, indeed. However, when viewed in the context of the kinds of tasks one has to perform in one's everyday life, the difference can be seen as rather small. People no more go around solving testlike analogies (except on tests) than they go around pressing buttons in response to lights or sounds. Although such tasks are not unheard of in the everyday world, they do not seem particularly representative of the kinds of things people normally do in their lives. The same, of course, can be said for most of the tasks that have been used in differential theorizing, although here the level of task seems, on the average, to be somewhat higher than that of many of the experimental tasks in the cognitive literature. If one's goal is to understand intelligence in terms of performance on extremely basic (and some might say, impoverished) tasks, then these low-level tasks are fine. But it is not immediately obvious that performance in real-world settings is ultimately going to be capable of reduction to components of task performance on very simple tasks.

Validation of explicit theories of intelligence

Two basic forms of validation have been used to test explicit theories of intelligence. These forms are internal and external validation.

Internal validation. Internal validation involves determining how well a theory accounts for the data from the task domain to which the theory is addressed. For example, a differential theorist might address the question of what proportion of the individual-differences variance in a set of test scores is accounted for by a particular set of structural factors postulated in his or her theory; an information-processing theorist might address the question of what proportion of the stimulus variance in a set of item means is accounted for by the particular set of process parameters postulated in his or her theory.

The theorist using internal validation to test a theory of intelligence usually defines the scope of intelligence in terms of that which is accounted for by the theory. The theorist may claim that the theory specifies the whole domain of behaviors to be labeled intelligent but is more likely to claim that the theory specifies an interesting subset of this domain (e.g., Anderson, 1976; Newell & Simon, 1972; Sternberg, 1981k). Although the theory determines the choice of tasks to be studied, in practice the theory has often been derived from prior analysis of the tasks whose selection it now specifies.

This approach to defining the scope of a theory of intelligence has the advantage of being theoretically based: One chooses tasks to study on the basis of a prior theory of which tasks matter and of what is involved in the performance of these tasks. Acceptance of the specified domain of tasks, however, depends upon acceptance of the theory. Although a successful demonstration of internal validity is certainly a necessary condition for acceptance of a theory of intelligence, it is not a sufficient condition; others may argue that whether or not the theory gives a good account of task performance, the tests or tasks under consideration form either an incomplete or incorrect basis for the formation of a theory of intelligence.

External validation of explicit theories. The theorist using external validation to test a theory of intelligence usually defines the scope of intelligence in terms of whatever correlates with external measures of intelligent functioning. The researcher thereby hopes to isolate critical aspects of intelligence – ones that are important in central measures or in many measures of intelligence. External validation involves determining the extent to which parameters (of whatever kind) of a theory account for data from a performance domain external to that encompassed by the theory but in which performance should be predictable from the parameters of the theory. For example, a differential theorist might correlate scores on factors such as "reasoning" or "verbal comprehension" with grades in school; or an information-processing theorist might correlate scores on process parameters such as "lexical access time" or "inference time" with scores on psychometric tests.

External validation is of two kinds. Convergent validation seeks to show high correlations between the task or parameter of interest and other measures with which the task or parameter should be correlated. For example, one would want to show a high correlation between an information-processing component alleged to underlie verbal ability and scores on a test such as the verbal section of the Scholastic Aptitude Test. Discriminant validation seeks to show a low correlation between the task or parameter of interest and other measures with which the task or parameter should not be correlated. For example, the information-processing component alleged to underlie verbal ability should not be highly correlated with a measure of perceptual speed.

Reliance on external validation in the absence or near-absence of internal validation is probably what gave research on intelligence a reputation for being atheoretical. Items for some psychometric tests of intelligence have been chosen primarily on the basis of their correlations with each other or with external criteria (such as grades in school), without reference to an internally validated theory of intelligent performance. A better procedure is to supplement external validation with internal validation.

Internal plus external validation of explicit theories. The theorist using internal plus external validation to define the scope of a theory shows not only that parameters of a given theory account for performance on tasks in the domain encompassed by the theory, but that individual differences in these parameters are related to individual differences in other tasks that are indicative of intelligent functioning. Often an attempt is made to choose "other" tasks that are more ecologically valid than those falling within the scope of the theory, even if this means that these other tasks involve aspects of performance other than intelligence.

This approach to defining the scope of a theory of intelligence has the advantage not only of being theoretically based but of demonstrating sensitivity to performance beyond the range of any single theory, which almost certainly will not include within its scope all tasks that might involve intelligent performance. A successful demonstration of external validity, like a successful demonstration of internal validity, would seem to be a necessary condition for an adequate theory of intelligence, in that probably no one would want to claim that intelligent behaviors are limited to those studied in the task domain under investigation. A demonstration of external validity, however, eventually encounters the same problem as a demonstration of internal validity – the need to accept some theoretically prespecified definition of intelligence. Many people would argue that neither grades in school, performance on psychometric tests, nor any of the external criteria commonly used in investigations of intelligence are adequate standards against which to test the parameters of a theory. It is often not clear that the external criteria are any better than, or qualitatively different from, the internal ones (see, e.g., the studies of Hunt et al., 1975, and of Sternberg, 1977b, where standard psychometric ability tests are used as criteria for external validation). In addition, in using external criteria as a basis for justifying the scope of the theory, one still runs the risk of eventual circularity – that is, that one will justify the theory on the basis of the correlations with external criteria, only later to justify the choice of external criteria on the basis of the theory.

Evolution of explicit theories

Explicit theories of intelligence, like theories of any other psychological construct, undergo an evolutionary process that theorists believe, or at least

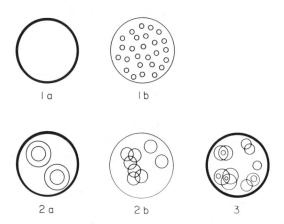

Figure 1.1. Schematic representations of the three stages of theory evolution. The unit of analysis within a given approach to intelligence is represented by a circle. Circles with heavy outer borders show emphasis upon a highest-order unit. Diagrams show alternative principles of organization for units in theories. The number of circles and placement of circles is meant to be illustrative only. (From "The evolution of theories of intelligence," by Robert J. Sternberg, 1981, *Intelligence, 5*, p. 211. Copyright 1981 by Ablex Publishing Corporation. Reprinted by permission of the publisher.)

hope, brings us to successively deeper levels of understanding of the psychological constructs under investigation. Although it is not clear that there is any potentially definitive end state toward which this evolution is proceeding, it is likely that newer theories represent advancements in definable ways (see Kuhn, 1970). It seems that theories of intelligence within a given world view for understanding intelligence follow a certain course of evolutionary development and that this course is closely parallel across approaches. In particular, it is proposed that the evolution of theories of intelligence can be conceptualized in terms of a three-stage model that seems to capture certain aspects of theory development in the differential and cognitive–experimental approaches to the study of intelligence (Sternberg, 1981c; for an alternative view of the evolution of differential theories, see Eysenck, 1967).

Overview of the evolutionary model. The three stages of the model of theory development represent successive degrees of complexity, as shown in Figure 1.1. The first two stages include two alternative instantiations of a given level of complexity. The two instantiations essentially compete with each other, generating a tension that is responsible for theory development within a given stage and for the eventual passage of theorizing about intelligence from one stage to the next. Each new stage helps to diffuse tension created by the preexisting stage, and at the same time it generates new tension of its own. Tension in Stages 1 and 2 is generated by the two competing instantiations and by competing theories within each instantiation. Tension in Stage 3 is generated by the lack of competing instantiations; this tension creates a feeling among investigators that no qualitatively new level of advancement in understanding the nature of intelligence is possible within a given approach.

Figure 1.1 shows the two competing views that characterize Stages 1 and 2 and the single view that characterizes Stage 3. The model depicts a given unit of analysis in the study of intelligence as a circle of the kind found in Euler diagrams. The identity of the particular unit depends upon the world view being considered. This unit might, for example, be a factor, an elementary information process, a schema, or some other kind of entity. The model specifies only the existence of units and the nature of their interrelations. It should be emphasized that the model also makes no claims about how long theorizing remains within a given stage: It claims only that the order of the stages of evolutionary development is fixed. Moreover, the model applies to the spirit rather than to the letter of a given theory. Discussion of the model will be accompanied by examples of its application to the differential and cognitive – experimental approaches.

Stages of the model. Consider now each of the three stages of the proposed model.

Stage 1. In Stage 1, two competing kinds of theories characterize thinking about the nature of intelligence. One kind of theory (labeled 1a in the figure) is essentially monistic: A single instantiation of the given unit of analysis dominates thinking about intelligence. Other instantiations may exist, but they are of little or no consequence. The other kind of theory (1b) is essentially pluralistic: Many independent instantiations of the given unit dominate thinking about intelligence. The fundamental tension in this stage is between monism and pluralism – between the one and the many. Tension may exist within as well as between these general views; that is, there may be alternative monistic and pluralistic theories. The fundamental tension to be resolved, however, is between the notion of intelligence as emanating from a single latent source of task and person differences in intelligent performance and the notion of intelligence as emanating from multiple, independent sources. The conflict between these two viewpoints is never resolved in favor of either of the original conceptualizations. Rather, the two points of view are eventually merged in Stage 2, but in two ways that again compete with each other.

Consider the application of Stage 1 to the development of differential theories of intelligence. Two very early theories seem to be especially appropriate examples: those of Spearman (1904, 1923, 1927) and of Thomson (Brown & Thomson, 1921; Thomson, 1939). Spearman's theory of general intelligence, or g, is prototypical of monistic theories and is certainly the most famous one. In this theory, a single structural factor, referred to as the general factor, permeates performance on all of the various tests and tasks used to assess intelligent behavior. Spearman's theory of g is a good example of one in which the letter and the spirit of the theory may be seen as differing. Spearman explicitly contrasted his "two-factor" theory of intelligence, which allowed for both a general factor and for specific factors, with a monarchic theory, which allowed for only a single controlling entity. My characterization of the theory as largely monistic derives from the fact that in both the bulk of Spearman's own work and of that which followed, the general factor received the lion's share of the attention and was viewed as critical to an understanding of the nature of intelligence. Specific factors were perceived as of minor significance.

Thomson's theory of general intelligence is prototypical of the pluralistic theories that characterize Stage 1. Thomson proposed that general intelligence can be conceived as comprising a very large number of independent structural "bonds," including reflexes, habits, learned associations, and the like. Performance on any one task would activate a large number of these bonds. Related tasks, such as those used in mental tests, would sample overlapping subsets of independent bonds. A factor analysis of a set of tests might give the appearance of a unitary general factor, but in Thomson's view, the communality among tests is attributable not to a unitary source of individual differences, such as mental energy, but rather to a multiplicity of sources, namely, those bonds that overlap across all tests. Thomson thus did not quibble with the validity of Spearman's mathematical discovery of a general factor but rather with Spearman's psychological interpretation of that factor.

Stage 1 can also be applied to the development of experimentally based theories of intelligence, such as the Gestalt theories (Koffka, 1935; Köhler, 1927, 1947; Wertheimer, 1959) and stimulus–response (S-R) theories (Guthrie, 1935; Thorndike, 1931; Watson, 1930). The Gestalt concept of *insight*, introduced in Köhler's (1927) work on the mentality of apes, is the key to an understanding of the Gestalt conception of intelligence. According to Köhler,

We can, in our experience, distinguish sharply between the kind of behavior which from the very beginning arises out of a consideration of the structure of a situation, and one that does not. Only in the former case do we speak of insight, and only that behavior of animals definitely appears to us intelligence which takes account from the beginning the lay of the land, and proceeds to deal with it in a single, continuous, and definite course. (P. 190)

In Köhler's view, then, insight is very closely linked to intellectual performance; indeed, only insightful behavior appears to us to be intelligent. In
Wertheimer's (1959) terms, intelligent behavior is characterized primarily
by productive (insightful) thinking rather than by reproductive (memorial)
thinking. Thus, "insight" seems, in Gestalt psychology, to correspond to *g* in
differential psychology: It is the one primary source of intelligent behavior.
Gestalt psychology, therefore, represents experimental psychology's monistic Stage 1a. Note that whereas in the psychometric conception of Stage 1a
the unit for understanding intelligence is a cognitive structure, in the experimental conception the unit is a cognitive process. This difference between
the two approaches continues to manifest itself throughout the stages.

The stimulus–response view of intelligence is particularly well stated by
the noted associationist Thorndike and his colleagues (1926):

> The hypothesis which we present and shall defend asserts that in their deeper nature
> the higher forms of intellectual operation are identical with mere association or
> connection forming, depending upon the same sort of physiological connections but
> requiring *many more of them*. By the same argument the person whose intellect is
> greater or higher or better than that of another person differs from him in the last
> analysis in having, not a new sort of physiological process, but simply a large number
> of connections of the ordinary sort. (P. 415)

According to Thorndike's view, therefore, intelligence is a function of the
number of S-R connections one has formed. In the terminology of the
evolutionary model, this conception is an example of Stage 1b. The S-R
connections of Thorndike are closely analogous to the bonds of Thomson. In
each case, intelligence is viewed as a function of the number of independent
units (bonds or connections) that a person has formed and brings to bear
upon the problems that confront him or her. Again, as in the differential
stream of research, Stage 1b theorizing stresses the pluralistic nature of the
sources of intelligent behavior.

Stage 2. Stage 2 of the model posits that a resolution of the struggle
between proponents of monistic and pluralistic theories is achieved by ac-
commodating both conceptions of the nature of intelligence. Yet two forms
of this resolution appear, which are again represented by two competing
kinds of theories. One kind of theory (2a in the figure) is essentially hierarchical: A single instantiation of the given unit of intelligence dominates others,
but in fact, other instantiations of the unit are nested within each other. In
general, instantiations of successively lower orders are nested within instantiations of successively higher orders. This view represents an integration of
the two views of Stage 1 in that one instantiation of the unit of analysis clearly
dominates all others, but there is at least one lower-order (and hence less
important) instantiation of the unit as well. At each level, a higher-order

instantiation dominates a lower-order one. This integration of Stages 1a and 1b emphasizes the "one" rather than the "many." The other kind of theory (2b) is essentially overlapping but nonhierarchical in nature: Multiple instantiations of the given unit are nonindependent of each other. They may overlap each other in any number of ways (functionally, structurally, causally, etc.), but they are always somehow interdependent in their functioning within a given theory. To the extent that any degree of overlap is common to all instantiations of the unit, the instantiations may be seen as giving rise to a higher-order instantiation that represents this overlap. However, this higher-order instantiation of the unit is seen as secondary to the nature of the system and may even be viewed as epiphenomenal. This view represents an integration of the two views of Stage 1 in that there are multiple instantiations of a given unit, but these multiple interdependent instantiations may give rise to a less important second-order unit. This integration of Stages 1a and 1b emphasizes the "many" rather than the "one."

On the whole, Stage 2a is a closer descendant of Stage 1a than it is of Stage 1b in that Stage 2a theories emphasize the "one"; contrarily, Stage 2b is a closer descendant of Stage 1b than it is of Stage 1a in that Stage 2b theories emphasize the "many." Both Stages 2a and 2b may be viewed as more complicated and at the same time more sophisticated developments emanating out of the conflict that arose between the two views characterizing Stage 1. The conflict between Stages 2a and 2b, like that between Stages 1a and 1b, is never resolved in favor of either of the original conceptualizations. Rather, the two points of view are merged in Stage 3.

According to the present view, the hierarchical theories of intelligence (e.g., Burt, 1940; Cattell, 1971; Holzinger, 1938; Horn, 1968; Jensen, 1970; Royce, 1973; Vernon, 1971) represent one kind of resolution of Stage 1 conflict. In each of these theories, Spearmanian g, or a close relative of it, dominates all other factors of intelligence, which are hierarchically nested under g. Usually, the general factor dominates group factors (which may themselves be of several orders), which in turn dominate specific factors (Burt, 1940; Holzinger, 1938; Vernon, 1971). The identities of these factors differ across theories. For example, in the Cattell–Horn theory, g is divided into subfactors, g_f and g_c (i.e., fluid and crystallized abilities); in the Vernon theory, g is divided into the two major group factors of practical–mechanical and verbal–educational ability (which are close in their conceptions to fluid and crystallized abilities, respectively). Despite their differences, however, all of these theories are hierarchical, as specified by Stage 2a of the evolutionary model.

Competing with the hierarchical theories of Stage 2a are the theories of primary mental abilities that characterize Stage 2b. In these theories of unordered factors, overlap is derived from correlations between individual differences in patterns of the various mental abilities. Correlation is not attributed to a higher-order factor, as in the hierarchical theories, but to direct relationships between abilities. Historically, the first such theory was Thurstone's (1938) theory of primary mental abilities. Although Thurstone did later concede the existence of a general factor, he never viewed his theory as hierarchical. Similarly, although Guilford (1980, 1982) has acknowledged the existence of higher-order factors (although not a general one), he has never viewed his theory as primarily hierarchical in nature.

Stage 2 can be applied also to the development of experimentally based theories of intelligence. Two classes of theories especially exemplify this stage: hierarchical, executive-based theories and nonhierarchical theories that do not specify executive processes that differ in kind from other processes. Note that, as in Stage 1, the existence or nonexistence of a hierarchy pertains to kinds of processes, rather than to kinds of structures.

Hierarchical theories of intelligent behavior present a plausible strategy for information processing in task performance: An executive directs a sequence of elementary information processes. Sometimes the existence of the executive is implicit, although as Carroll (1976, p. 31) has noted, "the assumption of an executive process . . . seems an intuitive necessity if one is going to get the system in operation" (see also Carroll, 1981). At other times, the existence of the executive is explicit, as in the theory of Sternberg (1979b, 1980f), which distinguishes metacomponents (executive processes) from other kinds of components; similarly, Brown (1978) distinguishes between metacognitive processes, such as predicting, checking, monitoring, and reality testing, and cognitive processes, such as those used in visual scanning or memory retrieval. Indeed, explicitly "metacognitive" theorists, such as Brown, are those most likely to propose the existence of executive processes that differ in kind from nonexecutive processes.

In some theories, the distinction between the two kinds of processes, although not explicit, nevertheless seems to be there. For example, Atkinson and Shiffrin (1968) discuss only one kind of process – the control process – at any length in their article on human memory. Yet they seem to make the same kind of distinction as that made by Brown, Sternberg, and others when they say, "we believe that the overall memory system is best described in terms of the flow of information into and out of short-term storage and the subject's control of that flow" (p. 83). Similarly, Newell, Shaw, and Simon (1958) discuss only one kind of process, the primitive information process, which operates on information in memory; however, they present as a separate element of their theory "a perfectly definite set of rules for combining these processes into whole *programs* of processing" (p. 151). The formation of these rules and of the program that comprises them would seem, in their theory, to require some kind of executive processing.

In some cases, kinds of processes are further differentiated within a hierarchy. For example, Hunt (1978) follows the lead of Schneider and Shiffrin (1977) in dividing mechanistic (nonexecutive) processes into automatic and controlled ones. All of these theories, on the present view, exemplify Stage 2a in that there are different orders of processes: executive ones that control nonexecutive ones and, in some theories, various kinds of nonexecutive ones.

An alternative conception of information processing does not distinguish between executive and nonexecutive processing (see, e.g., Chi, Glaser, & Rees, 1982). A well-known class of examples involves the notion of a production system (see Newell, 1973; Newell & Simon, 1972). A production is a condition–action sequence. If a certain condition is met, then a certain action is performed. Sequences of ordered productions are called production systems. Flow of control in a production system passes down a list of productions until one of the conditions is met; the action corresponding to that condition is then executed, and control is returned to the top of the production list. Flow of control then passes down through the list again, trying to satisfy a condition. This sequence is repeated until a termination point is reached or until it is found that none of the conditions in a system of productions is satisfied. Production systems and other nonhierarchical systems differ from hierarchical ones in at least one key way: There is no executive or need for an executive. A separate, qualitatively distinct level of control is not seen as necessary. It is possible, for example, for production systems to create other production systems, to control other production systems, and to modify themselves (see Anderson, 1976; Klahr, 1979). Thus, a single unit of analysis is sufficient for understanding information processing: Production systems can handle in a unitary way what is handled in a dual way – by executive and nonexecutive processes – in a hierarchical theory. The productions in such a system are directly interdependent on each other: The one that is executed in a given pass through a list of productions depends in part upon its precedence in that list, and the ordering of the list is determined by those productions that created the given system. These generating productions do not differ in kind, however, from the productions they generate, and indeed, the generating productions may themselves be modified by the ones they create. The nonhierarchical nature of production systems combined with the direct interdependence of productions on each other lead me to classify production-system theories of intellectual functioning as Stage 2b theories.

Stage 3. In Stage 3, the two views of Stage 2 are essentially merged into a single, all-encompassing view. The notion of different orders of units (hierarchy) is combined with the notion of overlap in units (nonhierarchy), as shown in panel 3 of Figure 1.1: Instantiations of a given unit may overlap with other instantiations of the unit and at the same time nest within higher-order instantiations of the unit. The tensions between the one and the many, and between the hierarchical and the overlapping, are at least partly resolved by merging elements of all of these views into a single, integrated view. Subsequent tension, however, arises from the simultaneous realizations that (a) the questions that the approach was supposed to answer have still not fully been answered and (b) there is nowhere qualitatively new to go with the chosen approach. The investigator is left with three basic options. The first is stagnation: Research continues within the third stage but seems not to go very far or very fast. Inevitably, people begin to lose interest in the approach to the problem and perhaps in the problem as well. The second option is a new subapproach (i.e., interpretation of the current world view): A new way of thinking within the approach is conceived, and thus the original problems and any new ones that have arisen since the original problems were posed can be investigated from a relatively new point of view. In essence, this option involves cycling backward to either Stage 1 or Stage 2. The third option is a new approach: A new way of studying intelligence is adopted that either deals with the old problems in a wholly new way or deals with new problems in a new way. In this case, theorizing starts at Stage 1.

Stage 3 thus presents a challenge to the investigator to reconceptualize his or her approach to the study of intelligence. The view presented here should not be interpreted as suggesting that research on intelligence is futile or hopeless because it eventually ends up "stalling" in Stage 3. To the contrary, the evolution of theoretical accounts of intelligence shows that progress *is* being made, although it is always more clear whence theories have come than where they will go.

Consider the application of the Stage 3 notion to the development of differential theories of intelligence. I find only one such theory that fits in this stage: Guttman's (1954, 1965) radex theory.

A *radex* (briefly described earlier) or "radial expansion of complexity" unites two distinct notions in a single theory. One notion is that of a difference in kind between tests; the other notion is that of a difference in degree. A radex is thus a double-ordered system in that each of these notions generates a separate concept of structural order within a battery of tests. The double ordering corresponds to the union of the two kinds of ordering represented in Stage 2 of the proposed model through the integrated theoretical development of Stage 3. The application of Guttman's various notions to test data is clearly stated in his own words:

Within all tests of the same kind, say of numerical ability, differences will be in degree. We shall see that addition, subtraction, multiplication, and division differ among themselves largely in the degree of their complexity. Such a set of variables will be called a *simplex*. It possesses a simple order of complexity. The tests can be arranged in a simple rank order from least complex to most complex. (Guttman, 1954, p. 260)

In other words, simplicially ordered tests are tests that are strictly hierarchically ordered from most to least complex or vice versa (as in Stage 2a).

Correspondingly, all tests of the same degree of complexity will differ among themselves only in the kind of ability they define. We shall postulate a law of order here too, but one which is not from "least" to "most" in any sense. It is an order which has no beginning and no end, namely, a circular order. A set of variables obeying such a law will be called a *circumplex*, to designate a "circular order of complexity." Our empirical data will testify that different abilities such as verbal, numerical, reasoning, etc. do tend to have such an order among themselves. (Guttman, 1954, p. 261)

The radex, then, combining as it does the simplex and the circumplex, represents the combination of Stages 2a and 2b shown as Stage 3 in the evolutionary model.

I view Guttman's type of theory as a kind of culmination of differential theorizing about intelligence. I do not believe Guttman's theory is the only possible Stage 3 theory, although I have not actually found any others. I simply contend that this level of theorizing represents an end of the line for the evolution of differential theories within the traditional factorial interpretation of correlational analysis. (Of course, future differential theorizing may prove me wrong.) At this point, the choices open to investigators of individual differences are stagnation, a new subapproach, or a new approach. I have seen evidence of all three outcomes operating in parallel. First, during the 1960s and 1970s, some stagnation occurred in traditional factor-analytic studies of intelligence. Second, at the same time, some exciting new subapproaches of the individual-differences approach emerged, for example, latent-trait analysis (Whitely, 1980) and confirmatory maximum-likelihood analysis (Frederiksen, 1980; Geiselman, Woodward, & Beatty, 1982). Third and finally, some investigators switched their allegiance to methods of analysis that were more experimentally based, as considered in this chapter.

How might Stage 3 apply to experimentally based theories of intelligence? A Stage 3 theory of intelligence would in some way combine aspects of theories with and theories without qualitatively distinct executive processes. My evaluation of current experimental theories of intelligence does not lead me to believe that any of them are clearly Stage 3 theories. However, the evolutionary framework I have proposed leads to a rough sketch of what such a theory might look like. The theory proposed in this book is proposed as a Stage 3 theory or, at worst, a precursor of one. This theory will be considered in subsequent chapters.

Evaluation of explicit theories

The review of theories presented above should at least hint both at the questions that explicit theories of intelligence have addressed well and at the questions that these theories have either not addressed well or not addressed at all. Both of these classes of questions are considered here.

Strengths of explicit theories. Explicit theories of intelligence have several notable strengths. Consider some of the main ones.

1. *Detailed specification of mental structures and processes.* A particular strength of explicit theories of the kinds considered above is their fairly detailed specification of the structures and processes that might be involved in intelligent performance. Differential theories address questions of structure but generally have less to say about process (although there are exceptions; see, e.g., Guilford, 1967); cognitive theories address questions of process, but generally have less to say about structure (although again there are exceptions; see, e.g., Anderson, 1976). Thus, to the extent one's goal is to attain an essentially mechanistic (and molar) model of the mind, these theories have served well.

2. *Beyond operational definitions.* Explicit theories have enabled investigators to go far beyond the trivial operational definition of intelligence as what intelligence tests measure (Boring, 1923; Jensen, 1969). A common misconception about research on intelligence is that there have been two psychometric "schools" of thought: One, tracing back to Galton (1883), is alleged to be theoretically based; the other, tracing back to Binet and Simon (1905), is alleged to be atheoretical (Hunt et al., 1973). This view of the history of intelligence research is, I believe, incorrect. A review of Binet's numerous writings on intelligence (see, e.g., Binet & Simon, 1973) will reveal that Binet was highly theoretical, at least as much so as Galton. The tests Binet and Simon created were based on a theory of intelligence, albeit one that at times seems to have been forgotten or at least lost sight of by Binet's successors. The same point would apply equally well to the tests of Wechsler: He, too, had quite well-conceived notions as to the nature of intelligence (Wechsler, 1950). In any event, explicit theories have helped formalize some of Binet's notions and have provided a fairly specific account of what it is that IQ tests measure. The tendency of test creators and publishers to choose test items primarily or solely on the basis of statistical criteria does not negate the theoretical bases for the kinds of items used. And in recent years, at least some test creators and publishers have been paying careful attention to the theoretical bases for their tests (e.g., Feuerstein, 1979; Kaufman & Kaufman, 1983).

3. *Heuristic value.* Explicit theories have had a good track record in terms of the evolution of the field of intelligence research (see Sternberg & Powell, 1982). A review of the differential literature on intelligence will reveal that there was active theoretical debate and discussion at least from the early 1900s until the 1950s, when research under this paradigm certainly slowed down and, from some points of view, might be seen as having stagnated, to some extent. By the late 1960s and certainly the early 1970s, the banner of intelligence research had been actively carried forward by cognitive researchers, who have continued the vigorous debate on the nature of intelligence (see, e.g., Eysenck, 1982; Resnick, 1976; Sternberg, 1982a, 1982c; Sternberg & Detterman, 1979). Although it is never clear what constitutes "progress" in a field of endeavor, there has certainly been very active theory development in recent years in the study of intelligence.

4. *Practical value.* Some explicit theories have proven to be very useful for practical purposes, such as for diagnosis, prediction, and training. For example, Feuerstein's (1979, 1980) theories of mediated learning experience and of deficient cognitive functions, as well as his adaptation of Vygotsky's (1978) notion of the zone of potential development, have proven to be very useful both in the assessment and training of intellectual functions. Cognitive theories of information processing in memory-task performance, particularly those emphasizing executive processing, have been instrumental in increasing the performance of retarded individuals on intellectual tasks (see, e.g., Belmont & Butterfield, 1971; Borkowski & Cavanaugh, 1979; Brown, Campione, & Murphy, 1977; Campione, Brown, & Ferrara, 1982).

In sum, explicit theories of intelligence have made some notable contributions to our understanding, assessment, and training of intellectual functioning. Today, the field of intelligence is being actively researched, and there is every reason to believe that the research being done will contribute to the explosion of knowledge about intelligence that has been characteristic of research over the past decade or so (see Sternberg, 1982c).

Weaknesses of explicit theories. It will come as no surprise that for all their strengths, the explicit theories and the research that has been done on them tend to share some notable weaknesses. Consider some of the most salient ones.

1. *Difficulty of falsification.* Many of the theories have proven remarkably difficult to falsify, not because of their extraordinary empirical validity, but because of intrinsic characteristics that make falsification difficult or impossible. Nonfalsifiability has long been a bane of differential theories (see Sternberg, 1977b). One reason for this problem is that inferential statistics for exploratory factor analysis are not well developed. Another reason is that

it is exceedingly difficult to compare theories that differ primarily from each other in the form of rotation applied to an initial factor solution: Mathematically, the alternative solutions are equivalent. Although various psychological and heuristic criteria have been proposed for discriminating among theories (see, e.g., Carroll, 1980), there has been nothing approaching a consensus regarding acceptance of these criteria. Cognitive theories have fared better in some respects, but not in others. On the one hand, inferential statistics are available for strong tests of internal validity (see, e.g., Mulholland et al., 1980; Sternberg, 1977b, 1978b); on the other hand, what constitutes successful external validation has never been clear, and the assumptions underlying the theories appear to be essentially untestable. Thus, for example, investigators such as Hunt et al. (1973) and Sternberg (1977b) have correlated parameters of their models against external criteria, such as psychometric tests of intelligence. But what constitutes a "high enough" correlation? Hunt et al. (1973) make very clear that they are quite satisfied with correlations of the order of .3; Sternberg (1981g) makes it equally clear that he is not satisfied with correlations of this order of magnitude. When one moves from the question of statistical significance to the question of theoretical or practical significance, the guidelines seem to be become fuzzy, indeed. Regardless of what level of correlation one accepts, one is assuming that information-processing components of some kind are an appropriate unit of analysis for understanding intelligence. But this assumption has not been tested, and is probably untestable (see, e.g., Guilford, 1980; Keating, 1980; Royce, 1980). Similarly, the structural assumptions underlying much of the information-processing work, for example, those of the distributive memory model (Hunt, 1971) that has guided Hunt's (1978, 1980) work on intelligence, are also not clearly testable.

2. *Tasks of dubitable ecological validity.* The theories are generally based and tested on kinds of tasks that from any point of view are of dubitable ecological validity. There would seem to be a substantial gap between the kinds of real-world adaptation required for everyday functioning and the kinds of adaptations required for performing testlike and laboratory tasks (Sternberg, in press-b). Although the skills involved in testlike and laboratory tasks may well contribute to real-world functioning, only an extreme reductionist would claim that they are exactly the same skills, and even such a reductionist would probably grant a difference in the level of processing at which the skills are exercised. Skeptics might claim with some justification that what are purported to be theories of "intelligence" would better be called theories of laboratory-task or test cognition. If intelligence is indeed more than what is measured by IQ tests, then strong demonstrations of the validity of existing theories for real-world performance are needed. Regard-

less of the predictive validity of the tests for such situations, which is in dispute (see, e.g., McClelland, 1973; Schmidt & Hunter, 1981), the validities of the theories underlying the use of the tests need to be demonstrated.

3. *Inattention to the contexts in which intelligent behavior occurs.* In a related vein, explicit theories in the differential and cognitive traditions have been, almost without exception, insensitive to the interface between intelligence and the context in which it is exercised. Yet many psychologists, anthropologists, and others have questioned whether it is possible fully to understand intelligence without regard to the contexts in which it develops and is exercised (see, e.g., Berry, 1974, 1981; Charlesworth, 1976, 1979a, 1979b; Dewey, 1957; Keating, 1984; Laboratory of Comparative Human Cognition, 1982, 1983; Neisser, 1976, 1979; Sternberg, in press-a; Sternberg & Salter, 1982). I do not believe that the failure of differential and cognitive theories to consider contextual variables necessarily renders these theories wrong, but it does render them incomplete. Intelligence exists in a world that is much broader and more complex than are the testing situations and tasks of most psychologists.

4. *Failure to provide an explicit basis for selection of tasks.* Explicit theorists have failed to supply a rational basis for the selection of tasks on the basis of which to study intelligence. Consider each of the differential and cognitive approaches in turn.

The selection of tasks is of utmost importance to the differential psychologist, since the results of a factor analysis (and other forms of correlational analysis) are greatly affected by the choice of variables to be factor-analyzed. Differential psychologists have traditionally used one of two means for deciding which tasks should be included in an assessment battery. The first means is to sample widely from the universe of available tasks purported to be useful as measures of mental abilities. But this procedure places the burden of task selection on one's predecessors. How did they decide which tasks are useful for measuring mental abilities? If they used the same means, we find ourselves led into an infinite regress. The second means is to choose tasks on the basis of their correlations with other tasks. But what exactly does this mean? If the differential psychologist chooses only tasks that are perfectly intercorrelated with each other (across subjects), then the result will be trivial variation in task makeup and a guaranteed "unifactor" theory of intelligence, since all tests will be measuring exactly the same thing. If the differential psychologist chooses only tasks that are uncorrelated, then wide variation in task content will be bought at the cost of there being as many factors as there are tasks. Reduction of data, one of the ultimate goals of psychology and any other science, will be impossible. Therefore, the differential psychologist must want to choose tasks having some intermediate degree of correlation with each other. But the rules for specifying just what is meant by an intermediate degree of correlation have never been stated, and since such a degree of correlation includes all but three points ($r = -1, 0, 1$), such rules would seem to be needed in order to use this means of task selection intelligently.

Information-processing psychologists have not fared a whole lot better in devising means for task selection, as was pointed out by Newell (1973). Information-processing psychology has at times seemed to be the study of specific tasks whose primary basis or bases for selection have never been fully justified or even rationalized. Sometimes a task is investigated because an empirical phenomenon resulting from subjects performing the task serves to illustrate a theoretical point. What often seems to happen in research is that as the years go by, researchers remember the task but forget why it was theoretically important, and subsequent research becomes a study of the task for its own sake rather than of the task as a vehicle for testing one or more psychological theories (see discussion in Sternberg & Bower, 1974).

In sum, then, explicit theorizing about intelligence seems to be quite useful as far as it goes, but the question of concern is that of just how far it does, in fact, go. Implicit theorizing, as discussed below, seems to deal at least somewhat with some of the incompletenesses of explicit theorizing.

Implicit theories of intelligence

Implicit theories of intelligence are based, or at least tested, on people's conceptions of what intelligence is: Implicit theories need to be "discovered" rather than "invented" because they already exist, in some form, in people's heads. The goal in research on such theories is to find out the form and content of people's informal theories. Thus, one attempts to reconstruct already existing theories rather than to construct new ones. The data of interest are people's communications (in whatever form) regarding their notions as to the nature of intelligence. For example, a survey of questions might be administered to a large group of people and the data from this survey analyzed in order to reconstruct people's belief systems about intelligence. Although investigators working with implicit theories of intelligence might disagree as to the structure and possibly even the content of people's beliefs, they would agree that the data base from which the proposed constructs should be isolated should consist of people's stated or implemented beliefs regarding intelligent functioning (Sternberg, Conway, Ketron, & Bernstein, 1981).

The theorist who uses implicit theories defines the scope of a theory of intelligence in terms of what people say intelligence is. Intelligence is viewed as a stipulative concept, one that achieves its meaning as a result of people positing it to mean a certain thing. A major proponent of a closely related view, Neisser (1979) believes that intelligence does not exist except as a resemblance to a prototype, that is, as a degree of similarity between actual persons and some ideally intelligent person. Neisser notes that this view can be traced back at least to Thorndike (1924), who suggested that

> for a first approximation, let intellect be defined as that quality of mind (or brain or behavior if one prefers) in respect to which Aristotle, Plato, Thucydides, and the like, differed most from Athenian idiots of their day, or in respect to which lawyers, physicians, scientists, scholars, and editors of reputed greatest ability at constant age, say a dozen of each, differ most from idiots of that age in asylums. (P. 241)

Neisser believes that the task domain considered by standard intelligence tests, although too limited, does make sense as far as it goes, because these tests measure a person's resemblance to a prototypical intelligence test "smartie" who would get all the items right.

One question that arises in the implicit-theory approach is that of whose conceptions of intelligence should be used in determining the scope of theories of intelligence. The two most common answers are experts in the field of intelligence and laypersons in our culture, although some investigators have studied as well the conceptions of intelligence held by people in other cultures (e.g., Wober, 1974).

Implicit theories of experts

The most famous study of experts' conceptions of the scope of intelligent behavior is that done some time ago by the editors of the *Journal of Educational Psychology* ("Intelligence and Its Measurement," 1921). Fourteen experts gave their views on the nature of intelligence, with definitions such as the following:

1. The power of good responses from the point of view of truth or fact (E. L. Thorndike);
2. The ability to carry on abstract thinking (L. M. Terman);
3. Having learned or ability to learn to adjust oneself to the environment (S. S. Colvin);
4. Ability to adapt oneself to relatively new situations in life (R. Pintner);
5. The capacity for knowledge and knowledge possessed (V. A. C. Henmon);
6. A biological mechanism by which the effects of a complexity of stimuli are brought together and given a somewhat unified effect in behavior (J. Peterson);
7. The capacity to inhibit an instinctive adjustment, the capacity to redefine the inhibited instinctive adjustment in the light of imaginally experienced trial and error, and the volitional capacity to realize the modified instinctive adjustment into overt behavior to the advantage of the individual as a social animal (L. L. Thurstone);
8. The capacity to acquire capacity (H. Woodrow);
9. The capacity to learn or to profit by experience (W. F. Dearborn).

There have been many, many definitions of intelligence since these were presented in the journal symposium, and an essay has even been written on the nature of definitions of intelligence (Miles, 1957). A problem with using these various definitions as a basis for specifying the scope of theories of intelligence is that it is not clear how to combine the definitions. Should the scope of one's theory be the disjunction of the various definitions, the conjunction of these definitions, or some other function of them? Nor is it clear how one would compute any of these functions, even if a function could be decided upon. Certain themes do seem to run through the definitions, such as the capacity to learn from experience and adaptation to one's environment, but the perception of common themes is probably as much in the eyes of the perceivers as in the minds of the experts. Clearly, one would like a nonarbitrary means of combining the perceptions of the various experts.

A contemporary version of this kind of study that does provide a means of combining the conceptions of various experts was conducted by Sternberg, Conway, Ketron, and Bernstein (1981). These investigators had a large number of experts rate each of a large number of behaviors in terms of the extent to which they were either distinctively characteristic of or important in defining intelligence in an ideally intelligent person. The ratings were factor-analyzed, and the three factors that emerged – verbal intelligence, problem solving, and practical intelligence – were taken as characterizing experts' conceptions of intelligence.

Implicit theories of laypersons

If one views intelligence as a cultural concept, then one may use laypersons' views as a basis for specifying the scope of a theory of intelligence. Consider some examples of the use of this approach.

Neisser (1979) collected informal data from Cornell undergraduates regarding their conceptions of what intelligence is. More formal studies have been conducted by Cantor (1978), who asked adult subjects to list attributes of a bright person, and by Bruner, Shapiro, and Tagiuri (1958), who asked people how often intelligent people also display other personality traits. These authors found, for example, that intelligent people are likely to be characterized as clever, deliberate, efficient, and energetic, but not as apathetic, unreliable, dishonest, and dependent.

Siegler and Richards (1982) asked adult subjects to characterize intelligence as it applies to children of different ages. They found a trend toward people conceiving of intelligence as less perceptual-motor and as more cognitive with increasing age. Yussen and Kane (in press) asked children in the first, third, and sixth grades what their conceptions of intelligence are. They found that older children's conceptions were more differentiated than were younger children's; that with increasing age, children increasingly characterized intelligence as an internalized quality; that older children were less likely than younger ones to think that overt signs signal intelligence; and that older children were less global in the qualities they associated with intelligence than were younger children.

Wober (1974) investigated conceptions of intelligence among members of different tribes in Uganda as well as within different subgroups of the tribes. Wober found differences in conceptions of intelligence both within and between tribes. The Baganda, for example, tended to associate intelligence with mental order, whereas the Batoro associated it with some degree of mental turmoil. In terms of semantic-differential scales, Baganda tribespeople thought of intelligence as persistent, hard, and obdurate, whereas the Batoro thought of it as soft, obedient, and yielding.

Serpell (1976) asked Chewa adults in rural eastern Zambia to rate village children on how well they could perform tasks requiring adaptation in the everyday world. He found that the ratings did not correlate with children's cognitive test scores, even when the tests that were used were adapted so as to be seemingly culturally appropriate. Serpell concluded that the rural Chewa criteria for their judgments of intelligence were not related to Western notions of intelligence.

Super (1982) analyzed concepts of intelligence among the Kokwet of western Kenya. He found that intelligence seemed to mean a different thing when referring to children and adults. The word *ngom* was applied to children, and it seemed to carry a connotation of responsibility as well as highly verbal cognitive quickness, the ability to comprehend complex matters quickly, and management of interpersonal relations. The word *utat* was applied to adults, and it suggested inventiveness, cleverness, and sometimes wisdom and unselfishness. A separate word, *kwelat*, was used to signify smartness or sharpness.

Sternberg et al. (1981) found that laypersons' conceptions of intelligence are remarkably similar to those of experts. Ratings between experts and laypersons generally correlated in the .80s and .90s with each other. Thus, the two groups of individuals seem largely to agree in what behaviors are characteristic of and important in defining the ideally intelligent person. The views were not identical, however: First, the experts considered motivation to be an important ingredient of "academic" intelligence, whereas no motivational factor emerged in factor analyses of laypersons' ratings; second, the laypersons seemed to place somewhat greater emphasis on the everyday aspects of intelligence than did the experts.

Validation of implicit theories

Like explicit theories, implicit theories can and should be subjected to both internal and external validation. In most past research, they have been subjected to a minimum of internal validation and no external validation. Sternberg et al. (1981) made some attempt to perform validations of both kinds. Details of these validations will be presented later. The implicit theories of experts and laypersons were internally validated in part by assessing the extent to which the major factors uncovered by their analysis accounted for the matrices of correlations from which the factors were derived. A three-factor model accounted for 46% of the variance in the laypersons' data and for 51% of the variance in the experts' data. External validation was assessed in several ways. The major way was to examine the extent to which individuals used the proposed factors of intelligence in their evaluations of the intelligence of persons whose behaviors were described in a fashion similar to the descriptions of letters of recommendation. The factors of the laypersons' implicit theories accounted for 92% of the variance in laypersons' ratings of the intelligence of the described persons.

Evaluation of implicit theories

Implicit theories, like explicit ones, have both strengths and weaknesses. Some of each are considered below.

Strengths of implicit theories. Implicit theories, and the implicit-theoretical approach to research on intelligence, have several strengths that tend to complement the strengths of explicit theories.

1. *Contextual relevance.* Whereas explicit theories tend to ignore the context in which intelligence is manifested, implicit theories not only pay attention to it, but are essentially derived from it. Implicit theories are expressions of people's conceptions of what intelligence is in the context in which it occurs. There is no guarantee, of course, that either experts or laypersons will accurately reflect in their implicit theories the contexts in which they live. But their views are, for better or worse, about the most accurate reflections we now have.

2. *Breadth of conceptualization.* Many people who have been exposed to the content of typical IQ tests, which are fair reflections of the differential theories that motivated them, cannot help but be struck by the narrowness of the conception of intelligence that they represent. On the one hand, they provide a fairly broad sampling of higher-level cognitive skills; on the other hand, they fail to sample the kinds of noncognitive adaptive skills that people (at least in our studies) indicate form a part of intelligence in the real world. Implicit theories are broader in scope. For example, the ratings of both experts and laypersons in the Sternberg et al. (1981) studies revealed the kinds of verbal and problem-solving abilities that characterize typical explicit theoretical notions of intelligence. However, these ratings also revealed social-competence or practical-intelligence abilities as being important

characteristics of an intelligent person; few explicit theories touch upon these abilities (but see Guilford, 1967).

3. *Falsifiability*. It may seem odd that implicit theories, which tend to be more global and vague in their formulations than explicit theories, are nevertheless more easily falsifiable. The main reason for this greater ease of falsifiability stems from the difference in purpose the two kinds of theories serve. Whereas the study of explicit theories seeks to understand intelligence as it operates in task performance, the study of implicit theories seeks to understand intelligence as it is conceptualized in people's heads. An implicit theory would be falsified if it were shown not to represent the way people conceptualize intelligence. It is possible to use converging operations (e.g., multidimensional scaling of proximity ratings or sortings, factor analysis of characteristicness ratings, verbal protocols, etc.) to check whether a given implicit theory does provide a fair representation of people's views. Moreover, by asking people to make judgments about their own intelligence and that of others at the same time that they rate themselves or others on the behaviors that are alleged to contribute to their implicit theories, it is possible to assess (via multiple regression) whether people actually evaluate their own and others' intelligence on the bases of the behaviors that are alleged to constitute their implicit theories.

4. *Ecological validity*. In many respects, implicit theories enjoy a level of ecological validity that is missing from most explicit theories. The kinds of behaviors people view as important in intelligence (e.g., "displays common sense," "plans ahead," "displays awareness to the world around him or her") tend to be much more characteristic of people's interactions with the real world than do the kinds of behaviors that form the bases for some explicit theories (e.g., deciding whether two letters have the same name). One indication of this ecological validity is the focus of implicit theories upon typical rather than maximal performance. Explicit theories are based and tested on maximal task performance: Individuals are asked to perform at a level that scarcely typifies their customary interactions with the environment. Implicit theories, in contrast, are based and tested on typical task performance.

Weaknesses of implicit theories. Implicit theories have certain weaknesses that are at least as noteworthy as their strengths. Consider some of the major ones.

1. *Lack of specificity*. The kinds of behaviors that emerge from implicit theoretical analysis tend to be at a very high level of generality. For example, few people would question that people who "reason logically and well" tend to be more intelligent (Sternberg et al., 1981), but many people would see a major task of a theory of intelligence to be the specification of just what it means to reason logically and well. Similarly, "sizing up situations well" or

"reading with high comprehension" would certainly seem to be important aspects of intelligent performance, but it is by no means clear, psychologically, what it means either to size up situations well or to read with high comprehension.

2. *The gap between what intelligence is and what people think it is.* What experts or laypersons think intelligence is may be wrong (unless one operationally defines intelligence as what people think it is, which seems unpleasantly reminiscent of operational definitions of intelligence in terms of what IQ tests measure). Scientific truth is not necessarily reached by majority rule. It has often been the idiosyncratic opinions of small numbers of geniuses, such as Freud, Piaget, Chomsky, or Skinner, that have most shaped people's views of the nature of psychological phenomena. The views of single or multiple individuals may be consensually, but not empirically, valid. Consider as an illustration a rather extreme case. At one time, experts and laypersons alike believed that elements were all formed from varying combinations of fire, air, earth, and water. The consensus on this matter, like the consensus on the geocentric theory of the universe, did not make the view correct. Today, of course, these views are almost uniformly ridiculed. But it is quite conceivable that people 100 years from now will ridicule our beliefs much as we ridicule those of our predecessors.

3. *The normative group is unclearly defined.* To those who believe that intelligence may refer to somewhat different things across different sociocultural groups and even individuals within these groups, implicit theories have the advantage of being able to reflect these differences. But at some point, fractionation of the concept of intelligence must stop, and it is not clear what that point is. Is it the culture, the society, the ethnic group, the community, the individual, or what? Moreover, can each unit's assessment of itself be taken at face value? It seems unlikely that this is the case. Although each person is likely to have at least a slightly different conception of intelligence from each other person, this fact in itself seems insufficient to lead to the conclusion that intelligence is a different thing for each person (and similarly for any definable group). Moreover, some people's judgments will be of dubitable merit (e.g., the mentally ill or the mentally retarded), so that it would seem unlikely that their conceptions of intelligence would reflect what intelligence is for them. But if their judgments are not to be used, whose are? In general, then, the problem of finding a normative group is an extremely difficult one with no obvious solution.

4. *The theories provide a framework for, rather than an account of, intelligence.* Implicit theories tell the investigator what various people or groups of people think intelligence is. They may best be seen as providing a framework within which explicit theories of intelligence can operate. When investigators seek to make more of implicit theories than they can offer, the only

possible long-term result is disappointment. Much as I respect Neisser's (1979) outstanding contribution to our understanding of implicit theories of intelligence, I cannot agree with him that

there is no such quality as *intelligence*, any more than there is such a thing as *chairness* - resemblance is an external fact and not an internal essence. There can be no process-based definition of intelligence, because it is not a unitary quality. It is a resemblance between two individuals, one real and the other prototypical. (Neisser, 1979, p. 185)

It was a mistake for some investigators to believe that intelligence could be understood totally in terms of explicit theories without reference as well to implicit theories. But it is equally a mistake to believe that intelligence can be understood totally in terms of implicit theories without reference as well to explicit theories. Both types of theories are needed.

Relations between explicit and implicit theories

Both explicit and implicit theories of intelligence should be of interest to psychologists. Explicit theories are of interest (a) because the importance of intelligence to psychological theory and measurement, as well as to society, makes it worthwhile to know, insofar as we are able, what intelligence is; (b) because these theories can serve as the basis for the systematic and rational assessment and, eventually, training of intelligence; and (c) because these theories can suggest where people's conceptions are adequate and where they are inadequate, and thereby help shape these conceptions. Implicit theories are of interest (a) because the importance of intelligence in our society makes it worthwhile to know what people mean by *intelligence*; (b) because these theories do in fact serve as the basis of informal, everyday assessment (as in college or job interviews) and training (as in parent–child interactions) of intelligence; and (c) because these theories may suggest aspects of intelligent behavior that need to be understood but are overlooked in available explicit theories of intelligence.

The importance of implicit theories of intelligence has been underplayed in psychological research. Most assessment and training of intelligence that transpire in the real world are based on implicit rather than explicit theories of intelligence. For example, many more assessments of other people's intellectual abilities are made in the course of interviews and even everyday social interactions (such as cocktail parties, conversations at coffee breaks, and the like) than are made in the evaluations of scores from intelligence tests. Moreover, people (even psychologists!) seem ultimately to trust those measurements based on their implicit theories more than measurements based on explicit theories. Psychologists conduct interviews all the time, despite the notoriously low validity and reliability of interview assessments. Moreover, psychologists as well as others seem to believe in the outcomes of these interviews. I have much more often seen people express astonishment at mental test scores that are inconsistent with their informal assessments of the interviewee's intellectual capabilities than I have seen people express astonishment at their own "poor" judgment after finding out that the mental test scores were inconsistent with their personal assessments.

To summarize, implicit and explicit theories of intelligence are actually theories of different things. Implicit theories tell us about people's views of what intelligence is. They are theories of word meaning, and, in the case of *intelligence*, the word is one of interest to a large number and variety of people. Explicit theories tell us (we hope) what intelligence is; in real life, it is more likely they tell us what some aspects of intelligence are. None of the currently available explicit theories seem to do justice to the full scope of intelligence, broadly defined. Perhaps no one theory ever could, whether the theory is explicit or implicit. But theory construction has to start somewhere, and in the course of scientific evolution, it seems that implicit theories of experts give rise to the explicit theories of these experts, which are in turn tested on objective behavioral data. Explicit theories may thus be seen as formalizations of experts' implicit theories. Ideally, these formalizations should allow empirical tests of their validity. Because of this developmental relationship between implicit and explicit theories, there will almost certainly be considerable overlap between them. I believe that a study of this overlap, as well as of the overlap among theories of each of the two kinds, can inform and strengthen both kinds of theories and research.

Part II

The triarchic theory: subtheories

Part II contains three chapters, each of which presents one of the three subtheories that together constitute the triarchic theory of human intelligence.

Chapter 2, "The context of intelligence," presents the contextual subtheory of intelligence and some of the data – both experimental and anecdotal – that support it. The subtheory emphasizes the roles of adaptation to, selection of, and shaping of environments in attaining fit to the environmental contexts in which one lives. This subtheory specifies the kinds of behavioral contents that are appropriate for understanding and measuring intelligence within a given sociocultural setting. The chapter describes what a contextual account is, what some previous contextual accounts of intelligence have claimed, how the present contextual account is similar to and different from these past contextual accounts, and what the strengths and weaknesses are of both the present and past contextual accounts of intelligence. The chapter shows how implicit theories of intelligence can help counteract the vagueness that tends to characterize contextual theories and presents the results of research my colleagues and I have done on the implicit theories of intelligence of adults living in the context of mainstream U.S. culture.

Chapter 3, "Experience and intelligence," presents the experiential subtheory of intelligence and some of the experimental data that have been used to elaborate and test the subtheory. This subtheory deals primarily with the points in a person's experience with a task or situation that are most relevant to understanding the role of intelligence in the person's interaction with the task or situation. These points are those at which (a) a task or situation is relatively novel to an individual or (b) performance in a given task or situation is in the process of becoming automatized. Most of the data presented in the chapter demonstrate how the ability to deal with novelty is an important part of intelligence. The experiential subtheory is used to account for some of the puzzles and inconsistencies in the literature on intelligence, and some relations are pointed out between the ability to deal with novelty and the ability to automatize information processing.

Chapter 4, "Components of intelligence," presents the componential subtheory of human intelligence. This subtheory deals with the mechanisms by which intelligent behavior is accomplished. Three kinds of processes are proposed to be critical to intelligent behavior: metacomponents, which are used in the planning, monitoring, and evaluating of task performance; performance components, which are used in actually performing the tasks one faces; and knowledge-acquisition components, which are used in learning how to perform tasks. This subtheory attempts to specify the processes underlying the behaviors one engages in so as to attain fit with the environment. As the componential subtheory is the oldest part of the theory of intelligence (indeed, it used to be a whole theory of intelligence, rather than part of a larger theory), it has been subjected to far more empirical testing and elaboration than have the other two subtheories. Because of the amount of data that it has generated, descriptions of empirical work arising from this subtheory are generally deferred until Part III of the book.

2 The context of intelligence

Although many of us act as though intelligence is what intelligence tests measure (Boring, 1923; Jensen, 1969), few of us believe it. But if intelligence is not identical to what the tests measure, then what is it? In the preceding chapter, a number of alternative approaches to answering this question, and some of the proposed answers, were considered. The approach in this chapter is one of viewing intelligence partially in terms of the context in which it occurs. In particular, implicit theories of the kind discussed in the last chapter are used to establish a framework in which explicit theorizing can occur. Thus, according to the present view, implicit and explicit theories are viewed as wholly compatible: Implicit theories set the context in which explicit theorizing occurs, and indeed, as we saw earlier, explicit theorizing *always* occurs within the context of explicit theorists' implicit theories, whether or not the theorists acknowledge this fact. Thus, the present approach does no more than to bring this context out into the open. This approach is in no way mutually exclusive with differential and cognitive approaches (as discussed in the previous chapter), although it does view previous theorizing as socioculturally bound in ways previous theorists may have been, in some cases, reluctant to admit.

Consideration of the nature of intelligence will be limited here to *individual* intelligence. Although the intellectual level of group accomplishments may be measurable in some sense and has been shown to be important in a variety of contexts (see, e.g., Laboratory of Comparative Human Cognition, 1982), consideration of group functioning would take the present chapter too far afield from its intended purpose. Hence, group intelligence is not dealt with here.

Why propose a contextual framework for understanding intelligence and even theories of intelligence? I believe there are at least three important reasons.

First, such a view offers an escape from the vicious circularity that has confronted much past research on intelligence. In this research, an attempt is made to escape from old conceptions of intelligence (such as the psychometric one that gave rise to IQ tests) by creating new conceptions of intelligence (such as the information-processing one), but in which the new conceptions are then validated (or invalidated!) against these old conceptions for lack of any better external criteria (see Neisser, 1979). There is a need to generate some kind of external standard that goes beyond the view, often subtly hidden, that intelligence is what IQ tests happen to measure. For whatever its operational appeal, this view lacks substantive theoretical grounding. When IQ test scores are used as the "external" criterion against which new theories and tests are validated, one is essentially accepting this operational view.

Second, a contextual view of intelligence provides a perspective on the nature of intelligence that is frequently neglected in contemporary theorizing about intelligence. The bulk of contemporary intelligence research deals with intelligence in relation to the internal world of the individual (see, e.g., Resnick, 1976; Sternberg, 1982a, 1982c). Such research provides a means for understanding intelligence in terms of cognitive processes and structures that contribute to it. But the research has little or nothing to say about intelligence in relation to the individual's external world. If one views intelligence at least in part in terms of adaptive behavior in the real-world environment (as even psychometric theorists, such as Binet and Wechsler, have), then it is impossible fully to understand the nature of intelligence without understanding how this environment shapes and is shaped by what constitutes intelligent behavior in a given sociocultural context. "Internal" analyses can elucidate the cognitive and other processes and structures that help form intelligent behavior. "External," contextual analyses, on the other hand, can elucidate which behaviors or classes of behavior are intelligent in a given environment or class of environments. The two kinds of analyses thus complement each other.

Third, a contextual viewpoint is useful in countering the predictor-criterion confusion that is rampant in current thinking about intelligence on the part of both laypersons and experts. This confusion – epitomized by the view that intelligence is what IQ tests test – results when the intelligence tests (whether they are called intelligence tests, mental ability tests, scholastic aptitude tests, or whatever) come to be viewed as better indicators of intelligence than the criterial, real-world intelligent behaviors they are supposed to predict. Many of us are familiar with admission and selection decisions where performance in tasks virtually identical to the criteria for such decisions is neglected in favor of test scores that have, at best, modest predictive validity for the criterial behaviors. Oftentimes, lower (or higher) test scores color the way all other information is perceived. There seems to be a need to study intelligence in relation to real-world behavior if only as a reminder that it is this behavior, and not behavior in taking tests that are highly imperfect simulations and predictors of such behavior, that should be of central interest to psychologists and others seeking to understand intelligence.

Contextualist approaches to intelligence are not new, and the view presented here draws on or is compatible with the views of many others who have chosen to view intelligence in a contextual perspective, for example, Berry (1974, 1980, 1981), Charlesworth (1976, 1979a, 1979b), Cole and his colleagues (Laboratory of Comparative Human Cognition, 1982, 1983), Dewey (1957), Keating (1984), Gordon and Terrell (1981), and Neisser (1976, 1979). My purpose is to present my own contextualist view and to consider it in light of objections that might be raised against it. Although my own views are derivative from and draw upon the views of others, I of course make no claim to represent anyone else's position: Contextualist views, like other views, are subject to considerable variation and disagreement (see Sternberg & Salter, 1982).

A contextual subtheory of intelligence

I view intelligence as mental activity directed toward *purposive adaptation to, and selection and shaping of, real-world environments relevant to one's life.* This stipulation is, of course, extremely general, and further constraints will be placed upon it both in this chapter and in the next two chapters. Thus, this view is a starting rather than a finishing point for a contextual definition of intelligence.

It is important to note at the outset that the contextual subtheory deals with the mental activity involved in attaining fit to context, not with physical activity or with external or internal influences that may facilitate or impede activity in context. Thus, for example, an individual may have all the mental skills needed to adapt in an electrical storm, but be struck by lightning nevertheless. Or an individual's pleasing physical appearance may facilitate his or her adaptation to environmental circumstances. The contextual subtheory would deal not with whether or not adaptation to the electrical storm ultimately succeeded or failed, but with one's mental activity in seeking to adapt. Similarly, the contextual subtheory would deal not with an individual's good (or bad) looks, but with the mental activity involved in making the most of one's physical appearance, whether positive or negative.

The three processes of adaptation, selection, and shaping referred to in the preceding definition are viewed as roughly hierarchically related. Let us consider the nature of this relation.

Typically, the individual attempts to *adapt* to the environment in which he or she finds him- or herself. Adaptation consists of trying to achieve a good fit between oneself and one's environment. Such a fit will be obtainable in greater or lesser degree. But if the degree of fit is below what one considers satisfactory for one's life, then the adaptive route may be viewed, at a higher level, as maladaptive. For examples, a partner in a marriage may be unable to attain satisfaction within the marriage; or an employee of a business concern may have values so different from those of the employer that a satisfactory fit does not seem possible; or one may find the situation one is in as morally reprehensible (say, in Nazi Germany). In such instances, adaptation to the present environment presents an unviable alternative to the individual, and the individual is forced to try something other than adaptation to the given environment.

When adaptation is not possible or desirable, the individual may attempt to *select* an alternative environment with which he or she is able, or potentially able, to attain a better contextual fit. For example, the partner may leave the marriage; the employee may seek another job; the resident of Nazi Germany may attempt to emigrate. Under these circumstances, the individual considers the alternative environments available to him or her and attempts to select that environment, within the constraints of feasibility, with which he or she will attain maximal fit. But sometimes this option is infeasible. For example, members of certain religions may view themselves as utterly committed to their marriages, or an individual may decide to stay in the marriage on account of children, despite its lack of appeal; or the employee may not be able to attain another job, either for lack of positions, lack of qualifications, or both; or the individual wishing to leave a country may lack the resources or permission to leave that country. In cases such as these, a third option remains.

Environmental *shaping* is used in lieu of environmental reselection and may well be tried before reselection rather than after it. In this case, one attempts to reshape one's environment so as to increase the fit between oneself and that environment. The marital partner may attempt to restructure the marriage; the employee may try to convince his or her employer to see or do things differently; the citizen may try to change the government, either through violent or nonviolent means. In each case, the individual attempts to change the environment so as to increase his or her fit to the (new) environment rather than merely attempting to adapt to what is already there.

This view of intelligence has one strong, and perhaps unsettling, implication for the nature of intelligence across individuals and groups. It implies that, because what is required for adaptation, selection, and shaping may differ across persons and groups, as well as across environments, intelligence is not quite the same thing from one person (or group) to another, nor is it exactly the same thing across environments. Nor is intelligence likely to be exactly the same thing at different points in the life span, as what is required for contextual fit will almost certainly differ, say, both for children versus adults and for adults of one age level versus adults of another age level. The contextual aspect of intelligence, therefore, is idiographic in nature. It is not the case in the triarchic theory, however, that intelligence is wholly a relative construct. It is relative when looked at from the outside inward (as in the contextual subtheory), but not when looked at from the inside outward (as in the componential subtheory to be described later). The claim is therefore that those aspects of intelligence that are contextually bound are relative, and that those aspects of intelligence that are contextually invariant (the components of information processing) are fixed. Thus, to understand and assess intelligence across individuals or cultures, as well as across age levels, it would be necessary to consider intelligence both in its idiographic (contextual) aspects and in its nomothetic (componential) aspects. Most research on intelligence has concentrated on the latter (whether through information-processing analysis or indirectly through factor analysis) to the exclusion of the former; however, I do not believe any better purpose is served by ignoring the nomothetic aspects of intelligence and claiming that intelligence is wholly relative. Instead, it is both, each in a different aspect. The triarchic theory specifies which aspect is which: Attainment of contextual fit is by idiographic means that differ from one individual to the other; componential processing is nomothetic. Individuals may use different components or strategies in a given task, but they use components and strategies of some kind.

Consider now some of the constraints built into the proposed notion of intelligence as consisting, in part, of the attainment of fit between an individual and his or her environmental context.

Constraints on the contextual definition of intelligence

The real world. First, I define intelligence in terms of behavior in real-world environments. I do so deliberately in order to exclude fantasy environments, such as might be invented in dreams or such as might be constructed by and for the minds of certain of the mentally ill. I would include in the domain of real-world environments those found in laboratory settings and in certain testing situations that, no matter how artificial or trivial they may be, nevertheless exist in the real world. It is as much a mistake to exclude testlike behavior from one's view of intelligence as it is to rely upon it exclusively.

Relevance. Second, I define intelligence in terms of behavior in environments that are relevant or potentially relevant to one's life. The intelligence of an African pygmy could not legitimately be assessed by placing the pygmy into a North American culture and using North American tests, unless it were relevant to test the pygmy for survival in a North American culture and one wished to assess the pygmy's intelligence for this culture (as, for example, if the pygmy happened to live in our culture and had to adapt to it). Similarly, a North American's intelligence could not be verbally assessed in terms of his or her adaptation to pygmy society unless adaptation to that society were relevant or potentially relevant to the person's life. (See Cole, 1979 – 1980, and McClelland, 1973, for further perspectives on the importance of relevance to the understanding and assessment of intelligence.) There is one qualification upon the relevance criterion, however. As will be discussed in Chapter 3, tasks and situations serve as particularly apt measures of intelligence when they involve some, but not excessive, novelty. Thus, a task requiring a North American individual to adapt to aspects of a pygmy environment might well serve to measure the North American's intelligence, but only in comparison to other North Americans for whom the task is equally novel. Similarly, pygmies might be compared in their intelligence by their ability to adapt to certain aspects of North American culture. In this case, one is measuring ability to adapt to novelty, an important aspect of adaptation in any culture. A problem arises only when one attempts to compare individuals across cultures on the same task, but the task is not equally novel for them. In this case, the task is not measuring the same thing for the different individuals. Unfortunately, it is precisely this kind of cross-cultural comparison, which I believe to be invalid, that serves as the basis for much research that seeks to compare the levels of intelligence of various individuals and groups that are of different cultures.

An implication of this view is that intelligence cannot be completely understood outside a sociocultural context and may in fact differ for a given individual from one culture to the next. With respect to the attainment of contextual fit, our most intelligent individuals might come out much less intelligent in another culture, and some of our less intelligent individuals might come out more intelligent in another culture. Consider, for example, people who are deficient in the ability to negotiate a large-scale spatial environment. Such people are often referred to as lacking a good "sense of direction." Although they can usually navigate themselves through old, familiar terrain with little or no difficulty, they may find it difficult to navigate themselves through new and unfamiliar terrains. If someone comes from a sociocultural milieu where people spend their lives in highly familiar environments, such as their home town plus a few well-known surrounding towns and cities, the idea of large-scale spatial navigation would never enter into his or her conception of intelligence and would be an irrelevant and essentially unknown cognitive skill. Navigation in unfamiliar spatial terrains would simply be irrelevant to such people's lives, just as the ability to shoot accurately with a bow and arrow is irrelevant to our lives. Were such navigation to become relevant in the sociocultural milieu, then what is "intelligent" would change for that culture. In the Puluwat culture, for example, large-scale spatial navigational ability would be one of the most important indices of an individual's adaptive intelligence (Berry, 1980; Gladwin, 1970; Neisser, 1976).

One need not go to exotic cultures to find effective differences or changes in what constitutes centrally intelligent behavior. As Horn (1979) has pointed out, the advent of the computer in our society seems likely to change what constitutes intelligent performance in our society. For example, numerical computation was an important part of some intelligence tests, such as the Thurstone and Thurstone (1962) Primary Mental Abilities Test. But with the advent of cheap calculators and ever cheaper computers, the importance of numerical computation skill in intelligent behavior seems to be on the decline. At the same time, the predictive value of numerical computation for assessing other kinds of performance, such as performance in school, may or may not decrease in the near future. The predictive value of the skill thus remains an open question. Possibly, using numerical computation as one of five subtests measuring intelligence, or as the sole or main index of number skill, is inappropriate in this day and age, no matter how appropriate it may have seemed when the Thurstones devised their test and even a few years ago when numerical computation skill was a central part of people's lives, both in school and out (as for balancing checkbooks, keeping track of expenses, and so on). Thus, even within our own culture, we see changes over time, no matter how slow, in what constitutes adaptive intelligence.

Purposiveness. Third, intelligence is purposive. It is directed toward goals, however vague or subconscious those goals may be. These goals need not be the attainment of the maxima of the goods most valued by society, for example, money, fame, or power. Rather, one may be willing to strive for less of one commodity in the hope of attaining more of another.

Adaptation. Fourth, intelligence involves adaptation to the environment. It is defined in terms of the knowledge, skills, and behaviors that constitute adaptive performance within a given sociocultural milieu (which, as indicated earlier, will include the ability to adapt to changes and novelties in that milieu). What is adaptive in one environment may actually be maladaptive in another, and hence actions that are intelligent in one culture may be unintelligent in another.

Consider, for example, "Latin American time." In some Latin American cultures, it is customary for meetings and appointments to start at times grossly later than the times that are scheduled. Members of these cultures take these delays into account in their planning. North Americans transported into these cultures may not. For example, in a meeting in Venezuela on the topic of intelligence, only 5 out of nearly 100 participants arrived on time the first day (8 a.m. in the morning). What these 5 (including myself) had in common was that they were the only North Americans at the conference. The same on-time behavior that is quite adaptive for American meetings proved to be quite maladaptive in the Venezuelan setting.

Some research measuring adaptive skills in two kinds of jobs – academic psychology and business – is presented in Chapter 9. In this research, it was found possible to predict success in these jobs via questionnaires that yield scores uncorrelated with general intelligence, but correlated about .4 with typical criteria for job performance. This research helps further decompose just what constitutes adaptive performance.

Selection. Fifth, intelligence involves selection of environments as well as adaptation to them. To differing but usually nontrivial extents, people are able to select the environments in which they live (Kessen, 1968; Scarr, 1981). Obviously, no one has complete control over the environments that he or she inhabits; but most people have *some* control, probably more than they realize. I believe that a key aspect of intelligence is the active selection, where possible, of an environment that enables one, in Cronbach and Snow's (1977) terms, to capitalize upon one's strengths and to compensate for one's weaknesses. One can see these skills at work particularly among highly successful people in a given field of endeavor. Such people tend to share not any one particular ability (such as spatial ability or verbal ability) but rather a higher-order ability to capitalize upon whatever abilities they have in their work and to minimize the negative consequences of their weaknesses. Where possible, more intelligent people actively select environments that are more favorable for their adaptive skills, that is, environments in which they perform more intelligently. To the extent that there is any aspect of intelligence that transcends particular environments, this aspect would appear to be critical.

Consider, again, the example of selection of a career. Few individuals have available to them all possible career options, if only for reasons of financial or educational resources. But many individuals have some options, and these options may be broader than the individual realizes. For example, financial emergencies may be dealt with by obtaining loans or by seeking extra sources of income; educational deficiencies may be remedied by further study, even later in life. Often, our options are more varied than they appear at first glance. But given that an individual has some career options available, it is, I believe, a matter of intelligence to select one that will optimize, insofar as possible, one's opportunities for success in terms of both one's interests and one's abilities. A given individual can expect to be differentially successful –

with "success" broadly defined according to the things that matter to oneself and one's reference groups – in different careers. Self-knowledge in terms of one's abilities, interests, and motivations can make the difference between high intelligence as exhibited in one occupational environment and low intelligence as exhibited in another.

This discussion of environmental selection and career choice may become less abstract if one examines some real-world examples. A rather poignant set of real-world examples is provided by Feldman's (1982) account of *What Ever Happened to the Quiz Kids?* The book provides biographies of a subset of the child prodigies who were chosen to appear on the "Quiz Kids" radio (and later television) show. On this show, children were asked to provide rapid answers to difficult factual questions. The Quiz Kids were originally selected for the show on the basis of a number of intellectual and personal traits. Existing records suggest that all or almost all of them had exceptionally high IQs, typically well over 140 and in some cases in excess of 200. Now the Quiz Kids are all middle-aged adults. One cannot help but be struck by how much less distinguished their later lives have been than their earlier lives, in many cases even by their own standards. There are undoubtedly any number of reasons for this lesser later success, including regression effects. But what is striking in biography after biography is that the ones who were most successful were those who found what they were good at and were interested in and then pursued it relentlessly. The less successful ones had difficulty in finding any one thing that interested them and in a number of cases floundered while trying to find a niche for themselves.

Shaping. Sixth, intelligence involves shaping of the environment. Environmental shaping is used when one's attempts to adapt to a given environment fail and possibly after attempts to select an alternative environment fail. (It is also possible that an individual will attempt to shape the environment before deciding to select an alternative one.) The most successful people in a given field of endeavor are often those who have shaped the field in their own image. In psychology, for example, the mathematical modelers of the 1960s (such as Bower, Estes, Falmagne, Luce, and others) essentially shaped the field of experimental psychology so that it valued what they were good at and liked to do. In the 1970s, computer modelers such as Newell and Simon had a similar effect, although the dominance of computer modeling on contemporary cognitive psychology is far from complete. The general point, though, is that environmental shapers can end up shaping not only their own environments, but those of others as well.

Environmental shaping need not take place on such a large scale. In their everyday lives, people are constantly attempting to change things in their lives so as to make them better: their marriages, their eating habits, their interactions with others, and so forth. Successful attempts to change oneself often hinge more upon changing the environment than upon changing anything basic in oneself. Indeed, behavioral therapies are explicitly directed toward this end.

It is important to note that people are (at least) as much shaped by their environments as they are shapers of them. Shaping of people by environments and shaping of environments by people are interactive processes, neither of which can be fully understood without the other. A full contextual account would need to specify in detail the kinds of environmental forces that contribute to the shaping of people's intellects. The account proposed here does not specify these forces, and thus needs further development along these lines.

Criticisms of the contextual view: some responses and elaborations

I have outlined above some of the main features of a contextual view of the nature of an important aspect of human intelligence. Contextual views have been criticized in the past on a number of grounds, among them their relativism, their seeming reinforcement of the status quo and inability to accommodate cultural change, their vagueness and lack of empirical verification, and their seeming overinclusiveness, by which is meant their placing into the realm of intelligence mental and behavioral phenomena that many would place into other realms, such as those of personality and motivation. In this section, I will describe and respond to each of these criticisms.

Relativity. It has been argued that contextualist views give up too much (Jonathan Baron, personal communication, 1982) – that they leave one essentially with no firm foundation for understanding the nature of intelligence, because "everything is relative."

I do not believe that everything is, in fact, relative. As I will make clear in subsequent chapters, I believe that there are many aspects of intelligence that transcend cultural boundaries and that are, in fact, universal. Moreover, I am aware of no evidence to suggest that either the hardware (anatomy and physiology) of cognitive functioning or the potential software (cognitive processes, strategies, mental representations, and so on) of such functioning differs from one culture or society to the next. To the contrary, any evidence I have seen suggests that both the hardware and potential software of the cognitive system are the same across the known range of sociocultural milieus. What differ, however, are the weights, or importances, of various aspects of mental hardware and software as they apply to defining what constitutes intelligent behavior.

For example, the complex and interactive cognitive skills that are prerequisite for reading are to be found in varying degrees in all people in all sociocultural milieus, at least as far as we know. I include in such prerequisite skills not the knowledge that is taught to participants in literate cultures, but the skills such as pattern perception, articulatory ability, and comparison ability that can be developed but that exist in individuals, in some amount, whether or not they ever receive formal schooling. But whereas these skills may exist in some amount in members of every culture, their importance to intelligent behavior may differ radically from one culture to the next. The skills needed for reading, and especially those specifically relevant to reading but of little or no relevance to other tasks, will be much less important in a preliterate society than in a literate one. Contrariwise, coordination skills that may be essential to life in a preliterate society (e.g., those motor skills required for shooting a bow and arrow) may be all but irrelevant to intelligent behavior for most people in a literate and more "developed" society.

It is probably not the case that these skills exist in equal amounts across cultures: Some cultures are likely to put much more emphasis on developing certain kinds of skills than do other cultures, which will in turn place their emphasis on developing other kinds of skills. As a result, cultures may appear to show mean differences in levels of measured intelligence – but probably only when intelligence is measured in terms of the knowledge and skills required by one of the two (or more) cultures. This argument applies as well to multiple subcultures within a single culture. Even if one could find a set of test items that measured just those skills that are common to the adaptive requirements of members of the two cultures, the test would be incomplete because it failed to measure the aspects of adaptation that are specific to but nevertheless relevant in each of the individual cultures; moreover, the test would most likely be incorrectly scored in a way that assumed that the weights of the common elements in adaptation were the same across the two cultures.

Thus, whereas there is no reason at all why one cannot compare levels of cognitive abilities across cultures (albeit with difficulty), there are good reasons why one usually cannot directly compare mean levels of intelligence. Ultimately, intelligence will not mean quite the same thing across the cultures, so that one will be in the proverbial position of the person who believes he or she can compare apples and oranges because they are both fruits.

Stability and change. One might – incorrectly, I believe – interpret the contextualist position as being unable to accommodate culture change or as reinforcing the status quo. These objections are unfounded. According to the contextualist view presented here, the nature of intelligence can change within a single culture as well as between multiple cultures. In a rapidly developing culture, what constitutes intelligent performance may actually change over a relatively short span of time. It is not inconceivable, for example, that as Venezuela becomes more industrialized, promptness with respect to scheduled times will become a more adaptive behavior. As noted earlier, in our own culture it is likely that the logical skills needed for computer programming and management will become successively more important to intelligent performance in our society as computational skills become successively less important. Moreover, environmental shaping, part of the present subtheory, can very well result in a change as to what is relevant to future adaptation.

There is, then, nothing in the contextualist view that either supports or vitiates the status quo. The contextualist view simply recognizes the changing nature over space and time of what constitutes intelligent behavior.

One might feel uncomfortable with the lability this notion implies in the constitution of intelligence. Indeed, I feel uncomfortable with it. But as the dinosaurs presumably learned a long time ago, whatever abilities or skills are adaptive under certain circumstances do not necessarily remain adaptive, and when what is adaptive changes, so does the nature of intelligence.

It is important here to recognize hierarchically distinct levels of discourse. I would claim, for example, that environmental adaptation, selection, and shaping are always relevant to intelligence, regardless of the nature of the society or culture in which one lives. Thus, what changes is not the importance of these skills, but exactly what constitutes these skills. For example, a person who might be able to adapt to a given society at a particular time might not be able to adapt at another time. Indeed, such a person may feel chronologically "misplaced."

Vagueness and lack of empirical verification. Contextual views are vague and tend not to be empirically validated. But this vagueness is not a necessary property of such views. There is no reason, in principle, why notions of what constitutes environmental adaptation, selection, or shaping cannot be tested, and indeed, tests of some of the present notions are presented in this book. What cannot be tested, of course, is the definitional aspect of the contextual view: It is difficult to see, for example, how one could directly show that adaptation is *not* a part of intelligence. Such a demonstration could be made indirectly, however, through the use of implicit theories, if people characterized adaptive behavior as either unintelligent or as not particularly relevant to intelligence. The primary test of definitions is their heuristic generativity, rather than their rightness or wrongness per se. Definitions, like metatheories, stand or fall on their usefulness rather than on their empirical verifiability.

Overinclusiveness. The contextualist view presented here is certainly highly inclusive in the sense that it includes within the realm of intelligence characteristics that typically might be placed in the realms of personality or motivation (see also Baron, 1982). For example, motivational phenomena relevant to purposive adaptive behavior – such as motivation to perform well in one's career – would be considered part of intelligence, broadly defined (see also Scarr, 1981; Zigler, 1971).

Another element included in the present view of intelligence is environmental selection. Obviously, one's choice of environment will be limited by many factors of luck over which one has no control. Indeed, the role in life of chance factors such as time and place is almost always passed over lightly in analyses of intelligence (but see Jencks, 1972). One can scarcely fault someone for circumstances beyond his or her control. The only circumstances relevant to the evaluation of someone's intelligence are those under which the individual has some behavioral control and under which the individual has an adequate opportunity to express his or her intelligence. The more control the individual has and the greater the opportunity for expressing intelligence, the more relevant the circumstances are for evaluating the person's intelligence. It should be emphasized that I speak here of the control an individual *can* have: People often fail to realize the full extent to which they can control or at least influence their environments. Indeed, the recognition of what can and cannot be changed in one's environment is a part of one's ability to shape the environment, and hence of intelligence.

It is important to note that the contextual subtheory does not equate intelligence or any aspect of it with life success. Rather, life success is a measure, but clearly an imperfect one, of contextually directed intelligence, just as academic or test successes would provide imperfect measures. Intelligence is, in part, the ability to attain success in life contexts, but for a variety of reasons having nothing to do with intelligence, this ability may be only imperfectly realized. Various forms of bad luck – physical infirmities, political repression, financial or familial exigencies – may get in the way of the realization of intelligence as specified by the contextual subtheory. One must thus keep in mind that the various possible measures of contextually directed intelligence suffer from all the kinds of flaws to which other measures are subject as well. Intelligence, then, is, in part, the ability to succeed in context, not the success itself, which may be moderated by a host of variables (such as wealth or poverty) that are unrelated to intellectual ability.

I would like to say, in closing this section, that the contextualist view is in no meaningful sense warmed-over social Darwinism. The social Darwinist viewpoint has never seemed to be well suited to taking into account the life circumstances allotted to one that are beyond one's control. The present view, on the other hand, is "conditionalized" upon such circumstances. What is adaptive for the slum ghetto dweller may be different from what is adaptive for the wealthy suburbanite. They are from two different subcultures that may differ as much as two national cultures, and comparing their adaptations may, again, be like comparing apples and oranges. One could easily conceive of a ghetto resident adapting better to his or her subculture than the suburbanite does to his or hers. Moreover, social Darwinism usually ends up being quite absolutist: The adaptive norm is set up as that of the dominant social class. The present view, if anything, takes the opposite stance, namely, that of a pluralism of niches to which one may ultimately adapt, with the niche partly determined by one's own choice and partly determined by life circumstances beyond one's control.

Evaluation of contextual views

Some of the strengths and weaknesses (or at least incompletenesses) of contextual views have been considered above. It might be useful to summarize these strengths and weaknesses here.

Strengths of contextual views. Contextual views have several notable strengths.
  1. *Escape from vicious circularity.* Contextual views enable one to escape the vicious circularity that has characterized much past thinking about intelligence, where an attempt is made to go beyond the notion that intelligence is what IQ tests measure but where such tests are then used as the criteria against which to validate new notions.
  2. *External as well as internal perspective.* Contextual views enable one to look at the relationship between intelligence and the external world in which people live and which sets the framework for what constitutes intelligent behavior. Too often, conventional theorizing has looked inside the individual to the exclusion of looking at what occurs outside the individual. Intelligence must be seen in the context of the external world as well as in the context of an individual's mental states and processes.
  3. *Resolution of predictor–criterion confusion.* In many instances, tests that were originally intended only to be predictors of intelligence in the world have come to be viewed as the criteria for intelligent behavior. This view is clearly contrary to the views of the originators of the tests, such as Binet and Wechsler, who themselves couched their theories in contextual terms. Contextual views provide a needed balance to those who forget what is predictor and what is criterion.
  4. *Framework for internally directed theories.* Contextual views provide a framework within which differential, cognitive, and other theories can be placed. They are not mutually exclusive with such theorizing: To the contrary, each kind of conceptualization needs the other. Contextual views can suggest where to look for what is intelligent in a given sociocultural milieu. Differential, cognitive, and other theories then help us understand the identified classes of behavioral phenomena in psychological terms.

Weaknesses of contextual views. Contextual views are weakened when they are forced to serve functions they cannot serve. Thus, the weaknesses listed here are in the nature of things that contextual views cannot do.

1. *Nonfalsifiability.* Contextual views probably cannot be falsified. This fact in itself should show that they need supplementation.

2. *Vagueness.* Contextual views are vague. Again, this characteristic is typical of metatheories. But contextual views have been notably slow in supplementing their highly general accounts with details.

3. *Incompleteness.* Contextual views often leave many questions of detail unanswered. Indeed, proponents of such views often have viewed their accounts as opposing rather than complementing other kinds of accounts, such as differential and cognitive ones.

In sum, contextual views serve a valuable but limited function. They need supplementation by other things. One of these other things is a contextually derived implicit theory of intelligence in a given sociocultural milieu, along with a means for deriving such a theory. Such a theory is presented below.

A contextually derived implicit theory of intelligence

Basis for a contextually derived implicit theory

What basis does one use for formulating a contextually derived implicit theory of human intelligence that applies within a given sociocultural milieu? I propose that an apt way of formulating such a theory is by determining the implicit theories of intelligence in the sociocultural population of interest, including both the "experts" within the culture whose business it is to study intelligence and the laypersons who live in the culture but have no particular expertise in the field of intelligence. The reason that implicit theories provide an excellent basis for understanding how intelligence operates within a given context is that such theories are jointly determined by, and also determine, the context of intelligence within the culture. According to this view, the best way to discover the nature of intelligence in context is to ask the people who live in that context. There is no guarantee that people's conceptions of intelligence will accurately reflect the context in which they live. Thus, I would make no claim that implicit theories are the only, or even the best, way to proceed to understand intelligence in context. Certainly, people from outside the context can never attain the kind of understanding of the context that people living within the context have. If there is a consensus among the inhabitants of a given context as to what intelligence in that context is, then this consensus would seem to provide the kind of framework for explicit theories that implicit theories are supposed to provide (see preceding chapter). It would also seem to provide the kind of framework for internally oriented theories (which focus on mental structures and processes) that externally oriented theories (which focus on the interface between intelligence and the real world) are supposed to provide.

In sum, the proposed approach is to determine the implicit theories of persons within a sociocultural context and to assert that such theories provide one basis for an understanding of how intelligence operates in context. This approach does not provide a detailed account of the cognitive mechanisms involved in intelligent performance. Rather, it specifies the realm or content of mental and overt behaviors for which the underlying cognitive mechanisms need to be understood. Moreover, it should convey some sense of the kinds of behaviors that individuals see as being required for adaptation to environments. It seems less likely that implicit theories will address the issues of selection and shaping of environments. Thus, it sets the framework for an explicit theory of intelligence rather than substituting for such a theory.

Content of proposed contextually based implicit theory

Our studies of people's implicit theories of intelligence (Sternberg et al., 1981) indicate that intelligence in the modal sociocultural milieu in the United States involves three main factors, or constellations, of skills: *problem-solving ability, verbal ability, and social competence.* The nature of each of these constellations of skills may be clarified by listing behaviors highly associated with each:

1. *Practical problem-solving ability:* reasons logically and well, identifies connections among ideas, sees all aspects of a problem, keeps an open mind, responds thoughtfully to others' ideas, sizes up situations well, gets to the heart of problems, interprets information accurately, makes good decisions, goes to original sources of basic information, poses problems in an optimal way, is a good source of ideas, perceives implied assumptions and conclusions, listens to all sides of an argument, and deals with problems resourcefully.

2. *Verbal ability:* speaks clearly and articulately, is verbally fluent, converses well, is knowledgeable about a particular field, studies hard, reads with high comprehension, reads widely, deals effectively with people, writes without difficulty, sets time aside for reading, displays a good vocabulary, accepts social norms, and tries new things.

3. *Social competence:* accepts others for what they are, admits mistakes, displays interest in the world at large, is on time for appointments, has social conscience, thinks before speaking and doing, displays curiosity, does not make snap judgments, makes fair judgments, assesses well the relevance of information to a problem at hand, is sensitive to other people's needs and desires, is frank and honest with self and others, and displays interest in the immediate environment.

Deriving the contextual subtheory

From where do these factors and the behaviors that they comprise derive? Their origin is in a set of experiments on people's implicit theories of intelligence conducted by Sternberg, Conway, Ketron, and Bernstein (1981).

Derivation and internal validation of theory. In a series of experiments carried out over a year, we personally interviewed or questioned by mail 476 men and women, including students, railroad commuters, supermarket shoppers, and people who answered newspaper advertisements or whose names we selected at random from the phone book. To compare the ideas of our lay subjects with those of experts, we also sent questionnaires to 140 research psychologists specializing in intelligence.

We did not think it would be useful to ask laypersons directly for their definitions of intelligence. Such a request seemed less likely to elicit genuine convictions than to produce platitudes. We decided instead on an indirect approach. In our first experiment, for instance, we gave people a blank sheet of paper and asked them to list behaviors that they considered to be characteristic of "intelligence," "academic intelligence," "everyday intelligence," and "unintelligence."

We found our lay subjects in natural settings. Sixty-three of them were commuters about to board trains at the New Haven station; 62 of them were housewives and others about to enter a New Haven supermarket; and 61 were students studying in a Yale library. Almost no one had trouble with our request; people were apparently convinced that certain kinds of behavior indicated certain kinds of intelligence – or the lack of it.

From people's responses, we compiled a master list of 250 behaviors, 170 of which had been named as characteristic of intelligence (of one or more of the three kinds about which we queried) and 80 of which had been called signs of unintelligence. Some of the behaviors most frequently listed as intelligent were "reasons logically and well," "reads widely," "displays common sense," and "reads with high comprehension." For unintelligence, the most commonly listed behaviors included "does not tolerate diversity of views," "does not display curiosity," and "behaves with insufficient consideration of others." The great diversity of the behaviors cited showed that our subjects held eclectic views of intelligent and unintelligent behavior and suggested that people probably do not consider any one-dimensional scale adequate for measuring intelligence.

A study of this kind runs the risk of finding some idiosyncratic responses that reflect just one or two people's peculiar notions. For example, one person listed "bores people" as a characteristic of an intelligent person, whereas another person listed "is fun to be with" – almost the opposite. In order to deal with this problem, we had 28 people from the New Haven area

– nonstudents answering a newspaper advertisement – rate on a scale of 1 (low) to 9 (high) how characteristic they thought each of the 250 behaviors on the master list was of an ideally intelligent person, an ideally academically intelligent person, and an ideally everyday intelligent person. Another group of laypersons rated how important each behavior was to defining the nature of intelligence.

We then applied factor analysis to these ratings in order to analyze people's tendencies to view certain subsets of behaviors as related. The statistical method grouped together all the behaviors that people viewed as similar and grouped separately all those that they viewed as dissimilar and allowed us to determine the few basic factors underlying people's diverse and, in a few instances, highly unusual responses. The result was to give us, in effect, a simple characterization of intelligence as viewed by our subjects.

The three factors presented in the preceding section are those that evolved from this data analysis for ratings of an ideally intelligent person. The behaviors listed are those that had factor loadings of .60 or over on each of the factors. In other words, these are the behaviors that were highly associated with each of the factors. The three factors accounted for 46% of the variance in the intercorrelational data (between all possible pairs of listed behaviors).

Because we had asked people not only about intelligence in general but also about academic intelligence and everyday intelligence, we also factor-analyzed the behaviors that had been rated as highly characteristic of these two additional qualities. Our subjects, we learned, conceived of academic intelligence as composed of *verbal ability*, *problem-solving ability*, and *social competence*. These factors sound almost identical to the ones that emerged for intelligence in general; they were, in fact, quite similar, but the specific behaviors that had been listed reflected greater emphasis on academic skills, such as studying hard. The factors that emerged for everyday intelligence we called *practical problem-solving ability*, *social competence*, *character*, and *interest in learning and culture*. These, too, overlapped with those for intelligence in general, but less so, and had more of an everyday slant.

The resemblance between the views of psychologists and nonpsychologists is surprisingly clear. On the whole, the informal theories of intelligence that laypersons have – without even realizing that their ideas constitute theories – conform fairly closely to the most widely accepted formal theories of intelligence that scientists have constructed. The kinds of behaviors that constitute the problem-solving factor are very similar to what Cattell (1971) and Horn (1968) have referred to as "fluid ability"; the kinds of behaviors that constitute the verbal ability factor are very similar to what these investigators have referred to as "crystallized ability"; and the kinds of behaviors that constitute the social-competence factor are very similar to behaviors in explicit theories of intelligence that have included a social- or practical-competence factor (e.g.,

Guilford, 1967; Thorndike, 1920; see also Sternberg, 1981f, 1982h). This resemblance becomes all the more understandable when one compares the implicit theories of the laypersons with those of the experts.

The experts who received our questionnaires all hold doctorates in psychology and teach and do research in major American universities; each has published several articles, books, or book chapters on the subject of human intelligence. Experts were asked only to rate, not to generate, behaviors. Two different questionnaires were sent to the experts. One questionnaire asked respondents to rate how characteristic each behavior was of an ideally intelligent, ideally academically intelligent, and ideally everyday intelligent person. The other questionnaire asked respondents to rate how important each behavior was to defining the respondents' conceptions of each of these three kinds of people.

Taking into account both the characteristicness and the importance ratings for the three kinds of intelligence (general, academic, everyday), the median correlation between the response patterns of experts and those of laypersons was .82. Factor analyses revealed very similar factor patterns for the two groups.

There were two main differences between the groups. One was that the experts considered motivation to be an important ingredient in academic intelligence – an ingredient that did not emerge when we factor-analyzed the responses of the laypersons. Behaviors central to this motivational factor included "displays dedication and motivation in chosen pursuits," "gets involved in what he or she is doing," "studies hard," and "is persistent."

The second difference was that laypersons seemed to place somewhat greater emphasis on the social–cultural aspects of intelligence than did the experts. Behaviors such as "sensitivity to other people's needs and desires" and "is frank and honest with self and others" showed up in the "social-competence" factor for laypersons but not in the analogous "practical-intelligence" factor for experts.

In order to get a better sense of just how experts and laypersons differ in their views of intelligence, I went back to the original ratings of the importance of the various behaviors to people's conceptions of intelligence. I was particularly interested in the behaviors that received higher ratings from laypersons than from experts and in those that received higher ratings from experts than from laypersons. The pattern was clear. Consider first some of the behaviors that laypersons emphasized more than did the experts in defining intelligence: "acts politely," "displays patience with self and others," "gets along well with others," "is frank and honest with self and others," and "emotions are appropriate to situations." These behaviors, which are typical of those rated higher by laypersons, clearly show an emphasis upon *inter*personal competence in a *social* context. Consider next some of the behaviors that experts typically emphasized more than did laypersons in defining intelligence: "reads with high comprehension," "shows flexibility in thought and action," "reasons logically and well," "displays curiosity," "learns rapidly," "thinks deeply," and "solves problems well." These behaviors clearly show an emphasis on *intra*personal competence in an *individual* context. To the extent that there is a difference, therefore, it is clearly in the greater emphasis among laypersons on intelligence as an interpersonal and social construct.

External validation of theory. Several forms of external validation were performed in order to validate the ratings and the implicit theory derived from the factor analyses of laypersons' and experts' ratings of characteristicness of the set of behaviors of an ideally intelligent person.

1. *Correlations between rating patterns of laypersons and experts.* Experts' and nonexperts' response patterns were correlated with each other in order to determine the extent to which the two groups' perceptions of what is intelligent resembled each other. Correlations were computed across questionnaire responses averaged over subjects in each group. Correlations between experts' and laypersons' response patterns were .82 for intelligence, .89 for academic intelligence, and .81 for everyday intelligence. Clearly, then, experts and novices share similar but not identical views as to the nature of each of the three kinds of intelligence.

2. *Correlations between rating patterns for each of the three kinds of intelligence.* Correlations were also computed for experts and laypersons separately between rating patterns for each of the three kinds of intelligence. For experts, these correlations were .83 between intelligence and academic intelligence, .84 between intelligence and everyday intelligence, and .46 between academic intelligence and everyday intelligence. For laypersons, these correlations were .75 between intelligence and academic intelligence, .86 between intelligence and everyday intelligence, and .45 between academic intelligence and everyday intelligence. Two conclusions seem to emerge from these correlations. First, both experts and laypersons view intelligence as more similar to each of academic and everyday intelligence than they view these latter two kinds of intelligences as similar to each other. Second, and confirming inferences noted earlier, laypersons seem to view academic aspects of intelligence as less central to intelligence per se than do experts.

3. *Use of implicit theories in evaluating one's own intelligence.* Consider – for the questionnaire asking subjects to rate the characteristicness of each of a set of 250 behaviors in an ideally intelligent, academically intelligent, and everyday intelligent person – the meaning of a mean response pattern averaged over subjects, whether these subjects be experts or laypersons. One might view a mean response pattern as representing an approximation to the

population's prototype for what constitutes an ideally intelligent, academically intelligent, or everyday intelligent person. On the basis of the data collected in this study, three such prototypes could be formed for experts (one for each type of intelligence) and three such prototypes could be formed for laypersons. We did, in fact, form such prototypical response patterns (which, as noted above, were highly correlated between experts and laypersons).

Suppose one were to ask a subject to rate the characteristicness of each of the 250 behaviors for his or her own behavior and then to correlate this individual response pattern with the prototypical response pattern (as obtained from different subjects filling out a different questionnaire, namely, the questionnaire asking for characteristicness ratings for the "ideally intelligent" person rather than oneself). One might view the correlation between the individual's response pattern and the prototypical response pattern as measuring the degree to which a given subject resembles the prototype of an intelligent person. In effect, one has a resemblance measure of intelligence, based on a comparison between individuals' self-descriptions and others' descriptions of an ideal: Higher scores represent closer resemblance between the individual and the prototype. We computed the correlations between the self-ratings and prototypes, basing the correlations only on the 170 behaviors that were intelligent (as opposed to unintelligent).

The mean correlation of subjects' response patterns for themselves compared to the prototype response pattern for experts (results were practically identical using the prototype response pattern for laypersons) was .40 for intelligence, .31 for academic intelligence, and .41 for everyday intelligence. All of these correlations are highly statistically significant. On the average, then, people saw themselves as having a moderate degree of resemblance to each of the prototypes. The range in degrees of resemblance was quite large, though. For intelligence, for example, the range of correlations for individual subjects was from -.05 to .65.

Correlations were also computed between the prototypicality measures (i.e., the correlations between actual and ideal response patterns) and IQ. Mean correlations with IQ were .52 for the intelligence prototype score, .56 for the academic intelligence prototype score, and .45 for the everyday intelligence prototype score. All correlations were highly statistically significant. Clearly, people's self-rated resemblances to the prototypes provide quite good measurement of their IQs, particularly for academic intelligence and intelligence, and somewhat less so for everyday intelligence (as would be expected, since everyday intelligence is certainly less well measured by IQ tests than are the other two types of intelligences).

In sum, people's resemblances to the prototypes for the three kinds of intelligence are substantially related to their psychometrically measured IQ, suggesting at least some degree of overlap between people's evaluations of themselves in terms of their abstract implicit theories of intelligence and whatever it is that IQ tests measure.

4. *Use of implicit theories in evaluating the intelligence of others.* People seem to use their implicit theories in evaluating their own intelligence, and the evaluations people make are correlated with external criteria. But do people use these same theories in evaluating the intelligence of others? The evidence we collected suggests that they do.

To find out whether or not what people say intelligence is actually has any relation to their judgments of intelligence, we sent lay subjects a series of personal sketches of fictitious people, employing behaviors taken from our master list. These sketches in some ways resembled brief and telegraphic letters of recommendation one might get if one sought written evaluations of people's intelligence. Consider two typical sketches:

Susan:
She keeps an open mind.
She is knowledgeable about a particular field.
She converses well.
She shows a lack of independence.
She is on time for appointments.

Adam:
He deals effectively with people.
He thinks he knows everything.
He shows a lack of independence.
He lacks interest in solving problems.
He speaks clearly and articulately.
He fails to ask questions.
He is on time for appointments.

The respondents' task was to rate the intelligence of each person on a scale from 1 (low) to 9 (high). Our task was to find out whether or not respondents' ratings were consistent with laypersons' conceptions of intelligence. If they were, then behaviors that received higher characteristicness ratings for intelligence should lead to higher ratings of the intelligence of the fictitious persons; behaviors that received lower characteristicness ratings should lead to lower ratings of the intelligence of the fictitious persons. "Keeps an open mind," for example, had been rated 7.7, whereas "shows a lack of independence" had been rated just 2.7. Averaging the characteristicness ratings for each of the behaviors of each of the fictitious persons, we came up with a score of 6.0 for Susan and of 4.3 for Adam. By comparison, our respondents rated Susan's intelligence at 5.8 and Adam's at 4.3. Overall, when we calculated the correlation between the two sets of ratings (expected values on the basis of the average of the characteristicness ratings for the described person, on the one hand, and actual ratings of the described persons, on the other), we obtained a coefficient of .96. In other words, laypersons' ratings of other people's intelligence were indeed firmly grounded in their implicit theories about intelligence.

We also used multiple-regression techniques in order to determine the weights for each of the three factors in laypersons' implicit theories. As independent variables, we used approximation factor scores of each of the described individuals on each of the factors of the implicit theory (as well as on unintelligence). The multiple correlation, .97, was only slightly higher than the simple correlation noted above. The standardized regression (beta) weights for each of the three factors were .32 for problem-solving ability, .33 for verbal ability, and .19 for social competence (and -.48 for unintelligence). These weights indicate the psychological importance assigned to each of these factors by the subjects in the study. All weights were statistically significant, and all signs were in the predicted directions, with only unintelligent behaviors showing a negative weight. As expected, the unintelligent behaviors had the highest regression weight, since there was only one independent variable for such behaviors, as opposed to three for intelligent behaviors. Moreover, as anyone who has read letters of recommendation knows, even one negative comment can carry quite a bit of weight. Of the three kinds of intelligent behaviors, the two cognitive kinds (problem-solving ability and verbal ability) carried about equal weight, and the noncognitive kind (social competence) carried less weight.

To summarize, people use their implicit theories of intelligence in evaluating the intelligence of others as well as of themselves. Their evaluations of others, based on relatively brief behavioral descriptions of these others, can be predicted at a high level on the basis of their implicit theories. As in the self-ratings, people seem to weigh cognitive factors more heavily than noncognitive ones and to take into account negative as well as positive information. The implicit theories of experts and of laypersons are similar enough so that it makes little difference which is used in making predictions: Results are almost identical for each.

Conclusions

People have well-developed, implicit theories of intelligence that they use both in self-evaluation and in the evaluation of others. Although there are some differences in these theories across groups within our culture, there seems to be a common core that is found in the belief systems of individuals in all of the groups I have studied. The common core includes a problem-solving factor, a verbal-ability factor, and a social-competence factor.

A recent review of literatures covering different approaches to understanding intelligence – including the present implicit-theory approach as well as explicit-theory ones involving the differential, cognitive, and mental-retardation approaches – concludes that these three factors of intelligence plus a motivational one (which did, in fact, appear as a factor in the experts' ratings of academic intelligence) seem to emerge from a variety of approaches to intelligence (Sternberg, 1981f). Thus, the results of the implicit-theories approach seem to converge with research of other kinds in suggesting that intelligence (at least in our mainstream culture) is found to comprise certain kinds of behaviors almost without regard to the way in which it is studied.

An important qualification on this generalization is that the convergence of approaches applies only within the typical North American sociocultural milieu. The contextual subtheory presented earlier suggests that separate contextual accounts of intelligence must be derived for other milieux. These theories might well come out similarly or identically to the present one, but whether or not they do is an empirical question. A gross mistake of some early (and, unfortunately, not so early) cross-cultural research was to assume not only that our context could be carried over to other cultures, but that our instruments for measuring behavior in this context could be carried over as well. The appropriateness of our context and measures for assessing the intelligence of members of other cultures was assumed rather than demonstrated, so that the results obtained from much cross-cultural research must be interpreted with extreme caution. (See Cole & Means, 1981, for a detailed analysis of the pitfalls of comparative research.)

As noted throughout this chapter, the kind of contextual analysis proposed here only provides a start toward understanding the nature of intelligence, even within a single sociocultural milieu. The definition of intelligence presented at the beginning of the chapter was vague, to say the least, and needs further constraints. Moreover, the contextually based implicit theory presented here says nothing about the mental mechanisms by which the behaviors of problem solving, verbal ability, and social competence are carried out. These issues are considered in the next two chapters.

3   Experience and intelligence

All of the explicit-theoretical accounts presented in Chapter 1 – both differential and cognitive – suffer from a common flaw: They are post hoc. Investigators have started with a class of tasks and then claimed that intelligence is whatever it takes to do well on those tasks.

Consider first the differential theories. The "factors of intelligent behavior" that emerge from factor analysis are largely determined by the tasks that are entered into the factor analysis. For example, "spatial ability" can appear as a factor of intelligence only if spatial-type tasks are included in the test battery. If such tasks are not included, there is no way for a spatial factor to emerge. But how does one decide to include spatial tasks, or any other kinds of tasks, in one's test battery? Unfortunately, psychometric theorists never provided any a priori guidelines for task selection. Rather, they chose tasks that they thought would "work," in some sense of the word. As time progressed, the major basis for task selection seems to have become past use: Tasks were used that were similar or identical to tasks that had been used before. But tradition scarcely constitutes an a priori, theoretical basis for choosing tasks that measure intelligence.

Consider next cognitive theories. As Newell (1973) has observed, task selection in cognitive-psychological research has scarcely been theoretically motivated. To the contrary, it appears to have been at least as haphazard as task selection in differential research. Tasks have been selected for any number of reasons, but theoretical motivation does not appear to be among them. At times, cognitive psychology has seemed to be a psychology of tasks (Sternberg, 1979b) whose interrelationships have been only vaguely understood. Cognitive psychologists studying intelligence seem to have picked up well-worked standard tasks and then developed theories that happened to suit. For example, Hunt's (1978) early work was based on the standard tasks being used in cognitive psychologists' laboratories; my early work (Sternberg, 1977b) was based on standard tasks used in psychometric tests of intelligence.

The implicit-theoretical approach provides some independent motivation for task selection. The research presented in Chapter 2 suggests, for example, that the classes of tasks to be used in our own culture should be ones that measure problem-solving, verbal, and social-competence skills. But this specification of tasks needs further constraints. No one would believe that all problem-solving tasks are equally apt as measures of intelligence: Solving the problem of what to eat for lunch on a typical day scarcely seems to be in the same class as, say, solving the problem of identifying hidden assumptions in a persuasive communication as a measure of intelligence. Even within a given problem type, some problems seem to provide more apt measures of intelligence than do others. A verbal analogy that could be solved solely on the basis of knowing the meanings of the words in the analogy would seem to be a less apt measure of intelligence than a verbal analogy that required not only some vocabulary but also complex reasoning. In sum, some set of further constraints seems to be needed for assessing the extent to which a given task (or situation) requires intelligence. This chapter identifies how levels of experience in performance provide such constraints. Further constraints will be considered in the next chapter.

The subtheory presented below differs from previous accounts in starting with a specification of the attributes of tasks or situations that lead to the measurement of intelligence. No attempt is made here to specify the particular tasks or situations that should be used. Indeed, according to the present view, the proper choice of tasks and situations will vary across persons and groups of persons. Thus, what matters is not the particular tasks or situations used, but what they measure for a given individual. The facets of task and situational performance proposed here could, in fact, apply to almost any task or situation, given the right circumstances.

An experiential subtheory of intelligence

The experiential subtheory proposes that a task measures "intelligence" in part as a function of the extent to which it requires either or both of two skills: the ability to deal with novel kinds of task and situational demands and the ability to automatize the processing of information. Consider each of these skills in turn.

Ability to deal with novel task and situational demands

Novel tasks. The idea that intelligence involves the ability to deal with novel task demands is far from novel (see, e.g., Cattell, 1971; Horn, 1968; Kaufman & Kaufman, 1983; Raaheim, 1974; Snow, 1981; Sternberg, 1981d,

1982e, 1982f, in 1984a). Sternberg (1981d) has suggested, in fact, that intelligence is best measured by tasks that are "nonentrenched" in the sense of requiring information processing of kinds outside people's ordinary experience. The task may be nonentrenched in the kinds of operations it requires or in the concepts it requires the subjects to utilize. According to this view, then, intelligence involves

not merely the ability to learn and reason with new concepts but the ability to learn and reason with new kinds of concepts. Intelligence is not so much a person's ability to learn or think within conceptual systems that the person has already become familiar with as it is his or her ability to learn and think within new conceptual systems, which can then be brought to bear upon already existing knowledge structures. (Sternberg, 1981d, p. 4)

It is important to note that the usefulness of a task in measuring intelligence is not a linear function of task novelty. The task that is presented should be novel, but not totally outside the individual's past experience (Raaheim, 1974). If the task is too novel, then the individual will not have any cognitive structures to bring to bear upon the task, and as a result the task will simply be outside of the individual's range of comprehension. Calculus, for example, would be a highly novel field of endeavor for most 5-year-olds. But the calculus tasks would be so far outside their range of experience that they would be worthless for the assessment of 5-year-olds' intelligence. In Piagetian (1972) terms, the task should primarily require accommodation but must require some assimilation as well.

Implicit in the above discussion is the notion that novelty can be of two kinds, either or both of which may be involved in task performance. The two kinds of novelty might be characterized as involving (a) comprehension of the task and (b) acting upon one's comprehension of the task. Consider the meaning of each of these two kinds of novelty.

Novelty in comprehension of the task refers to the novelty that inheres in understanding the task confronting one. Once one understands the task, acting upon it may or may not be challenging. In essence, the novelty is in learning how to do the task rather than in actually doing it. Novelty in acting upon one's comprehension of the task refers to novelty in acting upon a problem rather than in learning about the problem or in learning how to solve it. The genre of task is familiar, but the parameters of the particular task are not. It is possible, of course, to formulate problems involving novelty in both comprehension and execution of a particular kind of task and to formulate problems that involve novelty in neither comprehension nor execution. The present account suggests that problems of these two kinds might be less satisfactory measures of intelligence than problems involving novelty in either comprehension or execution, but not both. The reason for this is that the former problems might be too novel, whereas the latter problems might not be novel enough to provide optimal measurement of intelligence.

Novel situations. The notion that intelligence is particularly aptly measured in situations that require adaptation to new and challenging environmental demands inheres both in experts' and laypersons' notions of the nature of intelligence (Intelligence and its measurement, 1921; Sternberg, Conway, Ketron, & Bernstein, 1981). The idea is that a person's intelligence is best shown not in run-of-the-mill situations that are encountered regularly in everyday life, but rather in extraordinary situations that challenge the individual's ability to cope with the environment. Almost everyone knows someone (perhaps oneself) who performs well when confronted with tasks that are presented in a familiar milieu, but who falls apart when presented with similar or even identical tasks that are in an unfamiliar milieu. For example, a person who performs well in his or her everyday environment might find it difficult to function in a foreign country, even one that is similar in many respects to the home environment. In general, some people can perform well, but only under situational circumstances that are highly favorable to their getting their work done. When the environment is less supportive, their efficacy is greatly reduced.

Essentially the same constraints that apply to task novelty apply to situational novelty as well. First, too much novelty can render the situation nondiagnostic of intellectual level. Moreover, there may exist situations in which no one could function effectively (perhaps as epitomized by the situation confronted by the protagonist in Sartre's *No Exit*). Second, situational novelty can inhere either in understanding the nature of the situation or in performing within the context of that situation. In some instances, it is figuring out just what the situation is that is difficult; in others, it is operating in that situation once one has figured out what it is.

Interactions among tasks, situations, and persons. It is important to take into account the fact that tasks or situations that are novel for some persons may not be novel for others. Thus, a given task or situation will not necessarily measure "intelligence" to the same extent for some people that it does for others. Similarly, people vary widely in the extent to which various kinds of situations are novel in their experience. Not only do task and situation interact with person, but they can interact with each other as well. A task that is novel in one situation might not be novel in another situation. Finally, at the level of "third-order" interaction, a task may be novel (or mundane) for some persons in one situation but not a second situation, whereas the same task would be novel (or mundane) for other persons in the second situation but not in the first. In sum, one needs to take into account interactions among these variables as well as their main effects.

Ability to automatize information processing

Automatization as a function of task. Many kinds of tasks requiring complex information processing seem so intricate that it is a wonder we can perform them at all. Consider reading, for example. The number and complexity of operations involved in reading is staggering, and what is more staggering is the rate at which these operations are performed (see, e.g., Crowder, 1982; Just & Carpenter, 1980). Performance of tasks as complex as reading would seem to be possible only because a substantial proportion of the operations required in reading are automatized and thus require minimal mental effort (see Schneider & Shiffrin, 1977, and Shiffrin & Schneider, 1977, for a discussion of the mental requirements of tasks involving controlled and automatized information processing). Deficiencies in reading have been theorized to result in large part from failures in automatization of operations that in normal readers have been automatized (LaBerge & Samuels, 1974; Sternberg & Wagner, 1982).

The proposal being made here is that complex tasks can feasibly be executed only because many of the operations involved in their performance have been automatized. Failure to automatize such operations, whether fully or in part, results in a breakdown of information processing and hence less intelligent task performance. Intellectual operations that can be performed smoothly and automatically by more intelligent individuals are performed only haltingly and under conscious control by less intelligent individuals.

As in the case of novelty, automatization can occur in either task comprehension, task execution, or both. Consider how each of these kinds of automatization operates in various tasks.

The standard synonyms test used to measure vocabulary is highly familiar to most middle-class students at or above the secondary school level. Indeed, when confronted with a multiple-choice synonyms test, about the only things the students need to check are whether the test is in fact one of synonyms (as opposed to, say, antonyms, which has a similar surface structure) and whether there is a penalty for guessing. But examinees can usually read the directions to such a test cursorily, and could probably skip them altogether if only they were told the name of the task. Comprehension of what is required is essentially automatic. But solution of individual test items may be far from automatic, especially if the test requires discriminating relatively fine shades of meaning. Students may find they have to give a fair amount of thought to the individual items, either because they need to discriminate shades of meaning or because they are unsure of particular words' meanings and have to employ strategies for guessing the best answers. In the standard synonyms task, comprehension of task instructions is essentially automatic (or nearly so), but solution of test items (beyond the simplest ones) probably is not.

In contrast, experimental tasks used in the cognitive psychologist's laboratory seem to present the opposite situation, in at least one respect. Tasks such as the Posner and Mitchell (1967) letter-matching task and the fixed-set S. Sternberg (1969) memory-scanning task are probably unfamiliar to most subjects when they enter the cognitive psychologist's laboratory. The subjects do not automatically know what is expected of them in task performance and have to listen reasonably carefully to the instructions. But after the task is explained and the subjects have had some practice in performing the tasks, it is likely that task performance becomes rapidly automatized. The tasks come to be executed almost effortlessly and with little conscious thought.

It is possible, of course, for task performance to be fully automatized or not to be automatized at all. When one gets hold of a mystery story to read, one knows essentially automatically what one is going to do and how one is going to do it. In contrast, learning how to solve a new kind of mathematics problem, such as a time – rate – distance problem, is probably not automatized with respect to either comprehension or task execution.

Automatization as a function of situation. Very little is known about how situations affect automatization of task performance. Clearly, one wishes to provide as much practice as possible on the task to be automatized. Presumably, one might wish to minimize distraction from the task in order to allow the individual to concentrate on learning the task and eventually automatizing it.

Interactions among tasks, situations, and persons. As was the case with response to novelty, interactions can exist, in the development of automatization, between tasks and situations; between tasks and persons; between situations and persons; and between tasks, situations, and persons. Much of the literature on aptitude – treatment interactions in task performance can be viewed as an attempt to understand how different kinds of environments promote or retard learning on specific classes of tasks as a function of aptitude characteristics of the learner. In general, replicable findings in the aptitude – treatment interaction literature are hard to come by (Cronbach & Snow, 1977). But sufficient evidence has been accumulated to suggest that such interactions do indeed exist.

In the domain of laboratory tasks, MacLeod, Hunt, and Mathews (1978) and Mathews, Hunt, and MacLeod (1980) found that optimal strategy for promotion of rapid performance on sentence – picture comparison items was a function of the individual's level of spatial ability: A spatial strategy worked better for some individuals, whereas a linguistic strategy worked better for others whose scores on spatial ability tests were relatively lower. Sternberg and Weil (1980) obtained a similar result for linear syllogisms: Optimality of a linguistic, spatial, or mixed strategy depended upon an individual's pattern of verbal and spatial aptitudes. In the domain of more commonly performed, real-world tasks, it seems highly likely that certain methods of teaching reading lead to better reading, including fuller skill automatization, than do other methods (Baron & Strawson, 1976; Cronbach & Snow, 1977; Crowder, 1982; Spache & Spache, 1973): The whole-word method seems better suited to certain ability patterns, and the phonics method to others. Similarly, different methods of foreign-language instruction seem to be differentially effective for individuals with different ability patterns but it is not yet clear just what the nature of the interaction is (Carroll, in press; Diller, 1978). Tentatively, one might venture that grammar-intensive and learning-from-context methods may work better for those with higher general intelligence but only average abilities specialized for language learning; mimicry and memorization methods may work better for those with higher specialized language-learning abilities but only average general intelligence.

Relationship between abilities to deal with novelty and to automatize processing

For many (but probably not all) kinds of tasks, the ability to deal with novelty and to automatize information processing may occur along an experiential continuum. When one first encounters a task or kind of situation, ability to deal with novelty comes into play. The more intelligent person will be more rapidly and fully able to cope with the novel demands being made upon him or her. As experience with the kind of task or situation increases, novelty decreases, and the task or situation will become less apt in its measurement of intelligence from the standpoint of processing of novelty. However, after some amount of practice with the task or in the situation, automatization skills may come into play, in which case the task will start to become a more apt measure of automatization skills. Moreover, processing resources allocated to novelty and to automatization can interact with each other: Greater automatization of information processing frees additional processing resources for attending to novelty. Thus, a given task or situation may continue to provide apt measurement of intelligence over practice, but for differing reasons at different points in practice: Early on in the person's experience, the ability to deal with novelty is assessed; later on in the person's experience, the ability to automatize information processing is assessed.

The various relationships discussed here and earlier in the chapter are

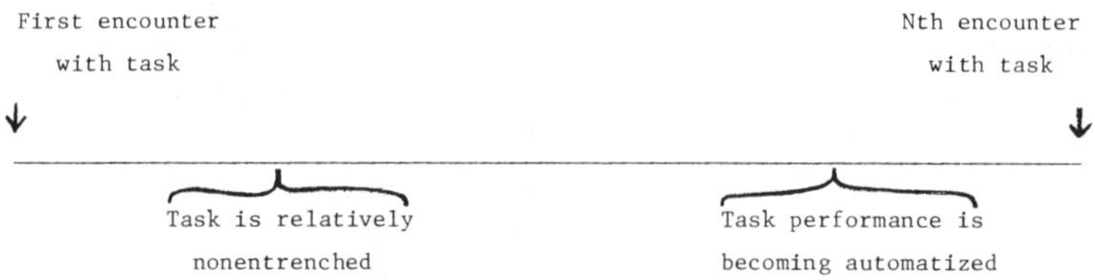

First encounter   Nth encounter
  with task   with task

↓   ↓
_____

                    ┌──────┴──────┐   ┌──────┴──────┐
                    Task is relatively   Task performance is
                     nonentrenched   becoming automatized

Figure 3.1. Course of experience with a task: Intelligence is best measured when the task is relatively nonentrenched or in the process of becoming automatized.

schematically summarized in Figure 3.1, which diagrams the various levels of experience that are important in the selection of tasks and situations that measure intelligence.

What tasks measure intelligence and why?

The proposed experiential subtheory suggests what properties of tasks and situations make them more or less useful measures of intelligence. Consider some of the tasks most frequently used and the implications of the subtheory for understanding why these tasks are more or less successful.

Laboratory tasks

A variety of laboratory tasks have been claimed to measure intelligence. According to the present view, the simpler tasks, such as simple reaction time, choice reaction time, and letter identification, have some validity as measures of intelligence because they measure primarily automatization of various kinds. For example, simple reaction-time tasks measure in part the extent to which an individual can automatize rapid responses to a single stimulus, and letter-identification tasks measure in part the extent to which access to highly overlearned codes stored in long-term memory is automatized. Speed is a reasonable measure of intellectual performance because it is presumably highly correlated with degree of automatization; however, it is only an indirect measure of this degree of automatization and hence provides an imperfect measure of it. One might expect some increase in correlation of task latencies with measured intelligence as task complexity increases, even at these very simple levels, because of the increased element of novelty in the higher levels even of simple tasks. Thus, choice reaction time introduces an element of uncertainty that is absent in simple reaction time, and the amount of uncertainty, and hence of novelty, increases as the number of response choices increases. In this argument, I am conjecturing that response to novelty contributes more to measured intelligence than does efficacy of automatization; this conjecture is in need of verification.

The more complex laboratory tasks, such as analogies, classifications, syllogisms, and the like, probably measure both degree of automatization and response to novelty. To the extent that subjects have had past practice on these item formats (such as in taking intelligence and aptitude tests, as well as in participating in experiments), their selection and implementation of strategies will be partially automatized when they start the tasks. But even if they have had little or no prior experience with certain item formats, the formats tend to be repetitive, and in the large numbers of trials typical of cognitive–psychological experiments, subjects are likely to automatize their performance to some degree while performing the tasks. The more complex items also measure response to novelty, in that the relations subjects have to recognize and reason with will usually be at least somewhat unfamiliar.

Psychometric tasks

The psychometric tasks found on ability tests are likely to measure intelligence for the same reasons as the complex laboratory tasks, in that they contain essentially the same kinds of contents. They are apt to be slightly better measures than the laboratory tasks for three reasons. First, the pencil-and-paper psychometric items tend to be harder, because laboratory tasks are often simplified in order to reduce error rates. Harder tasks will, on the average, involve greater amounts of novelty. Second, psychometric test items are usually presented en masse (subjects are given a fixed amount of time to solve all of them) rather than individually (subjects are given a fixed or free amount of time to solve each separate item). Presenting the items en masse requires individuals to plan an interitem as well as an intraitem strategy and hence requires more "executive" kinds of behaviors. Such behaviors may have been previously automatized in part, but are also responses to whatever novelty inheres in the particular testing situation confronted (content, difficulty, time limits, etc., for a particular test). Third, the psychometric test items found in most test batteries have been extensively validated, whereas the items used in laboratory experiments almost never have been.

Implications for task selection

The proposed subtheory carries with it certain implications for the selection of tasks to measure intelligence. In particular, one wishes to select tasks that involve some blend of automatized behaviors and behaviors in response to novelty. This blending is probably best achieved within test items, but may also be achieved by items that specialize in measuring either the one skill or the other. The blending may be achieved by presenting subjects with a novel task and then giving them enough practice with the task so that performance becomes differentially automatized (across subjects) over the length of the practice period. Such a task will thereby measure both response to novelty and degree of automatization, although at different times during the course of testing.

Resolution of some puzzles in the literature on intelligence

The proposed subtheory suggests resolutions to some of the puzzles that appear in the literature on intelligence. Consider four such puzzles.

Why do so many tasks measure intelligence? Almost any task one encounters is unfamiliar in some degree; thus, most tasks involve at least some coping with novelty. Similarly, almost any task that is not totally new has been encountered before, at least in part or in analogue; thus, most tasks involve at least some prior automatization in their performance. The result is that most tasks measure intelligence in greater or lesser degree. It is for this reason that it is so easy to find *some* degree of correlation between task performance and scores on tests specifically designed to measure intelligence. But not many tasks (including the tasks found in IQ tests) are exceptionally well suited to measuring either response to novelty or automatization of task performance. As a result, the number of tasks that provide highly valid measurement of intelligence is probably fairly limited. The present view suggests selecting tasks that are valid in the sense of measuring skills involved in coping with novelty and in automatizing performance.

At what point of practice on a task does it best measure intelligence? A lively debate has arisen over the point in practice at which a task best measures intelligence. Noble, Noble, and Alcock (1958) used tests from the Thurstone Primary Mental Abilities battery to predict individual differences in trial-and-error learning and found that prediction was higher for total correct scores than for initial correct scores, suggesting that the higher correlation came from performance in later trials. Fleishman and Hempel (1955) and Fleishman (1965) also found that the percentage of variance accounted for in motor tasks by traditional psychometric tests increases with practice. Results such as these have led Glaser (1967) to conclude that "the usual psychometric variables are correlated to a lesser degree with initial acquisition performance" (p. 12). These results, however, seem to be inconsistent with the idea that tasks measure intelligence to the extent that they are novel. The proposed subtheory, however, can account for these findings, as well as for the more common finding that correlations with intelligence remain about the same at all levels of practice (e.g., Guyote & Sternberg, 1981; Sternberg, 1980f). Indeed, psychometric tests are predicated on the idea that they are measuring intelligence to the same degree earlier and later during testing. According to the present view, a given task will tend more to measure novelty-coping skills earlier during practice and automatization skills later during practice. As a result, whether the correlation with intelligence as measured by psychometric tests will increase, remain the same, or decrease over practice will depend upon the extent to which the task successfully measures novelty and automatization at the various stages of practice. Some tasks may be more successful measuring the one or the other, so that they will tend to be more successful either earlier or later during practice. Thus, the overall correlation with measured intelligence may actually remain the same over practice, even while the skills that contribute to that correlation differ over time.

Can tests of intelligence be culture-fair? No test of intelligence can be *culture-free:* All tests require some degree of acculturation for their successful completion. But there is some question as to whether a test can be *culture-fair*. Can a given task measure intelligence to the same degree across cultures or even subcultures? According to the present view, a test will be culture-fair to the extent that it measures (a) coping with novelty and (b) automatization to an equal extent across (or even within) cultures. Unfortunately, people's experiences with tasks and classes of tasks tend to differ widely across cultures (and even, to a fairly large extent, within cultures). I doubt whether tests can be precisely equated in terms of the extent to which they measure each of coping with novelty and automatization across different groups. Consider, for example, the common finding that abstract, nonverbal items, which have often been proposed to be "culture-fair" (Cattell & Cattell, 1963), tend to show greater discrepancies across cultural groups than do verbal tests (Jensen, 1980)! According to the present view, this is because such tests can measure quite different skills across groups. For individuals who are familiar with these types of items (from taking tests or from everyday experiences with abstract kinds of materials), the nonverbal tests may hardly measure novelty-coping skills at all. For individuals unfamiliar with these types of items, the items may primarily measure the ability to cope with novelty. Thus, although the objective stimulus item is the same, the item measures different skills for the different individuals, and performance could not be compared fairly across these individuals.

Why do abilities tend to cluster into two groups, "fluid" and "crystallized"? Research using a variety of approaches has suggested that there are two main groups of abilities. These have been called "fluid" and "crystallized" abilities by Cattell (1971), Horn (1968), and Snow (1980), "practical – mechanical" and "verbal – educational" abilities by Vernon (1971), and problem-solving and verbal abilities by Sternberg et al. (1981). Fluid types of abilities are particularly well measured by reasoning items such as analogies and series completions, whereas crystallized abilities are measured particularly well by tests such as reading comprehension and vocabulary. On the present view, fluid ability tests tend to stress ability to deal with novelty, whereas crystallized ability tests tend to stress automatization of high-level processes. Laboratory tasks stressing response to novel demands measure fluid abilities. In contrast, laboratory tasks that stress automatization of higher-level codes, such as the letter-comparison task used by Hunt et al. (1975), are probably better understood as measures of precursors of crystallized abilities than of fluid abilities (see Hunt, 1978). Because of the extreme number of skills required in complex verbal tasks, such as reading, it is necessary to have a large number of operations automatized for their successful completion; if these operations are not automatized, specific disabilities in performance may result (Sternberg & Wagner, 1982).

In sum, it has been proposed that behavior is intelligent when it involves either or both of two sets of skills: adaptation to novelty and automatization of performance. This proposal has been used to explain why so many tasks seem to measure "intelligence" in greater or lesser degree as well as to account for other puzzling findings in the literature on human intelligence. Most importantly, the subtheory is an a priori specification of what a task or situation must measure in order to assess intelligence. It is distinctive in that it is not linked to any arbitrary choice of tasks or situations. Selection of tasks and situations follows from the subtheory, rather than the other way around.

A theory of response to novelty and automatization of information processing based upon the experiential subtheory of intelligence

The subtheory proposed here seeks to concretize some of the ideas presented above regarding novelty and automatization. Each of the two levels of experience will be considered in turn.

Response to novelty

The first part of the experiential subtheory deals with individuals' ways of responding to novelty. It was noted earlier that novelty can inhere primarily either in task performance or in understanding how to perform the task. Each of these two cases will be considered in turn.

Novelty in task performance: a model of insight. Novelty can inhere in task performance for any of a number of reasons. A particularly important class of tasks involving novelty in task performance is the class of insight tasks. Insight tasks require one to find a novel and unobvious solution to a problem that may or may not, on its face, seem difficult. Such tasks may be quite easy to understand, but quite difficult to perform. Conventional views of insight fall into two basic camps – the special-process views and the nothing-special views. Consider each of these views.

Conventional views of insight. According to "special-process" views, insight is a process that differs in kind from ordinary kinds of information processes. These views are most often associated with the Gestalt psychologists and their successors (e.g., Köhler, 1927; Maier, 1930; Wertheimer, 1959). Among these views are the ideas that insight results from extended unconscious leaps in thinking, that it results from greatly accelerated mental processing, and that it results from a short-circuiting of normal reasoning processes (see Perkins, 1981). These views are intuitively appealing, but seem to carry with them at least three problematical aspects. First, they do not really pin down what insight is. Calling insight an "unconscious leap in thinking" or a "short-circuiting of normal reasoning" leaves insight pretty much a "black box" of unknown contents. Even were one of these theories correct, just what insight is would remain to be identified. Second, virtually all of the evidence in support of these views is anecdotal rather than experimental, and for each piece of anecdotal evidence to support one of these views, there is at least one corresponding piece of evidence to refute it (Perkins, 1981). Finally, the positions are probably not pinned down sufficiently as they stand to permit empirical test. As a result, it is not clear that the positions are even falsifiable. It is this characteristic of nonfalsifiability that probably resulted in the death of Gestalt psychology: Its propositions were simply not testable.

According to the "nothing-special" views, insight is merely an extension of ordinary processes of perceiving, recognizing, learning, and conceiving. This view, most forcefully argued by Perkins (1981), would view past failures to identify any special processes of insight as being due to the (alleged) fact that there is no special process of insight. Insights are merely significant products of ordinary processes. We can understand the kind of frustration that would lead Perkins and others to this view: After repeated failures to identify a construct empirically, one can easily be tempted to ascribe the failure to the nonexistence of the construct. One cannot find what is not there! But I am not yet ready to abandon the notion that there is something special about insight, any more than I am ready, on the basis of Mischel's (1968) devastating critique of the trait literature, to abandon the notion of personality traits. Arguments for the "nothing-special" views are arguments by default – because we have not identified insight processes, they have no independent existence – and I do not accept such arguments because I believe we can create positive arguments for the existence of insight processes.

Proposed view of insight. Sternberg and Davidson (1982, 1983) have proposed that a main reason psychologists (and others) have had so much difficulty in isolating insight is that it involves not one but three separate but related psychological processes:

1. *Selective encoding.* An insight of selective encoding involves sifting out relevant information from irrelevant information. Significant problems generally present one with large amounts of information, only some of which is relevant to problem solution. For example, the facts of a legal case are usually both numerous and confusing: An insightful lawyer must figure out which of the myriad facts confronting him or her are relevant to principles of law. Similarly, a doctor or psychotherapist may be presented with a great volume of information regarding a patient's background and symptoms: An insightful doctor or psychotherapist must sift out those facts that are relevant for diagnosis or treatment. A famous example of what we refer to as an insight of selective encoding is Alexander Fleming's discovery of penicillin. In looking at a petri dish containing a culture that had become moldy, Fleming noticed that bacteria in the vicinity of the mold had been destroyed, presumably by the mold. In essence, Fleming encoded the information in his visual field in a highly selective way, zeroing in on that part of the field that was relevant to the discovery of the antibiotic.

2. *Selective combination.* An insight of selective combination involves combining what might originally seem to be isolated pieces of information into a unified whole that may or may not resemble its parts. Whereas selective encoding involves knowing which pieces of information are relevant, selective combination involves knowing how to put together the pieces of information that are relevant. For example, the lawyer must know how the relevant facts of a case fit together to make (or break!) the case. A doctor or psychotherapist must be able to figure out how to combine information about various isolated symptoms to identify a given medical (or psychological) syndrome. A famous example of selective combination is Darwin's formulation of the theory of evolution. It is well known that Darwin had available to him for many years the facts he needed to form the basis for the theory of natural selection. What eluded him for those years was a way to combine the facts into a coherent package.

3. *Selective comparison.* An insight of selective comparison involves relating newly acquired information to information acquired in the past. Problem solving by analogy, for example, is an instance of selective comparison:

One realizes that new information is similar to old information in certain ways (and dissimilar from it in other ways) and uses this information better to understand the new information. For example, an insightful lawyer will relate a current case to legal precedents; choosing the right precedents is absolutely essential. A doctor or psychotherapist relates the current set of presenting symptoms to previous case histories in his or her own or others' past experiences; again, choosing the right precedents is essential. A famous example of an insight of selective comparison is Kekulé's discovery of the structure of the benzene ring. Kekulé dreamed of a snake curling back on itself and catching its tail. When he woke up, he realized that the image of the snake catching its tail was a metaphor for the structure of the benzene ring.

Tests of the model of insight. Preliminary data testing the theory of insight are encouraging. Further, more experimentally based data will be presented later in the book when I discuss the role of insight in intellectual giftedness.

In one study (Sternberg & Davidson, 1982), we presented 30 adults from the New Haven area (who were not Yale-connected) with unlimited time to solve 12 insight problems chosen to require little background knowledge. Some examples are:

1. If you have black socks and brown socks in your drawer, mixed in the ratio of 4 to 5, how many socks will you have to take out to make sure of having a pair of socks the same color?
2. Suppose you and I have the same amount of money. How much must I give you so that you have 10 dollars more than I?
3. Water lilies double in area every 24 hours. At the beginning of the summer there is 1 water lily on a lake. It takes 60 days for the lake to become covered with water lilies. On what day is the lake half-covered?
4. A farmer has 17 sheep. All but 9 broke through a hole in the fence and wandered away. How many were left?

Of these particular problems, the first emphasizes selective encoding, the second emphasizes selective combination, and the third emphasizes both of these processes. The fourth emphasizes neither of these processes. Rather, it is a "trick" problem that requires one to read the problem and question very carefully. The difficulty of the problem is in encoding, but not in *selective* encoding of relevant versus irrelevant information. Incidentally, the answers to the problems are 3, 5, 59, and 9, respectively; proportions of subjects getting each of these particular problems correct were .43, .40, .40, and .57, respectively. Overall proportion correct for the full set of 12 problems was .37

Performance on the complete set of problems was correlated .66 with Henmon – Nelson IQ; .63 with inductive reasoning, as measured by "Letter

Sets" from the French Kit of Reference Tests for Cognitive Factors (French, Ekstrom, & Price, 1963); and .34 with deductive reasoning, as measured by "Nonsense Syllogisms" from the French Kit. In a second (as yet unpublished) study, performance of 30 different individuals (again not Yale-connected) on 20 insight problems such as the ones above was correlated .55 with Henmon – Nelson IQ, .51 with inductive reasoning (Letter Sets), and .42 with deductive reasoning (Nonsense Syllogisms). In both studies, an examination of point-biserial correlations between item scores and IQ revealed that the highest correlations tended to be for items that clearly measured either selective encoding, selective combination, or both. Trick problems, such as the "sheep" problem (no. 4 above), tended to have relatively lower correlations with IQ.

In the second study, we also investigated subjects' relative uses of the processes of selective encoding and selective combination. By far the most successful strategy was to use both of these processes in solving an insight problem. Using just selective encoding tended to result in a lesser degree of success, and using just selective combination resulted in the least degree of success. Unfortunately, this last strategy was used considerably more frequently than the other strategies (as determined by analysis of subjects' written protocols while they solved the problems).

A third study investigated the selective comparison process (Davidson & Sternberg, 1982). Subjects were again New Haven area adults who were not Yale-connected at the time of testing. Each subject was assigned to 1 of 4 experimental conditions and received 12 insight problems divided into 2 sets of 6 problems each. There were 4 types of conditions. In 1 of the 4 conditions, subjects received example problems that were relevant to solving half of the test problems prior to receiving the actual test problems. The relevance of the examples for the test problems was not pointed out, however. In a second condition, subjects received the same examples and test problems, except that the relevance of the samples for the test problems was pointed out to them. In a third condition, subjects received example and actual test problems, but the example problems were not directly relevant to the solution of the test problems. In the fourth condition, subjects received no example problems at all.

Subjects performed best when they received relevant example problems and the relevance of the examples was pointed out to them, second best when they received relevant problems but without the relevance of the problems being pointed out to them, and worst in the two conditions where there were no relevant examples. Moreover, the effect was isolated only in the particular half of the problems for which the examples had been relevant. Peformance on the problems for which the examples were not relevant was the same in all of the groups that received any examples, and these means did not differ from the nonexamples group either. These results indicate that subjects can perform an insight of selective comparison in solving the test problems, bringing to bear information from the examples when it is relevant. But as might be expected, subjects do even better when they are "given" the insight and told the examples are relevant rather than having to figure out this fact for themselves.

Performance in all kinds of conditions was highly correlated with psychometric test scores, as in the preceding two studies. The median correlation with IQ was .77; with inductive reasoning, it was .70; and with deductive reasoning, it was .56. Insight problems thus appear to overlap with whatever it is that IQ tests measure but to measure other skills as well that are not measured by the IQ tests.

From these three studies, we drew four primary conclusions that are relevant here. First, subjects use selective encoding, selective combination, and selective comparison in the solution of insight problems. Second, insight problems measure skills that are highly related, but not identical, to what it is that IQ tests measure. "Trick" problems, however, do not provide good measurement either of insight or of IQ. Third, subjects differ in the extent to which they use the various kinds of insights in solving a given problem. Finally, failures in past research to isolate a process of insight may stem in part from failure to realize that insights can be of at least three kinds. Providing one kind of insight for subjects may not be sufficient for problem solution if other kinds of insights are needed as well.

Novelty in task understanding: a model of concept projection. From the standpoint of the comprehension of novelty, there are five critical processes in the understanding of a novel task in which an individual must mentally move from a conventional conceptual system to a novel one. The critical processes are:

1. *Encoding the expectation of a change in conceptual system.* This process entails recognition on the part of an individual that a novel conceptual system will be required that is different from the one the subject is using in his or her current information processing.

2. *Accessing a novel conceptual system.* This process requires an individual to go from the current and conventional conceptual system to a new and novel one.

3. *Finding an appropriate concept in a new conceptual system.* This process requires an individual to find the appropriate concept within the now-accessed novel conceptual system.

4. *Allowing for a nonentrenched relationship.* This process requires an

individual to process a concept in a new conceptual system that is different in kind from the kinds of concepts with which the individual is familiar in the conventional conceptual system.

5. *Responding to a violation of an expectation of a change in conceptual system.* On occasion, an individual may expect there to be a change in conceptual system, but this expectation proves to be incorrect. This process requires recovery from this incorrect expectation so that the individual is again able to function in the conventional conceptual system.

The concept projection task. I have studied people's responses to novelty in understanding or learning how to perform a new kind of task through a "concept projection task" (Sternberg, 1981d, 1982e). In order to understand the model of concept projection, it is necessary to understand something about the kind of task used to measure this skill. The task is quite complicated, but this complication is deliberate. Remember that the goal here is for the task to require response to novelty in task understanding, although not necessarily in task performance.

The main novel or "nonentrenched" task I have studied is one that requires the individual to make a projection that characterizes the state of an object at some future time on the basis of incomplete information about the state of the object both at that time and at some earlier time. The projection task was studied with four different "surface" structures having very similar "deep" structures. Consider the first instantiation of the task, which requires projection of the color an object will appear to be at a future time.

In the first instantiation of the task, subjects were presented with a description of the color of an object in the present day and in the year 2000. The description in each case could be either pictorial – a green dot or a blue dot – or verbal – one of four color words, namely, *green, blue, grue,* and *bleen.* An object was defined as green if it appeared physically green both in the present and in the year 2000. An object was defined as blue if it appeared physically blue both in the present and in the year 2000. An object was defined as grue if it appeared physically green in the present but physically blue in the year 2000 (i.e., it appeared physically green until the year 2000 and physically blue thereafter). An object was defined as bleen if it appeared physically blue in the present but physically green in the year 2000 (i.e., it appeared physically blue until the year 2000 and physically green thereafter). (The terminology is based upon Goodman, 1955.)

Because each of the two descriptions (one in the present and one in the year 2000) could take one of either two pictorial forms or four verbal forms, there were 36 (6×6) different item types. The subject's task was to describe the object in the year 2000. If the given description for the year 2000 was a pictorial one, the subject had to indicate the correct verbal description of the object; if the given description for the year 2000 was a verbal one, the subject had to indicate the correct physical description of the object. There were always three answer choices from which the subject had to choose the correct one.

Subjects were alerted to a complexity in the projection task that applies to the real world as well. When one observes the physical appearance of an object in the present day, one can be certain of its current physical appearance but not of what its physical appearance will be in the year 2000. Hence, all descriptions given for the present day could be guaranteed to be accurate with respect to physical appearance in the present, but they could not be guaranteed to be accurate with respect to their implications, if any, regarding physical appearance in the future. For pictorial descriptions of objects as they appear in the present, this complexity presents no problems, since the pictorial description of an object (a green dot or a blue dot) carries no implications regarding the future physical appearance of the object. For verbal descriptions of objects as they appear in the present, however, this complexity does present a problem. The verbal descriptions *green* and *blue* imply constancy in physical appearance (*steady-state words*), whereas the verbal descriptions *grue* and *bleen* imply change (*variable-state words*). Unfortunately, all one can infer with certainty from these verbal descriptions is the current physical appearance of the object. The implication for the future physical appearance of the object can only be a guess, which may be right or wrong. This complexity ceases to exist for the observer in the year 2000 because at this point all of the evidence is in. The observer in the year 2000 knows for certain what the physical appearance of the object is in 2000 and also knows for certain what the physical appearance of the object was in what was once the present. Hence, the second description, that of the object in the year 2000, is guaranteed to be correct both with respect to the object's appearance in 2000 and the object's appearance in what was once the present. (The one exception to this guarantee is a certain problem type referred to as "inconsistent," as described below.)

To summarize, pictorial descriptions, which carried no implications for what an object would look like at another time, were always accurate in all respects. Verbal descriptions, which did carry an implication for the appearance of an object at another time, were always accurate with respect to the physical description they implied for the object at the time at which the description was given (except for inconsistent items), but in the present, they might not be accurate with respect to the physical description they implied for the year 2000.

Some examples of actual items will illustrate a few item types. (See Sternberg, 1981d, 1982e, for further examples.) In these examples, the letters G and B are used to represent the colored dots (green or blue) that were used to indicate the physical appearances of the actual objects. The letter I stands for "inconsistent." Recall that items could consist of either two verbal descriptions, a pictorial description and a verbal description, a verbal description and a pictorial description, or two pictorial descriptions.

Blue Blue   G B I

In this example, an object is described verbally as blue in the present and as blue in 2000. Clearly, its physical appearance in 2000 is B. This was an easy item, with a mean response latency of 1.5 seconds.

Blue Green   I B G

In this example, an object is described verbally as blue in the present but as green in 2000. These two items of information are inconsistent with each other, and hence the correct answer is the letter I. If the physical appearance of the object changes from blue in the present to green in 2000, the appropriate verbal description of the object in the year 2000 is bleen. If the physical appearance of the object does not change, the appropriate verbal description in the year 2000 is blue. But an object cannot correctly be described as green in the year 2000 if its physical appearance was formerly blue. This item was moderately difficult, with a mean response latency of 2.5 seconds.

G Grue   G B I

In this example, an object is described as physically green in the present but as verbally grue in the year 2000. The object thus must have appeared physically green in the present and physically blue in 2000. The correct answer is B. This item was also moderately difficult, with a mean solution latency of 3.1 seconds.

Bleen B   Green Bleen Blue

In this example, an object is described verbally as bleen in the present and physically as B in 2000. One can infer that its physical appearance remained in 2000 what it was in the present, blue. The prediction that the object would change in its physical appearance was incorrect. The correct answer is blue. This was a very difficult item, with a mean solution latency of 4.3 seconds.

B G   Bleen Green Grue

In this example, an object is described physically as B in the present and as G in 2000. The correct verbal description of the object in 2000 is bleen. This was a difficult item, with a mean solution latency of 3.5 seconds.

Consider the second instantiation of the projection task, which was seen by subjects different from those participating in the first experiment (instantiation). In this experiment, based on appearances of objects on the planet Kyron, an object was described as plin if it appears solid north of the equator and solid south of the equator, as kwef if it appears liquid north of the equator and liquid south of the equator, as balt if it appears solid north of the equator but liquid south of the equator, and as pros if it appears liquid north of the equator but solid south of the equator. In each case, subjects were told that knowledge about an object was obtained first regarding its state north of the equator and then regarding its state south of the equator. Hence, "north of the equator" corresponds to "the present" in the first experiment, and "south of the equator" corresponds to "the year 2000" in the first experiment. Pictorial representations of objects were either a filled dot (for solid physical appearance) or a hollow dot (for liquid physical appearance). Two experiments were conducted with this instantiation. The second one was added to the first because some subjects had difficulty with the complexity of the instructions in the first of the two experiments using this instantiation.

In the third instantiation of the projection task, which was seen by still different subjects, the words *plin, kwef, balt,* and *pros* were again used, but their meanings were different. Four types of persons were alleged to live on the planet Kyron. A person was described as plin if the person was born a child and remained a child throughout his or her life span. A person was described as kwef if the person was born an adult and remained an adult during the course of his or her life span. A person was described as balt if the person was born a child but became an adult during the course of his or her life span. And a person was described as pros if the person was born an adult but became a child during the course of his or her life span. A stick figure of a little person was used for the pictorial representation of a child; a stick figure of a big person was used for the pictorial representation of an adult.

In the fourth instantiation of the projection task, which was seen by a new set of subjects, the same four words were again used, but their meanings were different again. Subjects were told that a chemist had discovered four new chemicals that look and smell exactly the same. He had found, however, that each chemical had a different effect on the freezing (or melting) point of H_2O (the chemical formula for both water and ice). To test these effects, he added each chemical to a sample of H_2O at Time 1 and then placed the H_2O in either a warm oven (in one condition) or in a cold ice box (in the other condition). Subjects received items only in one of the two conditions. One day later, at Time 2, the chemist examined the H_2O. He learned that when the chemical plin is added to ice at Time 1, the H_2O is still ice at Time 2; when the chemical kwef is added to water at Time 1, the H_2O is still water at Time 2; when the chemical balt is added to ice at Time 1, the H_2O becomes water at Time 2; and when the chemical pros is added to water at Time 1, the H_2O becomes ice at Time 2. In these experiments, the chemist never added kwef or pros to ice, nor plin nor balt to water, because he had previously found that doing so produced a volatile reaction, resulting in a dangerous explosion. For pictorial descriptions, a filled circle was used to represent ice and a hollow

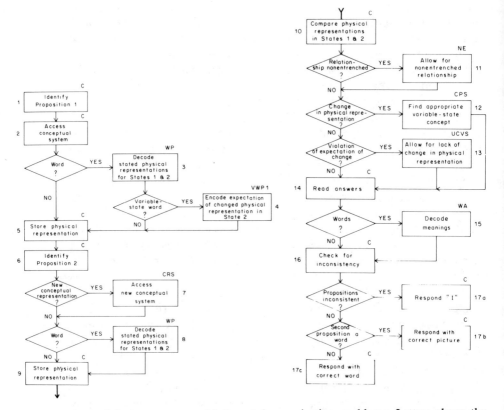

Figure 3.2. A strategy model for solving projection problems. Letters above the upper-right-hand corner of a box refer to latency parameters. Numerals to the right or left of each box correspond to the numerals in Figure 3.3. (From "Natural, unnatural, and supernatural concepts," by Robert J. Sternberg, 1982, *Cognitive Psychology*, *14*, pp. 460–461. Copyright 1982 by Academic Press, Inc. Reprinted by permission of the publisher.)

circle was used to represent water. Note that this surface structure has a certain ecological validity lacking in the previous experiments: It deals with the here and now on earth rather than the distant future or an indeterminate time, whether on earth or some other planet.

Model of concept projection. The proposed model will be described with reference to the following problem from the child–adult task, *balt plin C A I* (where I stands for "inconsistent"). Figure 3.2 shows a schematic flowchart for the model to be described, and Figure 3.3 shows the states through which the subject progresses in solving the sample problem.

	BALT PLIN C A I	PLIN C BALT KWEF PLIN
1	BALT	PLIN
2	[VARIABLE-STATE WORDS]	[STEADY-STATE WORDS]
3	C,A	C,C
4	C → A	---
5	⟨ C → A ⟩	⟨ C,C ⟩
6	PLIN	C
7	[STEADY-STATE WORDS]	[PICTURES]
8	C,C	---
9	⟨C,C⟩	⟨ -,C⟩
10	⟨C → A⟩ ⟨C,C⟩	⟨C,C⟩ ⟨-,C⟩
11	⟨C ⟩⟨ C⟩ OK	⟨C ⟩⟨ C⟩ OK
12	---	---
13	⟨ A⟩⟨ C⟩ OK	---
14	C A I	BALT KWEF PLIN
15	---	C,A A,A C,C
16	⟨C ⟩⟨C ⟩ OK	⟨C ⟩⟨- ⟩ OK
17	⟨C ⟩⟨ C⟩ ↓ C	⟨C ⟩⟨ C⟩ PLIN

Figure 3.3. Outputs from each process of the strategy model for each of two sample problems. In both examples, *C* represents a picture of an individual in the childlike state, and *A* represents a picture of an individual in the adultlike state. Memory representations are enclosed by brackets. A dash (– – –) in one of the two locations of each memory representation refers to the possibility of either a *C* or an *A* in that location. Numerals in the first column correspond to the numerals to the right or left of each box in Figure 3.2. Square brackets, [ ], indicate verbal descriptions; angular brackets, < >, indicate states for symbols. (From "Natural, unnatural, and supernatural concepts," by Robert J. Sternberg, 1982, *Cognitive Psychology, 14*, p. 462. Copyright 1982 by Academic Press, Inc. Reprinted by permission of the publisher.)

According to the proposed model, subjects initiate problem solution by *identifying Proposition 1*, which is *balt* (born a child and becomes an adult) in the sample problem. Next, they *access the conceptual system* appropriate for understanding this proposition, which is [*variable-state words*] in the case of the example. The other two possible states in the present set of problems are [*steady-state words*] and [*pictures*]. If the first proposition is a word, subjects *decode the stated physical representations for states 1 and 2*, which in the sample item are *C, A* (where *C* refers to a picture of a Kyronian in the childlike state and *A* refers to a picture of a Kyronian in the adultlike state). If the word is a variable-state word, subjects *encode the expectation of a changed physical representation in state 2: <C → A>* in the sample item. Next, regardless of whether or not the first proposition was a word, and, if so, whether or not it was a variable-state word, subjects *store the physical representation* of the first proposition in working memory, for example, *<C → A>*.

Now, subjects *identify Proposition 2*, which is *plin* in the example item (born a child and remaining a child). If this proposition uses a *new conceptual representation*, that is, a conceptual system different from the one required by the first proposition, subjects *access the new conceptual system*, which is *steady-state words* in the present example; otherwise, subjects stay with the same conceptual system that they had previously accessed (which would have been [*variable-state words*] in the example). If the second proposition takes the form of a word, subjects *decode the stated physical representations for states 1 and 2* as implied by the second proposition. Next, subjects *store the physical representation* implied by the second proposition, *C, C* in the present example.

Now, subjects are ready to *compare the physical representations in states 1 and 2*. This comparison involves the first item in the first representation, *C* in the example, and the second item in the second representation, also *C* in the example. If the relationship between these two items is nonentrenched with respect to subjects' experience, then subjects *allow for a nonentrenched relationship*. This is the case in the example because retention of the childlike state over a long period of time is nonentrenched with respect to our experience. If there is a *change in physical representation* between these same two items, then subjects *find the appropriate variable-state concept* to describe the change. In the example, there is no change in physical state. A change can be recorded even for an inconsistent item if the physical state represented by the second term is different from that represented by the first. If there is no change in physical representation, subjects further query whether there is a *violation of an expectation of change*, that is, whether the first proposition led one to expect a change that did not in fact occur. If there is a violation, subjects *allow for lack of change in the physical representation*. In the example, there is such a violation. *Balt* leads one to expect a change (from the childlike state to the adultlike state), but in fact no change occurred. Thus, the retention of the childlike state (indicated by the second item in the representation of the second proposition) is allowed despite the expectation of a change to the adultlike state (indicated by the second item in the representation of the first proposition).

Regardless of the outcomes of the previous tests, subjects are now ready to *read the answers* presented for the problem. In the example, these are *C, A,* and *I.* If the answers are words, which they are not in the example, the subject *decodes the meanings* of the words. Subjects now *check their representations for inconsistency* by comparing the first item in the representation for the first proposition with the first item in the representation for the second proposition. If these items do not match, subjects *respond with "inconsistent."* If the representations are consistent, subjects query whether the *second proposition is a word.* If so, subjects *respond with the correct picture,* which is the picture that matches the second item in the second representation. If the second proposition is not a word, subjects *respond with the correct word,* which is the word that corresponds to the conjunction of the first item in the first representation and the second item in the second representation. Note that in all cases, the final representation is sufficient to determine whether the problem is consistent and, if so, which picture or word provides the correct response.

Tests of the model of concept projection. Each of approximately 25 adult subjects was tested in each of 5 experiments. Testing consisted of a number of projection-task items followed by standardized tests of inductive reasoning ability from widely used tests of general intelligence. In the last experiment, deductive reasoning tests were also used. Each subject in each experiment saw each of the 36 item types 3 times, once with the correct answer in each of the 3 possible ordinal positions. Subjects also received tests of inductive reasoning ability in all of the 5 experiments and received a test of deductive reasoning ability in the last experiment.

Mean latencies were 3.02 seconds for the green–blue task, 5.44 and 3.89 seconds for harder and simpler versions of the liquid–solid task, 4.15 seconds for the child–adult task, and 5.54 seconds for the water–ice task. These means differed significantly. Latencies were highly correlated across experiments (using item types as observations), suggesting that similar information processing was involved in all four instantiations. The information-processing model of task performance accounted for .94, .92, .91, .92, and .84 of the variance (as measured by squared multiple correlations, or R^2) in the green–blue, liquid–solid (two versions), child–adult, and water–ice tasks, respectively. RMSDs (root-mean-square deviations) for the respective tasks were

.20, .43, .30, .29, and .42 second. Residuals were significant only in one variant of the second (liquid – solid) task and in the water – ice task, indicating that the model did an exceptionally good job of accounting for the task latencies.

Global correlations of task scores with psychometrically measured induction scores (averaged over psychometric tests) were -.69, -.77, -.61, -.48, and -.62 for the 5 respective experiments. These correlations are not only significant, they are somewhat higher than those obtained for any of the other cognitive tasks currently being studied in my laboratory (and possibly many other laboratories as well). The correlations are thus consistent with the notion that performance on nonentrenched tasks is related to intelligence in a particularly central way. Moreover, the task appears primarily to measure inductive rather than deductive reasoning skills. In the last experiment, the correlation with deductive reasoning was -.43. When deductive reasoning was held constant in a partial correlation of task scores with inductive reasoning, the first-order partial was a significant -.50. When inductive reasoning was held constant in a partial correlation of task scores with deductive reasoning, however, the first-order partial was a nonsignificant -.10. Patterns of correlations of parameter scores with the psychometric scores also made sense. Parameters representing dealing with novelty were the ones that tended to be responsible for the high levels of correlation with the global scores, whereas parameters representing operations dealing with conventional concepts were only trivially correlated with psychometric test scores.

Summary. To summarize, models have been presented for how subjects deal with novelty in performing a task (insight) and for how they deal with novelty in understanding the nature of a task (conceptual projection). Obviously, these models do not exhaust the possibilities for dealing with novelty in either task performance or understanding. However, they indicate that it is possible to understand at some level the processes individuals use in dealing with novel kinds of information. The models for the two types of tasks have been subjected to both internal and external validation with reasonable success, and they do, in fact, appear to provide insights into intelligence that go beyond the kinds of insights we have obtained from many of the more standard kinds of tasks.

Unfortunately, there do not exist at present models of how individuals respond to *situational* novelty, that is, novelty where the task is conventional but the situation is not.

In conclusion, then, response to novelty does appear to be an important facet of intelligence. In the next section, I will consider the other facet of the experiential subtheory of intelligence, automatization of information processing.

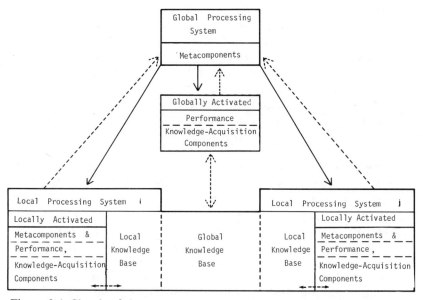

Figure 3.4. Sketch of the proposed control system for controlled and automatic processes. The designations *i* and *j* represent two arbitrary local processing systems. Global processing is controlled; local processing is automatic. Solid arrows represent passage of control (activation). Broken arrows represent passage of feedback. Metacomponents in the global processing system are able to instantiate themselves and other kinds of components in each of the local processing systems, and local processing systems are able to return control to the global processing system when their productions are unable to handle a problem. (From "The evolution of theories of intelligence," by Robert J. Sternberg, 1981, *Intelligence, 5*, p. 224. Copyright 1981 by Ablex Publishing Corporation. Reprinted by permission of the publisher.)

Automatization of information processing

The proposed model of automatization of information processing proposes that controlled information processing is under the conscious direction of the individual and is hierarchical in nature, with executive processes (processes used to plan, monitor, and revise strategies of information processing) directing nonexecutive processes (processes used actually to carry out the strategies that the executive processes select, monitor, and revise). Automatic information processing is preconscious and not under the conscious direction of the individual, and it is nonhierarchical in nature: There is no functional distinction between executive and nonexecutive processes. Instead, task execution occurs through a production system, where all kinds of processes function at a single level of analysis. The proposed view is represented and elaborated in Figure 3.4.

In processing information from new domains (and especially novel ones of the kind considered above), the individual relies primarily upon controlled, global processing. A central executive directly activates nonexecutive processes and receives direct feedback from them. Information processing is of strictly limited capacity, and attention is focused upon the task at hand. The total knowledge base stored in long-term memory is available for access by the processes used in the given task and situation.

In processing information from old domains or domains that are entrenched by nature, the individual relies primarily upon automatic, local processing. A central executive initially activates a system consisting of locally applicable processes and a locally applicable knowledge base. Multiple local systems can operate in parallel. Performance in these systems is automatic and of almost unlimited capacity; attention is not focused upon the task at hand. Only knowledge that has been transferred to the local knowledge base is available for access by the processes utilized in a given task and situation. A critical point is that activation is by executive processes in the global system to the local system as a whole. The executive processes can instantiate themselves as part of this local system; when used in this instantiation, they do not differ functionally from processes of any other kind.

In the domains where one has little expertise, processing is largely focused in the global processing and knowledge system. As expertise develops, greater and greater proportions of processing are transferred to (or packed into) a given local processing system. The advantage of using the local system is that activation is of the system as a whole, rather than of individual processes within the system, so that the amount of attention that needs to be devoted to use of the domain is much less than it is under global control. Indeed, attention allocation for a whole local system is comparable to that for a single lower-order process activated by the global system as part of the global system's functioning. The disadvantages of using the local system are that it is able to call upon only a limited knowledge base – in particular, that knowledge base that has been packed into that local system – and that the local system is able to call upon only those processes that have been packed into the local system. Experts are able to handle a wide variety of situations through the use of the local system, because they have packed tremendous amounts of information into the local system. Novices can hardly use local systems at all, because these systems have as yet acquired relatively few processes and relatively little knowledge.

Control passes to a local processing system when an executive process recognizes a given situation as one for which a local system is potentially relevant. The local system is presumed to be of the nature of a production system, with a set of productions ready to act upon the problem at hand. The productions comprise functions that are executive in nature, as well as functions that are not. But all of these functions are integrated into a single, nonhierarchical system. Control is passed back to the global processing system when, during task performance, none of the productions in a system is able to satisfy a given presented condition. When the bottom of the production list is reached and no given condition is satisfied, global processing is necessary to decide how to handle the new task or situation. Once this task or situation is successfully handled, it is possible to pack what has been learned from global processing of the new experience into a given local processing system, so that the next time such a situation is encountered, there will be no need to exit from the local processing system.

According to this view, the extent to which one develops expertise in a given domain largely depends on the ability of the individual to pack new information, in a usable way, into a given local processing system and to gain access to this information as needed. This view contrasts with that of certain theorists who seem to believe in the primacy of knowledge itself in intelligent functioning (e.g., Chi, Glaser, & Rees, 1982; Keil, 1984). I believe these investigators place too much stress on the knowledge base itself and not enough on the ability of the individual to pack this knowledge into an effective and efficient local processing system. According to the present view, the reason that, of two people who play chess a great deal, one may become an expert and the other remain a duffer is that the first has been able to exploit information in a highly efficacious way whereas the latter has not. The greater knowledge base of the expert is the result, rather than the cause, of the chess player's expertise, which derives from the expert's ability to organize effectively information he or she has encountered in many, many hours of play.

The expert is at an advantage in the domain of his or her expertise because his or her ability to stay for longer amounts of time in the better-developed local processing system enables the expert to free global processing resources for dealing with new situations. The novice is overwhelmed with new information and must engage global resources so frequently that most of the new information that is encountered is quickly lost. Therefore, the expert is more competent in handling familiar tasks within the domain of expertise. He or she is also more proficient at learning new tasks, because global processing resources are more readily available for the intricacies of the task or situation confronted. In essence, a loop is set up whereby packing more information and processes into the local system enables one to automate more processing and thus to have global resources more available for what is new in a given task or situation. The expert is also able to perform more distinct kinds of tasks in parallel, because whereas the global processing system is conscious and serial in its processing, multiple local processing systems can operate in parallel. For a novice, for example, driving a car consumes almost all of his or her available global resources. For an expert, driving a car consumes local resources and leaves central resources available for other tasks, unless a new situation (such as a road block) is confronted that is unfamiliar and requires redirection of control to one's global resources.

To summarize, the present view essentially combines hierarchical and nonhierarchical viewpoints by suggesting that information processing is hierarchical and controlled in a global processing mode and is nonhierarchical and automatic in local processing modes. Expertise develops largely from the successively greater assumption of information processing by local resources. When these local resources are engaged, parallel processing of multiple kinds of tasks becomes possible. Global resources, however, are serial and of very limited capacity in their problem-solving capabilities.

The view of automatization described here, as well as the view of response to novelty, assumes internal processing structures and mechanisms the nature of which has not yet been made explicit. Yet a complete theory of intelligence must specify in some detail the nature of these structures and mechanisms. This specification is the topic of the next chapter.

4 Components of intelligence

A theory of intelligence ought to specify the mechanisms by which intelligent performance is generated. Many kinds of theories do not specify these mechanisms. Consider two examples. Contextual theories may specify the kinds of behaviors that are intelligent (e.g., behaviors that are adaptive), but they fail to specify the mental processes that underlie contextually appropriate behaviors. Factor theories generally specify mental structures, but not mental processes (with some exceptions, such as Guilford, 1967). The purpose of this chapter is to present a componential subtheory specifying the mental mechanisms underlying intelligent performance.

The unit of analysis

Theories of human intelligence have traditionally relied upon some basic unit of analysis for explaining sources of individual differences in intelligent behavior (see Sternberg, 1980f, 1982b). Theories have differed in terms of (a) what is proposed as the basic unit; (b) the particular instantiations of this unit that are proposed somehow to be locked inside our heads; and (c) the way in which these instantiations are organized with respect to each other. Differences in basic units have defined "paradigms" of theory and research on intelligence; differences in instantiations and organizations of these units have defined particular theories within these paradigms. Some of the units that have been considered have been the factor, the S-R bond, and the TOTE (Test – Operate – Test – Exit). The present subtheory designates the information-processing component as the basic unit of analysis.

What is a component?

A component is an elementary information process that operates upon internal representations of objects or symbols (Sternberg, 1977b, 1980f; see

97

also Newell & Simon, 1972). The component may translate a sensory input into a conceptual representation, transform one conceptual representation into another, or translate a conceptual representation into a motor output. What is considered elementary enough to be labeled a component depends upon the desired level of theorizing. Just as factors can be split into successively finer subfactors, so can components be split into successively finer subcomponents. Thus, no claim is made that any of the components referred to later in this book are elementary at all levels of analysis. Rather, they are elementary at a convenient level of analysis. The same caveat applies to the proposed typology of components. Other typologies could doubtless be proposed that would serve this or other theoretical purposes as well or better. The particular typology proposed, however, has proved to be convenient in at least certain theoretical and experimental contexts.

A number of theories have been proposed during the past decade that might be labeled, at least loosely, "componential" (e.g., Butterfield & Belmont, 1977; Campione & Brown, 1979; Carroll, 1976, 1981; Hunt, 1978, 1980; Jensen, 1979; Pellegrino & Glaser, 1979; Snow, 1979). These theories share the cognitive focus of the present view, but differ somewhat in details. To the extent that the differences are metatheoretical (e.g., ways in which components can be parsed into different kinds), they are probably not addressable empirically.

Properties of components

Each component has three important properties associated with it: *duration*, *difficulty* (that is, probability of being executed erroneously), and *probability of execution*. Methods for estimating these properties of components are described in Sternberg (1978a) (see also Sternberg, 1977b; appendix to this book; Sternberg & Rifkin, 1979). The three properties are, at least in principle, independent. For example, a given component may take a rather long time to execute but may be rather easy to execute, in the sense that its execution rarely leads to an error in the solution; or the component may be executed quite rapidly and yet be rather difficult to execute, in the sense that its execution often leads to an error in solution (see Sternberg, 1977b, 1980f). Consider "mapping," which is one of the components used in solving analogies such as "LAWYER is to CLIENT as DOCTOR is to (a) PATIENT, (b) MEDICINE." Mapping calls for the discovery of the higher-order relation between the first and second halves of the analogy. The component has a certain probability of being executed in solving an analogy. If executed, it has a certain duration and a certain probability of being executed correctly.

Kinds of components

Components can be classified by function and by level of generality.

Function. Components can serve (at least) three kinds of functions. *Metacomponents* are higher-order executive processes used in planning, monitoring, and decision making in task performance. *Performance components* are processes used in the execution of a task. *Knowledge-acquisition components* are processes used in learning new information. In the preceding chapter, metacomponents were referred to as executive processes, whereas performance and knowledge-acquisition components were referred to as nonexecutive processes, in controlled information processing. In automatized information processing, all three kinds of components are nonexecutive (in that there is no longer any hierarchy of kinds of processes).

Metacomponents. Metacomponents are specific realizations of control processes that are sometimes collectively (and loosely) referred to as the "executive" or the "homunculus." I have identified seven metacomponents that I believe are quite prevalent in intellectual functioning (Sternberg, 1981e).

1. *Decision as to just what the problem is that needs to be solved.* Anyone who has done research with young children knows that half the battle is getting them to understand what is being asked of them. Their difficulty often lies not in actually solving a problem, but in figuring out just what the problem is that needs to be solved (see, for example, Flavell, 1977; Sternberg & Rifkin, 1979). A major feature distinguishing retarded persons from normal ones is the retardates' need to be instructed explicitly and completely as to the nature of the particular task they are solving and how it should be performed (Butterfield, Wambold, & Belmont, 1973; Campione & Brown, 1977, 1979). The importance of figuring out the nature of the problem is not limited to children and retarded persons. Resnick and Glaser (1976) have argued that intelligence is the ability to learn in the absence of direct or complete instruction. Indeed, distractors on intelligence tests are frequently chosen so as to be the right answers to the wrong problems. In my own research, as noted earlier, I have found that the sheer novelty of a task is an important determinant of the task's correlation with measured intelligence (Sternberg, 1982e): In the conceptual projection task described in the preceding chapter, a major difficulty individuals face is figuring out just what the nature of the problem is.

An example of the power of task understanding in determining empirical outcomes emerged out of research we did on analogy solution in children (Sternberg & Rifkin, 1979). In a pictorial analogies experiment, certain second-graders consistently circled as correct one or the other of the first two analogy terms rather than one or the other of the last two terms that constituted the answer options. We were puzzled by this systematic misunderstanding until we put together three facts: First, we were testing children in a Jewish parochial school; second, the children normally did their lessons in English in the morning and in Hebrew in the afternoon; and third, we happened to be doing our testing in the afternoon. Apparently, some of these young children persevered in their normal afternoon right-to-left visual scanning, even in a task presented in English where it was explicitly stated that the options were at the right. Similarly, in a verbal analogies experiment (Sternberg & Nigro, 1980), some of the younger children (third and sixth grades) used word association rather heavily in solving analogy items, despite the fact that the task was presented as an analogical reasoning task.

2. *Selection of lower-order components.* An individual must select a set of lower-order components to use in the solution of a given task. Selecting a nonoptimal set of components can result in incorrect or inefficient task performance. In some instances, the choice of components will be partially attributable to differential availability or accessibility of various components. For example, young children may lack certain components that are necessary or desirable for the accomplishment of particular tasks, or they may not yet execute these components in a way that is efficient enough to facilitate task solution. Sternberg and Rifkin (1979), for example, tested children in grades 2, 4, and 6, as well as adults, in their abilities to solve simple analogy problems. They found that the performance component used to form the higher-order relation between the two halves of the analogy (mapping) was used by adults and by children in the fourth and sixth grades, but not by children in the second grade. The authors suggested that the second-graders might not yet have acquired the capacity to discern higher-order relations (that is, relations between relations). The unavailability or inaccessibility of this mapping component necessitated a rather radical shift in the way the youngest children solved the analogy problems. Sometimes the failure to execute the components needed for solving a task can be traced to a deficiency in the knowledge necessary for the execution of these components. Sternberg (1979a), for example, found that failures in reasoning with logical connectives were due, in large part, to incorrect encodings of these connectives. Had the meanings of these connectives been available to the subjects (and especially the younger ones), the components of reasoning might well have been correctly executed.

3. *Selection of one or more representations or organizations for information.* A given component can often operate on any one of a number of different possible representations or organizations for information. The choice of representation or organization can facilitate or impede the efficacy

with which the component operates. Sternberg and Rifkin (1979), for example, found that second-graders organized information about analogies differently from older children and adults, but that this idiosyncratic organization enabled them to solve the analogies in a way that compensated for limitations in their working memories and mapping abilities. Sternberg and Weil (1980) found that the efficacy of various representations for information (linguistic, spatial, linguistic and spatial) in a linear-syllogisms task (for example, "John is taller than Bill; Bill is taller than Pete; who is tallest?") depended upon individual subjects' patterns of verbal and spatial abilities. In problem solving, the optimal form of representation for information may depend upon item content. In some cases (for example, geometric analogies), an attribute-value representation may be best [e.g., one attribute and its corresponding value might be represented as CIRCLE (SHADED)]. In other cases (for example, animal-name analogies), a spatial representation may be best (e.g., a lion might be represented as having values on dimensions of size, ferocity, and humanness) (Sternberg & Gardner, 1983). Thus, the efficacy of a form of representation can be determined by either subject variables or task variables or by the interaction between them.

4. *Selection of a strategy for combining lower-order components.* In itself, a list of components is insufficient to perform a task. One must also sequence these components in a way that facilitates task performance, decide how exhaustively each component will be used, and decide which components to execute serially and which to execute in parallel. In an analogies task, for example, alternative strategies for problem solving differ in terms of which components are executed exhaustively and which with self-termination. The exhaustively executed components result in the comparison of all possible encoded attributes or dimensions linking a pair of terms (such as LAWYER and CLIENT, or DOCTOR and PATIENT). The components executed with self-termination result in the comparison of only a subset of the attributes that have been encoded.

In problem solving, the individual must decide which comparisons are to be done exhaustively and which are to be done with self-termination (Sternberg, 1977b). An incorrect decision can drastically affect performance. Overuse of a self-terminating strategy can result in a considerable increase in error (Sternberg, 1977b; Sternberg & Rifkin, 1979). Overuse of an exhaustive strategy can result in a considerable increase in solution latency (Sternberg & Ketron, 1982).

Bill Salter and I conducted an experiment whose primary goal was to isolate metacomponential strategy planning. In particular, we sought to isolate latencies for two forms of strategy planning, which we referred to as "global planning" and "local planning." Global planning refers to the formation of a macrostrategy that applies to a set of problems, regardless of the particular characteristics of a particular problem that is a member of a given set. The need for global planning can be largely a function of the context in which a set of problems is presented. Local planning refers to the formation of a microstrategy that will be sufficient for solving a particular problem within a given set. Whereas global planning is assumed to be highly sensitive to the context of the surrounding problems, local planning is assumed to be context-insensitive, applying to each item individually. It consists of the specific planning operations that are needed for a given item (e.g., tailoring the global plan to a specific item).

We studied these two metacomponents in the context of a complex analogical reasoning task (Sternberg, 1981d). The basic task was to solve verbal analogies correctly but in as little time as possible. The analogies differed from standard analogies, however, in that it was possible for from one to three analogy terms to be missing and for positions of missing terms to vary from one problem to another. Either two or three alternative answer options were substituted for each missing analogy term. In this respect, the problems were like ones used by Lunzer (1965) to study the development of analogical reasoning processes. An example of such a problem is MAN : SKIN :: (DOG, TREE) : (BARK, CAT). The correct answers are TREE and BARK. The complete set of formats included the following:

$$A_i : B :: C : D \qquad A_i : B :: C : D_i$$
$$A : B_i :: C : D \qquad A : B_i :: C_i : D$$
$$A : B :: C_i : D \qquad A : B_i :: C : D_i$$
$$A : B :: C : D_i \qquad A : B_i :: C_i : D_i$$

Terms with the subscript i are missing terms, with either two or three answer options substituted.

We manipulated the amount of global planning required by presenting sets of analogies in two conditions, one mixed and the other blocked. In the mixed condition, each analogy within a given set of 10 items was of a different one of the formats described above. Subjects in this condition were presumed to need considerable global planning to deal with the fact that problems within a given problem set were of a constantly shifting nature. Regardless of the particular item type encountered at a particular time, this item context is not conducive to rapid or automatic planning of a global strategy. In the blocked condition, all analogies within a given set of 10 items were of the same format (i.e., were the same with respect to the positions of the missing terms). Subjects in this condition were presumed to need less global planning, because all items within a given set were of the same structural format. Once a strategy was planned, it could be used for all problems with minimal or no revision.

We manipulated the amount of local planning required by presenting analogies in the various formats described above. More "difficult" formats were assumed to require more local planning; less "difficult" formats were assumed to require less local planning. Difficulty of a format was defined in terms of a strategic complexity index. The complexity of an item type was determined by the number of performance components disrupted by the placement of a multiple option (according to the componential theory of analogical reasoning presented in the next chapter).

In addition to solving analogies tachistoscopically, subjects also solved items presented in paper-and-pencil format. These items were from the Raven Progressive Matrices and from two letter-series completion tests. The first letter-series test was from the Science Research Associates Primary Mental Abilities; the second was homemade.

Mean solution latency for 20 adult subjects on the 20 different complex analogy types (10 formats × 2 different numbers of answer options) was 9.00 seconds. Mean error rate was 14%. A simple additive model with four parameters – global strategy planning, local strategy planning, performance component execution, and a regression constant representing response and other processes constant across item types – accounted for .97 of the variance in the mean latency data. As the reliability of the latency data was .98, the fit of the model was considered to be quite good. The model also provided good fits to individual data. Values of R^2 for individual subject data ranged from .71 to .92, with a mean of .85.

All parameters of the model were statistically significant at the .05 level. Standardized parameter estimates (beta weights) were more interpretable than unstandardized estimates (raw weights) because one of the independent variables that was used to estimate local planning time was not formulated as a real-time index (i.e., in terms of the number of times the corresponding operation is executed in real time). The standardized parameter estimates were .43 for the performance components, .04 for global planning, and .19 for local planning. Unstandardized weights showed the same pattern. Apparently and expectedly, subjects spent most of their time actually solving the problems. A relatively substantial amount of time went into strategy planning for each individual problem, however. Much less time went into global planning, as would be expected, since the blocked condition required much less global planning than the mixed condition, whereas the need for local planning was constant across conditions.

Latency scores for individual subjects were correlated with scores from the two kinds of ability tests (matrix problems and letter-series completions for the two letter-series tests combined). Since performance on the matrix problems was not correlated with either latency scores or performance on the letter-series tests, the matrix problems were removed from further consideration. Correlations with a composite of the letter-series tests were -.54 for all stimulus items combined, -.54 for items presented in the blocked condition, and -.53 for items presented in the mixed condition. The mean correlation between the composite of the letter-series tests and the average of the parameter estimates was -.42 for the execution of performance components, .43 for global planning, -.33 for local planning, and -.40 for the regression constant. All correlations were statistically significant at the .05 level, except that for local planning, which was only marginally significant at the .10 level. The multiple correlation between the letter-series composite score and an optimal combination of the four parameters was .64.

These correlations suggest several conclusions. I shall deal here only with those things relevant for understanding metacomponential functioning.

First, global planning is moderately related to scores on the psychometric reasoning test composite. Of particular interest is the fact that this correlation is positive, indicating that relatively longer global planning latencies were associated with higher reasoning scores. This result is strongly reminiscent of previous findings (see Sternberg, 1977b; Sternberg & Rifkin, 1979) indicating that better reasoners tend to spend more time encoding the terms of a problem than do poorer reasoners but tend to spend less time operating on these encodings than do poorer reasoners. Similarly, it now appears that the better reasoners tend to spend relatively more time in global planning of a strategy for problem solution but relatively less time in local planning than do poorer reasoners.

Second, local planning is at least weakly related to scores on the reasoning test composite. The measure of local planning difficulty was not a real-time-based one, and it is possible that the correlation of local planning and psychometrically measured reasoning skill might increase with a more sophisticated measure of local planning.

Third, the fact that the regression constant correlated significantly with psychometric test scores suggests the possibility that there were other metacomponential latencies that were not isolated by our parameter estimation procedures (indeed, it seems highly likely that this would be the case). For example, issues of problem definition, representation formation, and allocation of attentional resources were not dealt with in our partitioning of task variance. But we felt justified in concluding that at least some metacomponential latencies can be isolated fairly directly through procedures such as the ones we used.

5. *Decision regarding allocation of attentional resources.* All tasks and components used in performing tasks can be allocated only a limited proportion of the individual's total attentional resources. Greater limitations may result in reduced quality of performance. In particular, one must decide how much time to allocate to each task component and how much the time restriction will affect the quality of performance of the particular compo-

nent. One tries to allocate time across the various components of task performance in a way that maximizes the quality of the entire product. Even small changes in error rate can result in sizable changes in solution latency (Pachella, 1974). I have found in the linear-syllogisms task, for example, that a decrease in solution latency of just 1 second (from a mean of about 7 seconds to a mean of about 6 seconds) results in a sevenfold increase in error rate (from about 1% to 7%; see Sternberg, 1980d).

6. *Solution monitoring.* As individuals proceed through a problem, they must keep track of what they have already done, what they are currently doing, and what they still need to do. The relative importance of these three items of information differs across problems. If things are not progressing as expected, an accounting of one's progress may be needed, and one may even have to consider the possibility of changing goals. Often, new, more realistic goals need to be formulated as a person realizes that the old goals cannot be reached. In solving problems, individuals sometimes find that none of the available answer options provides a satisfactory answer. The individual must then decide whether to reperform certain processes that might have been performed erroneously or to choose the best of the available options. In the solution of linear syllogisms, the best strategy for most subjects is a rather nonobvious one, and hence subjects not trained in this strategy are unlikely to realize its existence until they have had at least some experience solving such problems (Quinton & Fellows, 1975; Sternberg & Weil, 1980).

7. *Sensitivity to external feedback.* External feedback provides a valuable means for improving one's task performance. The ability to understand feedback, to recognize its implications, and then to act upon it is thus a key skill in task performance. Consider, for example, the presentation of a lecture to an audience with whose background one is relatively unfamiliar. Novice lecturers will generally come with a prepared lecture and have great difficulty departing from it. A skilled lecturer, however, will be sensitive to cues from the audience and modify the lecture as he or she goes along, attempting to fine-tune it to the knowledge and interests of the audience. As any lecturer knows, sensitivity to the audience can mean the difference between success and failure in communicating the material to the audience.

Performance components. Performance components are used in the execution of various strategies for task performance. Although the number of possible performance components is quite large, many probably apply only to small or uninteresting subsets of tasks and hence deserve little attention.

I have suggested recently that performance components tend to organize themselves into stages of task solution that seem to be fairly general across tasks (Sternberg, 1981k). These stages include encoding of stimuli, combination of or comparison between stimuli, and response. In the analogies task, for example, I have separated encoding and response components (each of which may be viewed as constituting its own stage) and inference, mapping, application, comparison, and justification components (each of which requires some kind of comparison between stimuli).

1. *Encoding components.* Encoding components are those concerned with initial perception and storage of new information. Qualitative and quantitative changes in encoding seem to constitute a major source of intellectual development. For example, encoding (a) tends to become more nearly exhaustive with increasing age (Brown & DeLoache, 1978; Siegler, 1978; Sternberg & Nigro, 1980; Sternberg & Rifkin, 1979; Vurpillot, 1968); (b) tends to be executed more slowly per encoded attribute with increasing age (Sternberg & Rifkin, 1979); and (c) often operates on different representations of information with increasing age (Sternberg & Rifkin, 1979). The change in the rate at which encoding is executed in timed tasks tends to be fairly large in magnitude. For example, most of the difficulty in at least one complex deductive task, reasoning with logical connectives, turns out to be due to difficulty in encoding the connectives rather than difficulty in combining (reasoning with) them (Sternberg, 1979a).

2. *Combination and comparison components.* These components are involved in putting together or comparing information. Whereas encoding seems to be a critical source of intellectual development in almost all of the tasks I and at least some others have studied, the importance of development in combination and comparison components is much more variable. An example of a combination component can be found in the strategy people use to solve linear syllogisms, such as "John is taller than Bill; Bill is taller than Pete; who is tallest?" People represent each of the premises spatially, usually as one mental array depicting John above Bill and another mental array depicting Bill above Pete. These two mental arrays then need to be combined into a single array. An example of a comparison component can be found in the strategy people use in solving analogies. In solving an analogy such as BOY : MALE :: GIRL : ? people need to compare the attributes of BOY and MALE in order to determine in what ways these two terms are analogous (and disanalogous).

3. *Response component.* In my own research as well as that of others studying quite different kinds of intellectual abilities (e.g., Kail, Pellegrino, & Carter, 1980; Keating & Bobbitt, 1978), substantial decreases have been observed with increasing age in the latencies of components represented by the intercept of the regression equation used to estimate parameters. Moreover, strong correlations have been observed between the intercept and ability tests within age groups as well (Mulholland, Pellegrino, & Glaser, 1980; Sternberg, 1977b). I am inclined to attribute these effects to the confounding of metacomponent with response-component latency. Presum-

ably, latency for executing at least some metacomponents is constant across the various item types that form the data points of the regression and hence becomes part of the regression constant that is normally labeled "response."

To summarize, performance components are potentially important sources of intellectual development and individual differences, but a joint analysis of their role with that of the metacomponents leads me to believe that metacomponential processes are more fundamental sources of consequential individual and developmental differences. Changes in metacomponential functioning lead almost inevitably to changes in the functioning of performance components, but one can understand the latter changes only by looking for their metacomponential sources.

Knowledge-acquisition components. Knowledge-acquisition components are processes used in gaining new knowledge. It is proposed that three components are relevant to acquisition of declarative and procedural knowledge in virtually all domains of knowledge. These components are the same as those described earlier in the formation of insights, and indeed, according to this view, learning always requires at least minor insights.

1. *Selective encoding.* Selective encoding involves sifting out of relevant from irrelevant information. When new information is presented in natural contexts, relevant information for one's given purposes is embedded in the midst of large amounts of purpose-irrelevant information. A critical task for the learner is that of sifting the "wheat from the chaff": recognizing just what information among all the pieces of information presented is relevant for one's purposes (see Schank, 1980).

2. *Selective combination.* Selective combination involves combining selectively encoded information in such a way as to form an integrated, plausible whole. Simply sifting out relevant from irrelevant information is not enough to generate a new knowledge structure: One must know how to combine the pieces of information into an internally connected whole (see Mayer & Greeno, 1972).

3. *Selective comparison.* Selective comparison involves relating newly acquired or retrieved information to information acquired in the past. In the case of newly acquired information, a relation is seen between something just encoded and something that was encoded in the past. In the case of newly retrieved information, an item already stored in memory is related to some other item and thereby comes to be understood in a new way. Deciding what information to encode and how to combine it does not occur in a vacuum. Rather, encoding and combination of new knowledge are guided by retrieval of old information. New information will be all but useless if it cannot somehow be related to old knowledge so as to form an externally connected whole (see Mayer & Greeno, 1972).

These knowledge-acquisition components will be discussed in much greater detail in Chapter 7.

Level of generality. Components can be classified in terms of three levels of generality. *General components* are required to perform all tasks within a given task universe; *class components* are required to perform a proper subset of tasks that includes at least two tasks within the task universe; and *specific components* are required to perform single tasks within the task universe. Tasks calling for intelligent performance differ in the numbers of components they require for completion and in the number of each kind of component they require.

Consider, again, the example of an analogy. "Encoding" seems to be a general component, in that it is needed in the solution of all problems of all kinds: A problem cannot be solved unless its terms are encoded in some manner. "Inference" seems to be a class component, in that it is required for the solution of certain kinds of induction problems, but it is certainly not required for all problems involving intelligent performance. No task-specific components seem to be involved in analogical reasoning, which is perhaps one reason why analogies serve so well in tests of general intellectual functioning.

Two points need to be emphasized with regard to the level of generality of components. First, whereas components with different functions are qualitatively different from each other, components at different levels of generality are not. Function is a property of a given component; level of generality is a property of the range of the tasks into which a given component enters. Second, whereas a given component serves only a single function, it may serve at any level of generality, with the level depending upon the scope of the set of tasks being considered. A component may be general in a narrow range of tasks, for example, but class-related in a very broad range of tasks. For example, the inference component is general across inductive reasoning tasks but is a class component across the range of all tasks involving fluid kinds of abilities. It is not needed, for example, in many spatial tasks. Levels of generality will prove useful in understanding certain task interrelationships and factorial findings; their primary purpose is to provide a convenient descriptive language that is useful for conceptualizing certain kinds of phenomena in componential terms.

Interrelations among kinds of components

Components are interrelated in various ways. I shall discuss first how components serving different functions are interrelated and then how components of different levels of generality are interrelated. Because levels of gener-

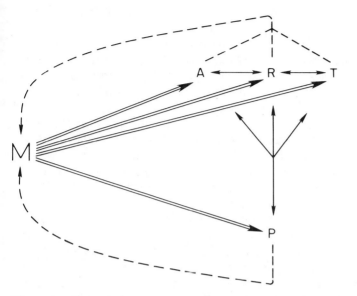

Figure 4.1. Interrelations among components serving different functions. In the figure, *M* refers to a set of metacomponents; *A*, *R*, and *T* refer to a set of knowledge-acquisition components as they function in the acquisition (*A*), retrieval (*R*), and transfer (*T*) of information; and *P* refers to a set of performance components. Direct activation of one kind of component by another is represented by solid double arrows. Indirect activation of one kind of component by another is represented by single solid arrows. Direct feedback from one kind of component to another is represented by single broken arrows. Indirect feedback from one kind of component to another proceeds from and to the same components as does indirect activation, and so is shown by the single solid arrows. (From "Sketch of a componential sub-theory of human intelligence," by Robert J. Sternberg, 1980, *Behavioral and Brain Sciences, 3,* p. 578. Copyright 1980 by Cambridge University Press.)

ality and functions are completely crossed, in principle, the interrelations among components of differing levels of generality apply to all of the functionally different kinds of components, and the interrelations among the functionally different kinds of components apply at all levels of generality.

Function. My speculations regarding the interrelations among the functionally different kinds of components are shown in Figure 4.1. The various kinds of components are closely related, as would be expected in an integrated, intelligent system. Four kinds of interrelations need to be considered. Direct activation of one kind of component by another is represented by double solid arrows. Indirect activation of one kind by another is represented by single solid arrows. Direct feedback from one kind to another is represented by single broken arrows. Indirect feedback proceeds from and to the same components, as does indirect activation, and so is shown by the single solid arrows. Direct activation or feedback refers to the immediate passage of control or information from one kind of component to another. Indirect activation or feedback refers to the mediated passage of control or information from one kind of component to another via a third kind of component.

In the proposed system, only metacomponents can directly activate and receive feedback from each other kind of component. Thus, all control passes directly from the metacomponents to the system, and all information passes directly from the system to the metacomponents. The other kinds of components can activate each other indirectly and receive information from each other indirectly; in every case, mediation must be supplied by the metacomponents. For example, the acquisition of information affects the performances that can be done on this information, but only via the link of knowledge-acquisition components and performance components to the metacomponents. Information from the performance components is filtered to the knowledge-acquisition components via the metacomponents.

Consider some examples of how the system might function in the solution of a word puzzle, such as an anagram (scrambled word). As soon as one decides upon a certain tentative strategy for unscrambling the letters of the word, activation of that strategy can pass directly from the metacomponent responsible for deciding upon a strategy to the performance component responsible for executing the first step of the strategy, and subsequently activation can pass to the successive performance components needed to execute the strategy. Feedback will return from the performance components indicating how successful the strategy seems to be. If the monitoring of this feedback signals lack of success, control may pass to the metacomponent that is "empowered" to change strategy; if no successful change in strategy can be realized, the solution-monitoring metacomponent may change the goal altogether.

As a given strategy is being executed, new information is being acquired about how to solve anagrams in general. This information is also fed back to the metacomponents, which may act upon or ignore this information. New information that seems useful is more likely to be directed back from the relevant metacomponents to the relevant knowledge-acquisition components for storage in long-term memory. What is acquired does not directly influence what is retained, however, so that "practice does not necessarily make perfect." Some people may be unable to profit from their experience because of inadequacies in metacomponential information processing.

The metacomponents are able to process only a limited amount of information at a given time. In a difficult task, and especially a new and different one, the amount of information being fed back to the metacomponents may exceed their capacity to act upon the information. In this case, the meta-components become overloaded, and valuable information that cannot be processed may simply be wasted. The total information-handling capacity of the metacomponents of a given system will thus be an important limiting aspect of that system. Similarly, the capacity to allocate attentional resources so as to minimize the probability of bottlenecks will be part of what determines the effective capacity of the system.

Figure 4.1 does not show the interrelations among various individual members of each single functional kind of component. These interrelations can be easily described in words, however. Metacomponents are able to communicate with each other directly and to activate each other directly. It seems likely that there exists at least one metacomponent (other than those described earlier) that controls communication and activation among the other metacomponents, and there is a certain sense in which this particular metacomponent might be viewed as a "meta-metacomponent," although I think such a concept is best avoided, as it seems to be a sure invitation to infinite regress. Other kinds of components are not able to communicate directly with each other, however, or to activate each other. But components of a given kind can communicate indirectly with other components of the same kind and can activate them indirectly. Indirect communication and activation proceed through the metacomponents, which can direct information or activation from one component to another of the same kind.

Level of generality. Components of varying levels of generality are related to each other through the ways in which they enter into the performance of tasks. Figure 4.2 shows the nature of this hierarchical relationship. Each node of the hierarchy contains a task, which is designated by a roman or arabic numeral or by a letter. Each task comprises a set of components at the general (g), class (c), and specific (s) levels. In the figure, g refers to a set of general components, and c_i and c_j each refers to a set of class components, whereas c_{ij} refers to a concatenated set of class components that includes the class components from both c_i and c_j; s_i refers to a set of specific components. The levels of the hierarchy differ in terms of the complexity of the tasks assigned to them. More complex tasks occupy higher levels of the hierarchy; simpler tasks occupy lower levels. Relative complexity is defined here in terms of the number and identities of the class components contained in the task: The more sets of class components that are concatenated in a particular task, the more complex the task is.

At the bottom of the hierarchy are very simple tasks (IA1, IA2, IB1, IB2), each of which requires a set of general, class, and specific components for its execution. At one extreme, the general components are the same in all four tasks (and in all of the tasks in the hierarchy), in that a general component is

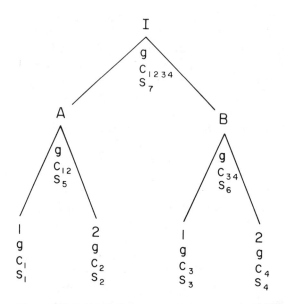

Figure 4.2. Interrelations among components of different levels of generality. Each node of the hierarchy contains a task, which is designated by a roman or arabic numeral or by a letter. Each task comprises a set of components at the general (g), class (c), and specific (s) levels. In the figure, g refers to a set of general components; c_i and c_j each refer to a set of class components, and c_{ij} refers to a concatenated set of class components that includes the class components from both c_i and c_j; s_i refers to a set of specific components. (From "Sketch of a componential subtheory of human intelligence," by Robert J. Sternberg, 1980, *Behavioral and Brain Sciences, 3*, p. 579. Copyright 1980 by Cambridge University Press.)

by definition one that is involved in the performance of every task in the universe (here expressed as a hierarchy) of interest. At the other extreme, the specific components are unique to each task at this (and every other) level, in that a specific component is by definition one that is relevant only to a single task. The class components are also not shared across tasks at this level: Task IA1 has one set of class components, Task IA2 another, Task IB1 another, and Task IB2 yet another. As examples, Task IA1 might be series completions (such as 2, 4, 6, 8, ?), Task IA2 metaphorical ratings (How good a metaphor is "The moon is a ghostly galleon?"), Task IB1 linear syllogisms (N is higher than P; P is higher than L; which is highest?), and Task IB2 categorical syllogisms (All C are B; some B are A; can one conclude that some C are A?).

Consider next the middle level of the hierarchy, containing Tasks IA and IB. Tasks IA and IB both share with the lower-order tasks, and with each other, all of their general components but none of their specific components. What distinguishes Tasks IA and IB from each other, however, and what places them in their respective positions in the hierarchy, is the particular set of class components involved in each. The class components involved in the performance of Task IA represent a concatenation of the class components involved in the performance of Tasks IA1 and IA2; the class components involved in the performance of Task IB represent a concatenation of the class components involved in the performance of Tasks IB1 and IB2. Tasks IA and IB contain no common class components, however.

Finally, consider the task at the top level of the hierarchy, Task I. Like all tasks in the hierarchy, it shares general components with all other tasks in the hierarchy, but it shares specific components with none of these tasks (again, since these components are, by definition, task-specific). Performance on this task is related to performance on Tasks IA and IB through the concatenation of class components from these two tasks.

According to the present view, many kinds of tasks are hierarchically interrelated to each other via components of information processing. The proposed hierarchical model shows the nature of these interrelations. It should be made clear just what is arbitrary and what is not in this hierarchical arrangement. The arrangement does not prespecify the degrees of differentiation between the top and bottom levels of the hierarchy, nor where the hierarchy should start and stop. As was stated earlier, the level that is defined as "elementary" and thus suitable for specification of components is arbitrary: What is a component in one theory might be two components in another or a task in still another theory. The level of specification depends upon the purpose of the theory. Theories at different levels serve different purposes and must be justified in their own right. But certain important aspects of the arrangement are not arbitrary. The vertical order of tasks in the hierarchy, for example, is not subject to permutation, and although whole branches of the hierarchy (from top to bottom) can be permuted (the left side becoming the right side and vice versa), individual portions of those branches cannot be permuted. For example, IA and IB cannot be switched unless the tasks below them are switched as well. In other words, horizontal reflection of the whole hierarchy is possible, but horizontal reflection of selected vertical portions is not possible. These nonarbitrary elements of the hierarchy make disconfirmation of a given theory both possible and feasible. A given hierarchy can be found to be inadequate if the various constraints outlined above are not met. In many instances, the hierarchy may simply be found to be incomplete, in that branches or nodes of branches may be missing and thus need to be filled in.

The interrelational schemes described above are intended to provide a framework for explaining empirical phenomena rather than to provide a unified perspective for understanding empirical findings in the literature on intelligence.

Interrelations between components and other units of analysis

Consider how components relate to units of analysis proposed by other investigators operating within a variety of paradigms.

The differential approach

In most psychometric investigations of intelligence, the basic unit of analysis has been the factor (see Chapter 1). What, exactly, is a factor? There is no single, agreed-upon answer to this question. Thurstone (1947) noted that "factors may be called by different names, such as 'causes,' 'faculties,' 'parameters,' 'functional unities,' 'abilities,' or 'independent measurements'" (p. 56). Royce (1963) added to this list "dimensions, determinants, . . . and taxonomic categories" (p. 522), and Cattell (1971) has referred to factors as "source traits."

I do not believe there is any meaningful sense in which one can refer to either components or factors as "more basic" than each other: Each kind of unit involves a different kind of variance, and each can be related to the other. I tend to view factors as constellations of various kinds of components, but component scores can be factor-analyzed and factor scores can be predicted componentially. Interrelations between components and various kinds of factors will be considered shortly.

Information-processing approaches

Information-processing approaches to intelligent performance share the positing of some kind of elementary information process as a fundamental unit of behavior. It is assumed that all behavior of a human information-processing system can be understood in part as a result of the combination of these elementary processes. The various approaches differ from each other, however, in the units they have posited as being central to understanding behavior. I consider here some of the alternative units that have been proposed and how they relate to the component construct and the theory built upon it.

1. *The TOTE.* Miller, Galanter, and Pribram (1960) proposed as the fundamental unit of intelligent behavior the TOTE (Test–Operate–Test–Exit). Each unit of behavior starts with a Test of the present outcome against the desired outcome. If the result of the Test is congruent with the desired outcome (called an "Image"), an Exit is made. If not, another Operation is

performed in order to make the result of the next Test conform as closely as possible to the Image. If the result of the next Test is congruent with the Image, an Exit is made. Otherwise, still another Operation is performed, and this sequence continues until the Test result corresponds to the Image (which may have been modified along the way in order to make it conform more closely to the demands of reality). An individual TOTE, a hierarchy of TOTEs, or a sequence of TOTEs (which may include hierarchies) executed in order to realize an Image is called a Plan.

The TOTE and its derivative concepts are wholly compatible with the component and its derivative concepts. A TOTE would be viewed in my own system as a substrategy consisting of two comparison components (the Tests), one encoding or combination component (the Operation), and a response component (the Exit). A Plan is what I have referred to as a strategy, and an Image is the goal state the strategy is meant to realize. Miller et al. do not distinguish between higher-order types of metacomponential constructs, on the one hand, and lower-order types of componential constructs, on the other. Instead, they (1960) propose that

a central notion of the method followed in these pages is that the operational components of TOTE units may themselves be TOTE units. That is to say, the TOTE pattern decribes both strategic and tactical units of behavior. Thus the operational phase of a higher-order TOTE might itself consist of a string of other TOTE units, and each of these, in turn, may contain still other strings of TOTEs, and so on. (P. 32)

2. *The production.* A production is a condition–action sequence. If a certain condition is met, then a certain action is performed. Sequences of ordered productions are called production systems.

The flow of control for a production system is assumed to make its way down the ordered list of productions until one of the conditions is met. The action corresponding to that condition is executed, and control is returned to the top of the list. Control then passes down the list again, trying to satisfy a condition. When it does so, an action is executed, control returns to the top, and so on. Processing stops when none of the conditions in the list of productions are satisfied. The production construct was popularized in psychology by Newell and Simon (1972) (see also Newell, 1973) and has been used extensively in psychological theorizing by Anderson (1976), Klahr and Wallace (1976), and others. The rules for production systems may be elaborated as required. Anderson (1976), for example, has suggested rules for strengthening and weakening productions, and Hunt and Poltrock (1974) have suggested that productions may be probabilistically ordered so that the exact order in which the list of productions is scanned may differ across scannings of the list.

A particularly attractive feature of production systems is that they can be self-modifying (see, e.g., Anderson, Kline, & Beasley, 1980; Klahr, 1984). Anderson et al. (1980) have proposed four transition mechanisms by which modification could occur. A designation mechanism is one that simply has as its action the instructions to build a new production of a certain kind. A strengthening mechanism increases the probability that a production will be activated. A generalization mechanism weakens the specific conditions that activate a production so that the production is more likely to be executed under a broader variety of circumstances. Finally, a discrimination mechanism strengthens the specifications for activation of a production so that the production will be activated only when more specific conditions are met than was originally the case. Notice that a critical assumption underlying these last three mechanisms is that productions have differential strengths that affect the likelihood of the productions being executed if they are reached. A rough analogy would be to the eliciting conditions necessary to fire a neuron in the nervous system.

The production can easily be understood in componential terms. The test of the condition is analogous to a comparison component (or a Test in TOTE terminology). The action that is contingent upon meeting the condition is analogous to an encoding or combination component, or possibly even to another comparison component, where the comparison is between two new pieces of information rather than between a new and an old piece of information (or an Operation, in TOTE terminology), unless the action is a terminal one, in which case it is analogous to a response (or an Exit in TOTE terminology).

The componential system specifies two operating systems rather than just one. In contrast, the operating system for the production system is used only for automatized information processing. Executive-based processing is used for controlled information processing (see Chapter 3). Thus, whether the production control system is used is proposed to depend upon the kind of processing involved.

3. *The scheme.* The notion of a "scheme" proposed by Pascual-Leone (1970) and elaborated by Case (1974a, 1974b, 1978) is viewed as "neo-Piagetian," drawing as it does on the basic Piagetian notion of the "schema." What these investigators have done, however, is to specify the notion of a scheme more precisely than has Piaget.

There are three basic kinds of schemes – figurative, operative, and executive. All three kinds of schemes are internal representations, but they differ in the forms they take. Figurative schemes, according to Case (1974b), are "internal representations of items of information with which a subject is familiar, or of perceptual configurations which he can recognize" (p. 545). If, for example, a subject described a photograph as depicting a picture of his or her house, one could say that the subject assimilated the sensory input to a figurative "house scheme." Operative schemes, according to Case (1974b), are "internal representations of functions (rules), which can be applied to one set of figurative schemes, in order to generate a new set" (p. 545). If, for example, a subject looked at two different photographs of a house and judged them to depict the "same" house, one would describe the subject as applying an operative scheme representing a "sameness" function to the figurative schemes representing the features of each of the two photographs. Executive schemes, according to Case (1974b), are "internal representations of procedures which can be applied in the face of particular problem situations, in an attempt to reach particular objectives" (p. 546). The executive schemes are to a large extent responsible for determining which figurative and operative schemes a person activates in a particular problem situation. The figurative and operative schemes just suggested in the comparison of two photographs, for example, would presumably be activated only if they were part of some larger executive scheme that required the particular comparison.

Whether or not a subject actually solves a particular problem is assumed to depend on four basic factors. The first is the repertoire of schemes that a subject brings to the problem. The second is the maximum number of schemes that the subject's psychological system is capable of activating at a given time. The maximum mental effort a subject can apply to a problem is referred to as "M-power" and is assumed to vary both within and between age groups. M-power is essentially the same as what is usually referred to as "working memory capacity." M-power is viewed as at least one source of individual differences within and between age levels in overall general ability (*g*): It is assumed to increase linearly with age. The third factor is a subject's tendency to utilize the full M-power that is available; some subjects are assumed to be more willing than others to apply full M-power, and, in general, subjects differ in the proportion of M-power they typically exploit. Finally, a fourth factor is the relative weights assigned to cues from the perceptual field on the one hand and to cues from all other sources (e.g., task instructions) on the other.

Case (1974b) describes several ways in which new schemes may be acquired and hence learning and intellectual development can occur. First, new schemes can be acquired by modification of old schemes. Second, new schemes can be acquired by the combination or consolidation of multiple old schemes. These two ways of acquiring new schemes can be further subdivided, resulting in multiple means by which intellectual change can occur.

These various types of schemes can be viewed in componential terms. Figurative schemes are unitized internal representations, roughly equivalent to what Miller (1956) has called "chunks." Operative schemes are roughly equivalent to lower-order components (performance and knowledge acquisition), or to what Inhelder and Piaget (1958) have referred to as "transformations" and what Newell and Simon (1972) have referred to as "elementary information processes." Executive schemes are equivalent to strategies as formulated by higher-order metacomponents, or to what Miller et al. (1960) have referred to as "Plans" and what Newell and Simon (1972) have referred to as "executive programs."

An interesting feature of the system of Pascual-Leone and Case is the set of factors assumed to determine whether or not a given problem is actually solved. Again, these limiting factors can be understood in componential terms. First, the repertoire of schemes is simply a repertoire of strategies, which is assumed to increase with age. Second, what is referred to as "M-power" in the scheme system is referred to as processing capacity or channel capacity in the componential system and most other information-processing systems. Third, the subject's tendency to utilize full M-power would be viewed as a motivational variable in the componential and most other information-processing systems. Finally, componential analysis weighs the various kinds of inputs to the information-processing system through parameter estimates. These estimates tell how important each kind of information is in reaching a final solution to a given problem.

4. *The rule (or principle).* Rules (Siegler, 1981) and principles (Gelman & Gallistel, 1978) form the final unit that I consider here. According to Siegler (1981): "The basic assumption underlying the rule-assessment approach is that cognitive development can be characterized in large part as the acquisition of increasingly powerful rules for solving problems" (p. 3). Rules or principles emphasize knowledge rather than process as the basic unit of development. What Siegler refers to as a rule, however, is virtually identical to what I and others have referred to as a strategy, or to what Miller et al. (1960) have referred to as a Plan. As children grow older, the complexity of their rules increases, generally because earlier rules fail to take into account all of the relevant information in a given problem. The rules of older children tend to reflect more thorough encoding and more nearly exhaustive information processing than do the rules of younger children.

Relations between components and aspects of human intelligence

Consider some of the key phenomena described in the textbook literature on intelligence (for example, Brody & Brody, 1976; Butcher, 1970; Cronbach, 1970; Vernon, 1979) and how they would be explained within a componential framework. Some of these phenomena have actually appeared to be mutually incompatible, but they no longer appear so when viewed through the "lens" of the componential framework. None of these phenomena has been established beyond a doubt; indeed, some of them are subject to considerable controversy. Nevertheless, they are about as solid as any phenomena reported in the literature on intelligence, and they are ones that I, at least, am willing to accept tentatively until the evidence sways me to believe otherwise.

1. *There appears to be a factor of "general intelligence."* Various sorts of evidence have been adduced in support of the existence of a general intelligence factor (see Humphreys, 1979; Jensen, 1980; McNemar, 1964). Perhaps the most persuasive evidence is everyday experience: Casual observation in everyday life suggests that some people are "generally" more intelligent than others. People's rank orderings of each other may differ according to exactly how they define intelligence (see Chapter 2), but some rank ordering is usually possible. Historically, the evidence that has been offered most often in favor of the existence of general intelligence is the appearance of a general factor in unrotated factor solutions from factor analyses of tests of intelligence (for example, Spearman, 1927). In itself, this evidence is not persuasive, because factor analysis of any battery of measures will yield a general factor if the factors are not rotated: This is a mathematical rather than a psychological outcome of factor analysis. However, the psychological status of this outcome is bolstered by the fact that an analogous outcome appears in information-processing research as well: Information-processing analyses of a variety of tasks have revealed strong communalities in information-processing components across tasks with high internal and external validity for predicting intelligent performance (see Sternberg & Gardner, 1983; Chapter 5 of this book).

The strongest evidence that has been offered against the existence of general intelligence is that some rotations of factors fail to yield a general factor. But this failure to find a general factor in certain kinds of rotated solutions is as much determined by mathematical properties of the factorial algorithm as is the success in finding a general factor in an unrotated solution. Moreover, if the multiple factors are correlated, and if they are themselves factored, they will often yield a "second-order" general factor.

In componential analysis, individual differences in general intelligence are attributed to individual differences in the effectiveness with which general components are used. Since these components are common to all of the tasks in a given task universe, factor analyses will tend to lump these general sources of individual-difference variance into a single general factor. As it happens, the metacomponents have a much higher proportion of general components among them than do any of the other kinds of components, presumably because the executive routines needed to plan, monitor, and possibly replan performance are highly overlapping across widely differing tasks. Thus, individual differences in metacomponential functioning are largely responsible for the persistent appearance of a general factor.

Metacomponents are probably not solely responsible for *g*, however. Most behavior, and probably all of the behavior exhibited on intelligence tests, is learned. Knowledge-acquisition components may be general to a wide variety of learning situations and particularly novel situations, which also then enter into the general factor. Finally, certain aspects of performance – such as encoding and response – are common to virtually all tasks, and they, too, may enter into the general factor. Therefore, although the metacomponents are primarily responsible for individual differences in general intelligence, they are probably not solely responsible.

2. *Intelligence comprises a set of "primary mental abilities."* When a factorial solution is rotated to a Thurstonian (1947) simple structure, a set of primary mental abilities typically appears. The concept of simple structure is complexly defined, but basically it involves a factorial solution in which factors tend to have some variables loading highly on them, some variables loading only modestly on them, and few variables having intermediate loadings on them. As noted above, the appearance of one or another kind of factor set is largely a mathematical property of factor analysis and the kind of rotation used (see also Sternberg, 1977b). If one views factors as causal entities, as do many adherents to the traditional psychometric approach to intelligence (e.g., Cattell, 1971; Spearman, 1927), then one may become involved in a seemingly unresolvable debate regarding the "correct" rotation of factors. Mathematically, all rigid rotations of a set of factor axes are permissible, and there seems to be no agreed-upon psychological criterion for choosing a "correct" rotation. In componential analysis, the choice of a criterion for rotation is arbitrary – a matter of convenience. Different rotations serve different purposes. The unrotated solution considered above, for example, is probably ideal for isolating a composite measure of individual differences in the effectiveness of the execution of general components.

Consider next what is probably the most popular orientation of factorial axes among American psychometricians, that obtained by Thurstonian rotation to simple structure. In such rotations, primary mental abilities such as verbal comprehension, word fluency, number, spatial visualization, and so on (see Thurstone, 1938) may appear. The simple-structure rotation, like the unrotated solution, has somehow seemed special to psychometricians over the years, and I believe that there may well be a sense in which this rotation is special. Whereas the unrotated solution seems to provide the best composite measure of general components, my inspections of various rotated solutions have led me to believe that simple-structure rotations tend to provide the "best" measures of class components – best in the sense that there is minimal overlap across factors in the appearances of class components. A simple-structure rotation distributes the general components throughout the set of factors so that the same general components may appear in multiple factors: Such factors, therefore, will necessarily be correlated. But I believe the low to moderate correlations are due for the most part to overlap among general components: The class components found at a fairly high level of generality seem to be rather well restricted to individual factors. Given that the factorial model of primary mental abilities originally proposed by Thurstone was nonhierarchical, there will have to be some overlap across factors in class components; for theoretical and practical purposes, however, this overlap seems to be minimized. Thus, neither the unrotated solution of Spearman (1927) and others nor the simple-structure solution of Thurstone (1938) and others is "correct" to the exclusion of the other. Each serves a different theoretical purpose and possibly a different practical purpose as well: The factorial theory of Spearman is useful when one desires the most general, all-purpose predictor possible. The factorial theory of Thurstone is useful when one desires differential prediction, for example, between individuals' levels of spatial and verbal abilities.

3. *In hierarchical factor analyses, there seem to be two very broad group factors (or general subfactors), sometimes referred to as crystallized and fluid abilities.* The crystallized–fluid distinction has been proposed by Cattell (1971) and Horn (1968), and a similar distinction has been proposed by Vernon (1971), as noted earlier (Chapter 1). Crystallized ability is best measured by tests that measure the products of enculturation: vocabulary, reading comprehension, general information, and the like. Fluid ability is best measured by tests of abstract reasoning: abstract analogies, classifications, series completions, and the like. (Verbal items are also useful for this purpose if their vocabulary level is kept low.) Once again, I believe that there is something special about this hierarchical solution. Crystallized ability tests seem best able to separate the products of knowledge-acquisition components. I say "products," because tests of crystallized ability measure outcomes of these processes rather than the processes as they are actually executed. Fluid ability tests, on the other hand, seem most suitable for separating the execution of performance components. Thus, dividing factors along the crystallized–fluid dimension seems to provide a good distinction between the products of acquisition, on the one hand, and the current functioning of performance components, on the other. Crystallized and fluid factors will be correlated, however, because of shared metacomponents.

4. *Procrustean rotation of a factorial solution can result in the appearance of a large number of "structure-of-intellect" factors.* Procrustean rotation of a factorial solution involves rotation of a set of axes into maximum correspondence with a predetermined theory regarding where the axes should be placed. Guilford (1967, 1982; Guilford & Hoepfner, 1971) has used procrustean rotation to support his "structure-of-intellect" theory. According to this theory, intelligence comprises 150 distinct abilities (in the 1982 version of

the theory – see Chapter 1). Horn and Knapp (1973) have shown that comparable levels of support can be obtained via procrustean rotation to randomly determined theories. The validity of Guilford's theory is therefore open to at least some question (see also Cronbach & Snow, 1977). Nevertheless, I believe that there is probably a psychological basis for at least some aspects of Guilford's theory and that these aspects of the theory can be interpreted in componential terms.

A given component must act upon a particular form of representation for information and upon a particular type of information (content). The representation, for example, might be spatial or linguistic; the type of information (content) might be, for example, an abstract geometric design, a picture, a symbol, or a word. Forms of representations and contents, like components, can serve as sources of individual differences: A given individual might be quite competent when applying a particular component to one kind of content but not when applying it to another. Representation, content, and process have been largely confounded in most factorial theories, probably because certain components tend more often to operate upon certain kinds of representations and contents. This confounding serves a practical purpose, that of keeping to a manageable number the factors appearing in a given theory or test. But it does obscure any separable effects of process, representation, and content. Guilford's theory provides some separation, at least between process and content. I doubt the product dimension has much validity, other than through the fact that different kinds of products probably involve slightly different mixes of components. On the one hand, the theory points out the potential separability of process and content. On the other hand, it does so at the expense of manageability. Moreover, it seems highly unlikely that the 150 factors are independent. The correlations Guilford (1982) has found among them are probably due at least in part to shared metacomponents.

The distinction among process, content, and representation is an important one to keep in mind, because it is partly responsible for the low intercorrelations that are often obtained between seemingly highly related tasks. Two tasks (such as verbal and geometric analogies) may share the same information-processing components and yet show only moderate correlations because of content and representational differences. Guilford's finding of generally low intercorrelations between ability tests is probably due in part to the wide variation in the processes, contents, and representations required for solution of his various test items.

5. *One of the best single measures of overall intelligence (as measured by intelligence tests) is vocabulary.* This result (see, for example, Jensen, 1980; Matarazzo, 1972) has seemed rather surprising to some, because vocabulary tests seem to measure acquired knowledge rather than intelligent function-

ing. But the above discussion should suggest why vocabulary is such a good measure of overall intelligence. Vocabulary is acquired incidentally throughout one's lifetime as a result of knowledge-acquisition components. Moreover, to operate effectively, these knowledge-acquisition components must be under the control of metacomponents. Thus, vocabulary provides a good, although indirect, measure of an individual's lifetime operations of these various kinds of components. Vocabulary has an advantage over many kinds of performance tests, which measure the functioning of performance components only at the time of testing. The latter kinds of tests are more susceptible to the day-to-day fluctuations in performance that create unreliability and, ultimately, invalidity in tests. Because performance components are not as critical to individual differences in scores on vocabulary tests, one would expect vocabulary test scores to be less highly correlated with performance types of tests than with other verbal tests, and this is in fact the case (Matarazzo, 1972).

It was noted earlier that in some instances lack of knowledge can block successful execution of the performance components needed for intelligent functioning. For example, it is impossible to reason with logical connectives if one does not know what they mean or to solve verbal analogies if the meanings of words constituting the analogies are unknown. Thus, vocabulary is not only affected by operations of components, it affects their operations as well. If one grows up in a household that encourages exposure to words, then one's vocabulary may well be greater, which in turn may lead to a superior learning and performance on other kinds of tasks that require vocabulary. This is one way in which early rearing can have a substantial effect on vocabulary and on the behaviors vocabulary in turn affects.

6. *The absolute level of intelligence in children increases with age.* Why do children grow smarter as they grow older? The system of interrelations among components depicted in Figure 4.1 seems to contain a dynamic mechanism whereby cognitive growth can occur.

First, the components of knowledge acquisition provide the mechanisms for a steadily developing knowledge base. Increments in the knowledge base, in turn, allow for more sophisticated forms of knowledge acquisition and possibly for greater ease in executing performance components. For example, as the base of old knowledge becomes deeper and broader, the possibilities for relating new knowledge to old knowledge (selective comparison), and thus for incorporating that new knowledge into the existing knowledge base, increase. There is thus the possibility of an unending feedback loop: The components lead to an increased knowledge base, which leads to more effective use of the components, which leads to further increases in the knowledge base, and so on.

Second, the self-monitoring metacomponents can, in effect, learn from their own mistakes. Early on, allocation of metacomponential resources to varying tasks or kinds of components may be less than optimal, with a resulting loss of valuable feedback information. Self-monitoring should eventually result in improved allocations of metacomponential resources, in particular to the self-monitoring of the metacomponents. Thus, self-monitoring by the metacomponents results in improved allocation of metacomponential resources to the self-monitoring of the metacomponents, which in turn leads to improved self-monitoring, and so on. Here, too, there exists the possibility of an unending feedback loop, one that is internal to the metacomponents themselves.

Finally, indirect feedback from components other than metacomponents to each other, and direct feedback to the metacomponents, should result in improved effectiveness of performance. Knowledge-acquisition components, for example, can provide valuable information to performance components (via the metacomponents) concerning how to perform a task, and the performance components, in turn, can provide feedback to the acquisition components (via the metacomponents) concerning what else needs to be learned to perform the task optimally. Thus, other kinds of components, too, can generate unending feedback loops in which performance improves as a result of interactions between different kinds of components or between multiple components of the same kind.

There can be no doubt that the major variables in the individual-differences equation will be those deriving from the metacomponents. All feedback is filtered through these elements, and if they do not perform their function well, then it won't matter very much what the other kinds of components can do. It is for this reason that the metacomponents are viewed as truly central in understanding the nature of general intelligence and its development.

7. *Intelligence tests provide imperfect, but quite good, prediction of academic achievement.* A good intelligence test such as the Stanford–Binet will sample widely from the range of intellectual tasks that can reasonably be used in a testing situation. The wider this sampling, and the more closely the particular mix of components sampled resembles the mix of components required in academic achievement, the better the prediction will be. A vocabulary test, for example, will provide quite a good predictor of academic achievement, because academic achievement is strongly dependent upon knowledge acquisition and upon the metacomponents that control the components of knowledge acquisition. A spatial test will probably not be as good a predictor of general academic performance, because the performance components sampled in such a test will not be particularly relevant to general academic achievement, such as that required in English or history courses. An abstract reasoning test will probably be better than a spatial test in

predicting academic performance, because the particular performance components involved in these tasks seem to be general across tests involving inductive reasoning, including those found in academic learning environments. All intelligence tests will necessarily be imperfect predictors of academic achievement, however, because there is more to intelligence than is measured by intelligence tests and because there is more to school achievement than intelligence (see Chapter 2 of this book).

8. *Occasionally, people are quite good at one aspect of intellectual functioning, but quite poor at another.* Everyone knows of people who exhibit unusual and sometimes bizarre discrepancies in intellectual functioning. A person who is mathematically gifted may have trouble writing a sentence, or an accomplished novelist may have trouble adding simple columns of numbers. In the componential framework, the discrepancy can be accounted for in either of two ways. First, there may be inadequate functioning of, or inadequate feedback from, particular class components. The discrepancy cannot be in the general components, since they are (by definition) applicable to all tasks. Hence, the discrepancy must be found in those class components that permeate performance of a given set of tasks, such as mathematical tasks, verbal tasks, spatial tasks, or any of the other tasks that constitute measures of the "primary mental abilities." Differential ability to execute such class components might result, say, in a relatively high level of skill in dealing with novel situations but a relatively low level of skill in automatizing information processing, or vice versa; such a discrepancy in skills would in itself result in radically different levels of performance among kinds of tasks, particularly as a function of the levels of novelty and automatization involved. Note that in contrast, someone whose intellectual performance is generally depressed is more likely to be suffering from inadequacies in the execution of or feedback from general components (and possibly class components as well). Second, the discrepancy can be accounted for by difficulty in operating upon a particular form of representation. Different kinds of information are probably represented in different ways, at least at some level of information processing. For example, there is good reason to believe that linguistic and spatial representations differ in at least some respects from each other (MacLeod, Hunt, & Mathews, 1978; Paivio, 1971; Sternberg, 1980e). A given component may operate successfully upon one form of representation but not another, as discussed earlier.

9. *Intelligence is a necessary but not sufficient condition for creativity.* Creativity, according to the componential view, is due largely to the insightful use of knowledge-acquisition components and to extremely sensitive feedback between the various kinds of components. Such feedback is more likely to occur if, in knowledge acquisition, knowledge has been organized in a serviceable and richly interconnected way. But for interesting creative

behavior to occur, there must be a rather substantial knowledge base so that there is something to and from which transfer of information can occur. Thus, for creativity to be shown, a high level of functioning in the knowledge-acquisition components would seem to be necessary. These high levels of functioning are not in themselves sufficient for creativity to occur, however, since a sophisticated knowledge base does not guarantee that the knowledge base will be used with sophisticated feedback between kinds of components. This mechanism does not account for all creative behavior, of course, nor does it even give a full account of the creative behavior to which it can be applied. It does seem like a start toward a more detailed account, however.

This componential view is consistent with recent research on expert–novice distinctions that suggests that a major part of what distinguishes experts from novices is differences in the knowledge base and its organization (see, e.g., Chase & Simon, 1973; Chi, Glaser, & Rees, 1982; Glaser & Chi, 1979; Larkin, McDermott, Simon, & Simon, 1980). The view is also consistent with that of Horn (1979), who has suggested that creativity may be better understood by investigating crystallized ability than by investigating fluid ability. Our previous failures to isolate interesting loci of creative behavior may derive from our almost exclusive emphasis upon fluid abilities. The creativity tests that have resulted from this emphasis have measured what I believe to be rather trivial forms of creativity having little in common with the forms of creativity shown by creative novelists, scientists, artists, and the like. At the same time, it seems certain that high levels of crystallized abilities are not sufficient for creativity. Possession of knowledge does not guarantee creative use of that knowledge.

10. *Speed and accuracy (or quality) of intelligent performance may be positively correlated, negatively correlated, or uncorrelated.* The results of the "new wave" of intelligence research (e.g., Hunt et al., 1975; Mulholland, Pellegrino, & Glaser, 1980; Sternberg, 1977b) make it clear that speed and quality of performance bear no unique relation to each other. In the analogies task, for example, faster inference, mapping, application, and response component times are associated with higher intelligence test scores, but slower encoding seems to be associated with higher scores (Mulholland et al., 1980; Sternberg, 1977b). This finding and others like it can be explained at a metacomponential level: Individuals who encode stimuli more slowly are later able to operate upon their encodings more rapidly and accurately than are individuals who encode stimuli more rapidly. Faster encoding can thus actually slow down and impair the quality of overall performance. Similarly, individuals with higher intelligence tend to spend more time implementing the metacomponent of global strategy planning and less time implementing the metacomponent of local strategy planning (Sternberg, 1981d). Findings

such as these emphasize the importance of decomposing overall response time and accuracy into their constituent components, since different components may show different relations to intelligent performance. These findings also show the importance of seeking explanations for behavior at the metacomponential level. As important as it is to know what individuals are doing, it is even more important to know why they are doing it.

11. *Training of intelligent performance is most successful when it is at both the metacomponential and performance-componential levels.* Research on the training of intelligent performance has shown that the most successful approaches address metacomponential or metacognitive functioning as well as particular performance components and the strategies into which they combine (see, e.g., Borkowski & Cavanaugh, 1979; Brown & DeLoache, 1978; Butterfield & Belmont, 1977; Feuerstein, 1979, 1980; Sternberg, in press-c; Sternberg, Ketron, & Powell, 1982). This finding is consistent with the kind of framework shown in Figure 4.1. The interaction of metacomponents and performance components is such that training of just one kind of component will be fruitless unless there is at least some spillover into the other kind of component. The two kinds of components work in tandem and hence are most successfully trained in tandem. To obtain generalizability as well as durability of training, it may be necessary to train knowledge-acquisition components as well.

12. *Intelligence can mean somewhat different things in different cultures.* Cross-cultural research, as reviewed in Chapter 2, suggests that intelligence can mean somewhat different things in different cultures (Berry, 1974; Cole, Gay, Glick, & Sharp, 1971; Goodnow, 1976; Wober, 1974; see also Neisser, 1976, 1979). This view is consistent with the componential framework presented here. I interpret the available evidence as providing no support for the notion that the components of human cognition differ from one culture to another; the evidence, however, provides considerable support for the notion that the importances or weights of these components differ from one culture to another and that the kinds of task and situational instantiations that can successfully measure componential skills may also differ radically across cultures. Thus, components of cognitive functioning are viewed as an important part of intelligence in every culture, but which components are important and how they are best measured are viewed as differing.

The 12 findings on intelligence discussed above provide only a very partial list of empirical generalizations in the literature on intelligence; they cover sufficient ground, however, to convey some sense of how the componential view accounts for various phenomena involving intelligence. The componential view can account for a number of other phenomena as well, but it is important to remember that the view is incomplete: It must be supplemented by an account of the facets of intelligent behavior (Chapter 3) and of the contexts in which this behavior occurs (Chapter 2). According to the present view, then, components and their interactions are what enable individuals to deal with novelty and to automatize performance, and they function in the context of one or more given sociocultural milieux. *Intelligence is the mental capability of emitting contextually appropriate behavior at those regions in the experiential continuum that involve response to novelty or automatization of information processing as a function of metacomponents, performance components, and knowledge-acquisition components.* Behavior involves intelligence to the extent it partakes of more aspects of this definition of intelligent behavior. Taking into account all three of these aspects of intelligent performance can provide a rather powerful account of the phenomenon of intelligence, as I shall attempt to show in the next part of the book.

Part III

The triarchic theory: tests

Part III presents tests, as well as elaborations, of the triarchic theory of human intelligence. This part of the book is divided into five chapters. These chapters present theories of some, although certainly not all, of the constituent cognitive abilities that are involved in intelligent processing of information. The organization of chapters generally follows from the contextually derived, implicit theory of intelligence presented in Part II. According to this implicit theory, abilities are perceived as being of three major kinds: problem-solving or fluid abilities, knowledge-based or crystallized abilities, and social and practical abilities.

Chapter 5, "Fluid abilities: inductive reasoning," presents a componential theory of inductive reasoning and models of inductive task performance in analogy, series completion, classification, metaphorical, and causal inference problems. These componential models are closely interrelated, involving various combinations of the basic mechanisms specified in the general theory of inductive reasoning (i.e., reasoning in problems for which there is no uniquely defined answer that is a priori correct). Tests of general intelligence have traditionally placed a heavy emphasis on the kinds of induction problems discussed in this chapter, and hence the chapter may be viewed as providing an information-processing framework for many psychometric tests (as well as theories) of general intelligence. In terms of the triarchic theory, the emphasis in this chapter is on performance components, as specified by the componential subtheory.

Chapter 6, "Fluid abilities: deductive reasoning," presents a componential theory of deductive reasoning and models of deductive task performance in linear, categorical, and conditional syllogistic reasoning problems. Whereas the inductive problems described in Chapter 5 do not yield a uniquely determined a priori correct response, these items do yield such a response. Deductive reasoning problems have been less central in the psychometric literature on intelligence than have inductive reasoning problems, perhaps because they do not tend to load as highly on a general factor of intelligence (*g*) and because they appear to be factorially complex, involving spatial and memory abilities as well as pure reasoning ability. Nevertheless, they have been of considerable importance in the cognitive literature, and they form a necessary complement to the inductive tasks. In order to understand reasoning fully, one must understand both its inductive and deductive aspects. This chapter, like Chapter 5, emphasizes the role of performance components in reasoning.

Chapter 7, "Crystallized intelligence: acquisition of verbal comprehension," shifts the focus from abilities involved in problem solving to abilities involved in knowledge acquisition and application. This chapter presents a tripartite theory of how verbal comprehension skills – and particularly skills involved in vocabulary acquisition – develop and operate in the understanding of verbal information. The proposed theory may be viewed as an attempt to understand the origins of crystallized ability. It addresses questions such as why vocabulary provides such a good index of intelligence and why vocabulary level is so closely related to reading comprehension skills. Whereas Chapters 5 and 6 emphasize the role of performance components in intelligent behavior, this chapter emphasizes the role of knowledge-acquisition components, as specified by the componential subtheory.

Chapter 8, "Crystallized intelligence: theory of information processing in real time verbal comprehension," presents a theory of how certain kinds of verbal information are processed in real time. Whereas Chapter 7 emphasizes the origins and development of verbal abilities, this chapter emphasizes current verbal functioning. It addresses questions such as how people represent and compare the meanings of words (as on a synonyms test) and how people allocate their time when reading various kinds of written texts. Whereas Chapter 7 emphasizes the role of knowledge-acquisition components in verbal behavior, this chapter emphasizes the roles of performance components and metacomponents.

Chapter 9, "Social and practical intelligence," shifts the focus of Part III from academic abilities to social and practical abilities. Although the approach to theory and research is heavily influenced by the componential subtheory, the questions addressed are at least as relevant to the contextual subtheory as they are to the componential one. Indeed, the research described in this chapter elaborates upon the nature of what adaptive behavior is in our culture. Whereas the contextual subtheory (like other contextual accounts of intelligence) posits the importance of environmentally adaptive behavior, it does not specify just which behaviors are adaptive. Implicit theories of intelligence specify people's conceptions of what behaviors are adaptive; the accounts of social and practical intelligence presented in this chapter attempt to do the same, but with an explicit-theoretical rather than an implicit-theoretical base.

5 Fluid abilities: inductive reasoning

Those abilities that psychologists have referred to as "fluid" (see, e.g., Cattell, 1971; Horn, 1968; Snow, 1979, 1981; Sternberg, 1981k) correspond quite closely to the kinds of problem-solving behaviors identified by laypersons and experts alike as constituting an important aspect of intelligence. These behaviors include, for example, reasoning logically and well, identifying connections among ideas, seeing all aspects of a problem, posing problems in an optimal way, and getting to the heart of a problem (see Sternberg, Conway, Ketron, & Bernstein, 1981; see also Chapter 2 of this book). My collaborators and I have sought to understand the mental bases of these kinds of behaviors through componential analysis of the kinds of tasks that have been found in the differential and cognitive literatures and that have been believed to provide the best measurement of fluid abilities. These tasks, of course, differ in some ways among themselves, but virtually all of them have in common their key reliance upon what is known as *inductive reasoning.*

Inductive reasoning requires an individual to reason from part to whole or from particular to general *(Webster's New Collegiate Dictionary*, 1976). Inductive reasoning problems can be of various kinds, but the kinds most often used in psychometric tests and in experimental investigations of inductive reasoning ability are those that Greeno (1978) has referred to as problems of inducing structure. Problems of this kind include analogies (e.g., LAWYER is to CLIENT as DOCTOR is to a. MEDICINE, b. PATIENT), series completions (e.g., Which word should come next in the following series? PENNY, NICKEL, DIME, a. COIN, b. QUARTER), and classifications (e.g., Which of the two words at the right fits better with the three words at the left? CAT, MOUSE, LION, a. SQUIRREL, b. EAGLE). These problems are of particular interest because they have played a key role in both the psychometric and the information-processing literatures on reasoning and intelligence as well as in the recent literature attempting to integrate the psychometric and information-processing approaches (e.g., Pellegrino & Glaser, 1980; Sternberg, 1977b; Whitely, 1980).

131

Fluid abilities and intelligence: a capsule review of the literature

In the psychometric literature, problems of inducing structure have been considered important because they provide particularly good measures of fluid intelligence in particular and of g (general intelligence) in general. Spearman's (1923) theory of analogical reasoning provided the cornerstone for his theory of general intelligence. Thurstone (1938) used verbal and pattern analogies as bases for validating his theory of primary mental abilities. Also, Guilford (1967) used analogies of various kinds to measure a number of the structure-of-intellect abilities that constitute his model for intelligence. He manipulated the content, products, and processes required in order to tailor the test items to each of the targeted abilities. Thus, most of the major psychometric theories have drawn more or less heavily upon analogies as a basis for their evaluation and even formulation.

In the information-processing literature, problems of inducing structure have been considered important because the underlying processes involved in solving these problems seem to be basic to human cognition, both in laboratory and in real-world settings. These problems have served as the basis for a number of task analyses. Several computer programs, for example, have been devoted exclusively to the solution of analogies (Evans, 1968; Reitman, 1965) or series completions (Simon & Kotovsky, 1963), whereas other computer programs have dealt with analogies or series completions as well as other kinds of problems (Williams, 1972; Winston, 1974). Analogy problems have also been studied experimentally in a number of investigations with human subjects (e.g., Mulholland et al., 1980; Sternberg, 1977a, 1977b; Whitely & Barnes, 1979), as have series completions (e.g., Holzman, Glaser, & Pellegrino, 1976; Kotovsky & Simon, 1973). Information-processing analyses of the classification task have been conducted by Whitely (1980) and by Parseghian and Pellegrino (1980), and the literature on concepts and their attainment can be viewed as indirectly studying this sort of task (e.g., Bruner, Goodnow, & Austin, 1956; Rosch, 1978).

Several information-processing psychologists have claimed that the high intercorrelations obtained between subjects' performances on various kinds of problems of inducing structure are attributable to commonalities in information processing across the various kinds of problems (e.g., Greeno, 1978; Pellegrino & Glaser, 1979, 1980; Simon, 1976; Sternberg, 1977b, 1979b, 1982g). The theory and investigations described in this chapter represent an attempt to make this claim in a precise way and then to test the claim. Essentially, it is argued that the cognitive basis for "fluid ability" can be understood in terms of information-processing components that overlap between tasks that tap fluid ability.

Criteria for assessing commonalities in fluid (and other) tasks

Several criteria can be used for detecting commonalities in information processing, and before presenting theory and data it would be useful to summarize the main criteria that will be used in this chapter (and subsequent ones). Some of the theoretical sources of commonality include use of common (a) components, (b) strategies, (c) representations of information, and (d) knowledge base across tasks. The identification of such commonalities, however, depends upon empirical criteria for assessing these commonalities. Such empirical criteria include (a) comparable latencies and error probabilities across tasks for component processes alleged to be the same; (b) high correlations across tasks between problems subjected to the same experimental stimulus manipulation (e.g., increasing the number of times certain theoretically shared processes are executed and decreasing the number of times other theoretically shared processes are executed); (c) good fits of the same proposed theory to stimulus variations in the latency, error, or response probability data in the various tasks; (d) high correlations across subjects of global and comparable process scores on the various tasks; and (e) comparable correlations across subjects of task scores with psychometric ability test scores (i.e., scores on the various tasks should show the same patterns of correlation with external measures used for convergent and discriminant validation). The tasks used for convergent validation are ones that are predicted to show high correlations with the task scores; the tasks used for discriminant validation are ones that are predicted to show low correlations with the task scores. I have used all of these criteria at various times in the experiments to be reported. However, it is not possible to apply every criterion in every experiment, simply because the necessary data are unavailable in some data sets.

It should be noted that satisfaction of these criteria, singly or jointly, is not sufficient for concluding that two tasks measure exactly the same thing. One can never be sure of task comparability, if only because some future experimental manipulation of two tasks thought to be comparable may give divergent patterns of results for the two tasks and thus reveal that the tasks are not measuring quite the same thing, after all (see empirical criterion b above). At best, one can establish a highly plausible, if uncertain, case for the comparability of task performances.

Theory of inductive reasoning

The proposed theory of inductive reasoning is divided into two subtheories, one of which accounts for information processing in inductive reasoning, the other of which accounts for response choices in inductive reasoning. Each of these subtheories will be discussed in turn.

Componential theory of information processing in inductive reasoning

The proposed theory asserts that inductive information processing can be understood in terms of seven performance components that are common across inductive reasoning tasks: encoding, inference, mapping, application, comparison, justification, and response. Consider the generalized meaning of each of these components:

1. *Encoding*. A stimulus is translated into an internal representation upon which further mental operations can be performed. The translation process involves at least two subcomponents – perceiving the stimulus and accessing relevant information in long-term memory that enables one to interpret the stimulus. For example, encoding of the term LAWYER would involve perceiving the stimulus and recognizing, perhaps, that a lawyer is a person who renders professional legal services.

2. *Inference*. A rule is discovered that relates a given concept to another concept. For example, inferring the relation between LAWYER and CLIENT might involve recognition of the fact that a CLIENT is the person to whom a LAWYER renders his or her professional legal services.

3. *Mapping*. A higher-order rule is discovered that relates a given rule to another rule. For example, mapping might be used to recognize that the topic of the analogy that relates the LAWYER half to the DOCTOR half is professional renderers of services.

4. *Application*. A rule is generated that extrapolates to a new concept from an old concept on the basis of an analogy to a previously learned rule. For example, application might be used to recognize that it is, indeed, a PATIENT that receives professional services from a DOCTOR in much the same way that a CLIENT receives professional services from a LAWYER.

5. *Comparison*. The given answer options are compared to an extrapolated (and usually ideal) new concept in order to determine which option is closest in meaning to the extrapolated concept. For example, if the extrapolated concept is PATIENT, then comparison might be used to determine which of two options, SICK PATIENT and MEDICINE, is closer in meaning to PATIENT.

6. *Justification*. A preferred answer option is compared to the extrapolated (ideal) concept in order to determine whether the answer option is close enough in meaning to the extrapolated concept in order to justify its selection as the "correct" answer to a given problem.

7. *Response*. The chosen answer is communicated through an overt act.

For example, a button on a computer terminal might be pushed to indicate that SICK PERSON has been chosen as a correct answer to a problem.

Note that in terms of the stages of information processing discussed in the previous chapter, the encoding component occupies the encoding stage; inference, mapping, application, comparison, and justification occupy the comparison stage; and response occupies the response stage of information processing.

This componential theory needs to be supplemented by specific models that apply to particular inductive tasks. Whereas the theory specifies the components of information processing upon which the models draw, the models specify as well the way in which the set (or a subset) of performance components is combined into a strategy for task solution. Consider specific task models for three of the most commonly used and studied problems of inducing structure: analogies, series completions, and classifications. Note that each of these three kinds of problems can take a variety of forms and that the models have to be tailored to the particular form used for each task. Moreover, the models can be specified in various levels of detail. The unit of analysis in the present description of task models is the problem stimulus term (e.g., the A term in the analogy, $A:B::C:D$). For a more detailed description at the level of the stimulus term attribute, see Sternberg (1977b) (for analogies only).

Componential model of analogical reasoning. Solution of analogies of the form $A:B::C:(D_1, D_2)$ is theorized to require all seven of the information-processing components noted above. A schematic flowchart for the model is shown in Figure 5.1.

First, subjects *encode* the A and B analogy terms, storing possibly relevant attributes for analogy solution in working memory. Next, subjects *infer* a set of relations between A and B. Then, they encode the C term of the analogy. Next, subjects *map* the relation they inferred from A to B so as to carry it over to the second half of the analogy. Subjects then *apply* the relation they inferred from A to B, forming an ideal completion for the analogy. Next, subjects encode the two answer options, D_1 and D_2. Then, they *compare* each of the answer options to their extrapolated ideal, hoping to identify one of the options as identical to the ideal. If an identity is found, a response to the problem can be made. If the comparison fails to yield an answer option corresponding perfectly to the ideal, the subjects are assumed to *justify* one option as preferred but nonideal. Finally, subjects *respond*.

This generalized model applies to a number of different analogy forms and contents. The model does not apply in the above form to so-called "schematic-picture" analogies, however, in which the stimulus terms consist of

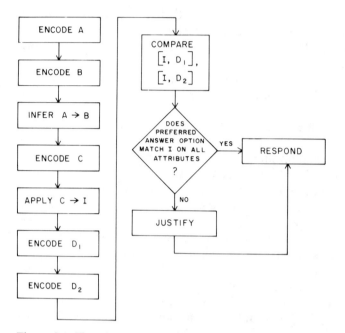

Figure 5.1. Flowchart representing the sequence of information processing during solution of analogies. (From "Unities in inductive reasoning," by Robert J. Sternberg and Michael K. Gardner, 1983, *Journal of Experimental Psychology: General, 112,* p. 101. Copyright 1983 by the American Psychological Association. Reprinted by permission of the publisher.)

pictures of objects with discrete and highly regular stimulus attributes . In schematic-picture analogies, subjects self-terminate in their performance of some component processes. Self-termination involves a subject's processing the minimal possible number of attributes of a given stimulus term in order to achieve problem solution (see Sternberg, 1977a, 1977b). If a given attribute turns out to provide a sufficient basis for falsifying one option (and hence confirming the other), the subject responds on the basis of this attribute and terminates information processing. If the attribute does not provide a sufficient basis for choosing between answer options, a second attribute is carried through the problem and an attempt is again made to falsify one answer option and thereby select the other on the basis of this attribute. This cycle is iterated until an attribute can be found that distinguishes between the better answer option and the worse one.

Componential model of series completions. The model described here applies to series completions of the form A B C :: D : (E_1, E_2), in which sub-

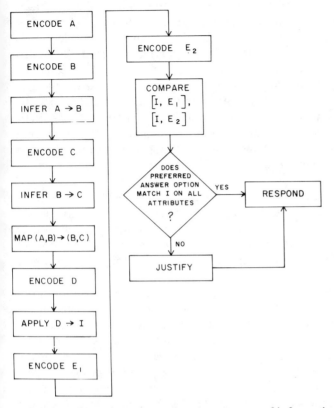

Figure 5.2. Flowchart representing the sequence of information processing during solution of series completions. (I = ideal point.) (From "Unities in inductive reasoning," by Robert J. Sternberg and Michael K. Gardner, 1983, *Journal of Experimental Psychology: General, 112,* p. 102. Copyright 1983 by the American Psychological Association. Reprinted by permission of the publisher.)

jects must recognize a series that relates A, B, and C, carry it over to D, and then extend the series to one of the two answer options. (Simplified versions of the model can be applied to simplified forms of the series completion problem, such as A B C (D_1, D_2), where the subject need simply continue a single series.) A schematic flowchart for the proposed model is shown in Figure 5.2.

First, subjects *encode* the A and B terms of a given series problem. Next, they *infer* a set of relations between the A and B terms. Then, they encode the C term of a given problem. Then, they infer a set of relations between the B and C terms. Next, they *map* the higher-order relation between the (A, B) relation, on the one hand, and the (B, C) relation, on the other, seeking out those relations that both relate to A and B and to C and D. Then, subjects encode the D term. With this term encoded, they *apply* from D to an ideal extrapolation that optimally completes the series completion problem. This ideal term is constructed from the attributes inferred earlier that have survived the mapping process (i.e., that are relevant in both the A-to-B and the B-to-C inferences). Next, subjects *compare* their self-constructed ideal to each of the answer options, attempting to find a perfect match between the ideal response and one of the given answer options. If a perfect match can be found, the subjects can respond. If neither of the options provides such a match, subjects *justify* one of the answer options as preferred, although nonideal. Finally, subjects *respond*.

Componential model of classification. The proposed model applies to classifications of the form A B, C D : E, in which the subject's task is to decide whether E fits better with A and B, on the one hand, or with C and D, on the other. Classification requires six separate performance components. A schematic flowchart illustrating the sequence of these components is shown in Figure 5.3.

First, subjects *encode* the A and B terms of the given classification problem. Next, they *infer* a set of relations between the A and B terms of the problem. Then, they encode the C and D terms. These encodings enable the subjects to infer a set of relations between the C and D terms of the problem. Then, subjects map the higher-order relation between relation (A, B), on the one hand, and relation (C, D), on the other, seeking in this problem type a subset of attributes that differentiate the (A, B) relationship from the (C, D) one. Then, subjects encode the E term of the classification. Now, subjects are able to *compare* the E term to each of the (A, B) and (C, D) relations, looking at all attributes but spending additional time on distinguishing attributes as determined earlier during the mapping process. If E perfectly matches either of (A, B) or (C, D) in both common and distinguishing attributes, the subject is then able to select that group as the correct response. If a perfect match is not found, then one of the two pairs (which here serve as answer options) – (A, B) or (C, D) – is *justified* as closer to the ideal, E. This pair serves as the basis for the subject's answer choice, making it possible for the subject to *respond*. Note that the application component does not enter into this model, because it is not necessary for the subject to construct an ideal. The function of the ideal is served in this problem type by E.

Theory of response choice in inductive reasoning

The proposed theory of response choice in inductive reasoning of the sort required by analogies, series completions, and classifications is an extension

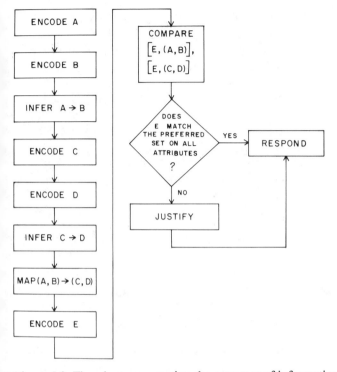

Figure 5.3. Flowchart representing the sequence of information processing during solution of classifications. (From "Unities in inductive reasoning," by Robert J. Sternberg and Michael K. Gardner, 1983, *Journal of Experimental Psychology: General, 112*, p. 103. Copyright 1983 by the American Psychological Association. Reprinted by permission of the publisher.)

of the Rumelhart–Abrahamson (1973) theory of response choice in analogical reasoning (see Sternberg & Gardner, 1983). Rumelhart and Abrahamson defined reasoning as the set of thought processes in information retrieval that operates on the structure, as opposed to the content, of organized memory. If information retrieval depends on specific content stored in memory, then retrieval is referred to as remembering. If, however, information retrieval depends on the form of one or more relationships among words, then it is referred to as reasoning.

Pursuing this definition of reasoning, Rumelhart and Abrahamson claimed that probably the simplest possible reasoning task is the judgment of the similarity or dissimilarity between concepts. They assumed that the degree of similarity between concepts is not directly stored as such but is instead derived from previously existing memory structures. Judged similarity between concepts is a simple function of the "psychological distance" between these concepts in the memory structure. The nature of this function and of the memory structure on which it operates is clarified by their assumptions (after Henley, 1969) that (a) the memory structure may be represented as a multidimensional Euclidean space and (b) judged similarity is inversely related to distance in this space.

According to this view, inductive reasoning may be considered as involving kinds of similarity judgments (such as the inference, mapping, comparison, and justification components described earlier), judgments in which not only the magnitude of the distance but also the direction is of importance. For example, we would ordinarily interpret the analogy problem $A:B::C:X_i$ as stating that A is similar to B in approximately the same way that C is similar to X_i. According to the assumptions outlined above, one might reinterpret this analogy as saying that the directed or vector distance between A and B is exactly the same as the vector distance between C and X_i. The analogy is imprecise to the extent to which the two vector distances are unequal.

The assumptions of the theory can be formalized (following Rumelhart & Abrahamson, 1973) as follows:

1. Corresponding to each stimulus term in an induction problem there is a point in an m-dimensional (psychological) space.

2. For any induction problem (involving extrapolation), there is an ideal point, I, in the multidimensional space that corresponds to the optimal solution of the problem.

3. The probability that any given alternative X_i is chosen as the best solution from the set of alternatives $X_1, \ldots, X_n$ is a monotonically decreasing function of the absolute value of the distance between the point X_i and I. In particular, the probability that any given alternative X_i is chosen from the set of alternatives is given by $P(X_i/X_1, \ldots, X_n) = p_i = v(d_i)/[\Sigma_j v(d_j)]$, where d_i denotes the absolute value of the distance between X_i and I, and $v(\ )$ is a monotonically decreasing function of its argument.

4. $v(X) = \exp(-\alpha X)$.

5. Subjects rank a set of alternatives by first choosing the rank 1 element according to assumption 3 above, and then, of the remaining alternatives, deciding which is superior by application of assumption 3 to the remaining set and assigning that rank 2. This procedure is assumed to continue until all alternatives are ranked.

Assumption 3 is an adaptation of Luce's (1959) choice rule to the choice situation in the induction problem. Assumption 4 further specifies that the monotone decrease in the likelihood of choosing a particular answer option as being the best choice follows an exponential decay function with increas-

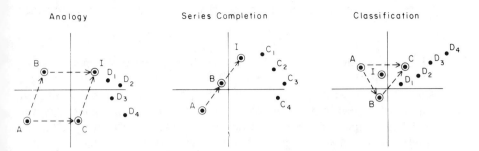

Figure 5.4. Schematic diagrams showing rules for arriving at ideal point *I* in each of three induction tasks. In analogies, *I* is located as the fourth vertex in a parallelogram having *A*, *B*, and *C* as the three given vertices. In series completions, *I* is located as the completion of a line segment that is at the same vector distance from *B* that *B* is from *A*. In classifications, *I* is the centroid of the triangle with *A*, *B*, and *C* as vertices. In each type of problem, four answer options are presented at successively greater Euclidean distances from the ideal point. (From "Unities in inductive reasoning," by Robert J. Sternberg and Michael K. Gardner, 1983, *Journal of Experimental Psychology: General, 112*, p. 84. Copyright 1983 by the American Psychological Association. Reprinted by permission of the publisher.)

ing distance from the ideal point. The model of response choice therefore requires a single parameter, α, representing the slope of the function.

We have extended the Rumelhart–Abrahamson model to account for response choices in series completions and classifications as well as in analogies. The response choice is assumed to occur during execution of the comparison component and, optionally, the justification component if the fit of the preferred option is nonoptimal. Consider each problem type, using Figure 5.4 as a referent.

Model of response choice in analogical reasoning. Consider an analogy problem of the form, $A : B :: C : (D_1, D_2, D_3, D_4)$ – for example, TIGER : CHIMPANZEE :: WOLF : (a. RACCOON, b. CAMEL, c. MONKEY, d. LEOPARD), in which the subject's task is to rank-order the answer options in terms of how well their relation to WOLF is parallel to the relation between CHIMPANZEE and TIGER. In an analogy problem such as this one, the subject must find an ideal point that is the same vector distance from WOLF as CHIMPANZEE is from TIGER. Having found this point, the subject rank-orders answer options according to their overall Euclidean distance from the ideal point. The probability of selecting any one answer option as best is assumed to follow an exponential decay function, with probability decreasing as distance from the ideal point increases. The same selection rule is applied in rank-ordering successive options, with previously selected options removed from consideration.

Model of response choice in serial reasoning. Consider next a series completion problem of the form, $A:B::(C_1, C_2, C_3, C_4)$ – for example, SQUIRREL : CHIPMUNK :: (a. RACCOON, b. HORSE, c. DOG, d. CAMEL), in which the subject's task is to rank-order the answer options in terms of how well they complete the series carried from SQUIRREL to CHIPMUNK. Here, the subject must find an ideal point that is the same vector distance from CHIPMUNK as CHIPMUNK is from SQUIRREL. Note that the difference between a series completion problem and an analogy problem is that whereas the terms of an analogy form a parallelogram in the multidimensional space, the terms of a series completion form a line segment in the space. The same principle would apply regardless of the number of terms in the item stem. Having found the ideal point, the subject rank-orders answer options with respect to the ideal point in just the same way that he or she would in an analogy problem.

Model of response choice in classificational reasoning. Consider finally a classification problem of the form, $A, B, C, (D_1, D_2, D_3, D_4)$ – for example, ZEBRA, GIRAFFE, GOAT, (a. DOG, b. COW, c. MOUSE, d. DEER), in which the subject's task is to rank-order the answer options in terms of how well they fit with the three terms in the item stem. In this type of problem, the subject must find an ideal point that represents the centroid in multidimensional space of ZEBRA, GIRAFFE, and GOAT. Having found this point, the subject rank-orders the answer options according to their overall Euclidean distance from the ideal point, in just the same way he or she would for analogies or series completions. Again, the same basic principle applies without regard to the number of terms in the item stem. The centroid of the points is theorized always to serve as the ideal point.

Tests of the theory of inductive reasoning

Tests of the componential theory of information processing

Initial tests of the theory of analogical reasoning processes. I initially tested the theory of analogical reasoning processes (minus the comparison component, which had not yet become part of the theory at the time) under the assumptions that (a) the components were combined sequentially and that (b) they acted upon an attribute – value mental representation for information, meaning that each analogy term could be decomposed into a set of

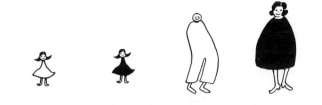

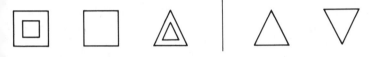

Figure 5.5. Examples of schematic-picture, verbal, and geometric analogies. The first two analogy types were true–false; the last was forced-choice. Subjects were told either to determine whether the analogy was true or false or to determine which of two answer options better completed the analogy. Subjects solving schematic-picture analogies were told that four binary attributes – height (tall, short), weight (fat, thin), sex (male, female), and clothing color (blue, red, in the actual stimuli) – were relevant to item solution.

attributes with some range of possible values on each attribute – for example, height: tall–short. Alternative models were tested that varied in terms of which components of the theory were exhaustive (all encoded attributes compared) and which self-terminating (only a proper subset of the encoded attributes compared), and alternative theories were also tested that varied in the numbers of components theorized to be needed for analogy solution.

Subjects in the first set of experiments (Sternberg, 1977a, 1977b) were Stanford undergraduates. One group of 16 subjects solved 1,152 schematic-picture ("People Piece") analogies and 68 verbal analogies; a second group of 24 subjects solved 90 geometric analogies. An example of each of the three kinds of items is shown in Figure 5.5. Note that the schematic-picture and verbal analogies were presented in a true–false format and the geometric analogies in a forced-choice format. The primary dependent variable was response time (with error rate serving as a secondary dependent variable), and the independent variables were manipulations of various aspects of item difficulty that were needed in order to separate parameters representing durations of the theorized component processes. Subjects were tested tachistoscopically, meaning that they sat in front of a large boxlike contraption that presented stimuli, measured response time, and recorded response choices. Tachistoscopic testing was followed by paper-and-pencil testing on psychometric measures of reasoning and perceptual – motor speed abilities.

Internal validation. Theory testing was accomplished via mathematical modeling. Each alternative theory and model was initially expressed as an information-processing flowchart representing each performance component as a box in the chart. These models were then quantified by assigning a mathematical parameter to represent the duration (or difficulty) of a given processing component. Multiple linear regression was used to predict the mean response time to each analogy item type from the appropriate set of independent variables representing the number of times a given component had to be performed in analogy solution. This model-testing procedure was possible because items had been systematically constructed so as to vary the sources of difficulty involved in their solution (see Sternberg, 1977a, 1977b, for further details).

Mean response times were 1.42 seconds for schematic-picture analogies, 2.42 seconds for verbal analogies, and 6.58 seconds for geometric analogies. Error rates were very low (ranging from 1% to 5% across tasks). The proposed theory provided the best fit to the latency data, accounting for .92, .86, and .80 of the variance in the schematic-picture, verbal, and geometric group – mean latency data. (These proportions are the squared correlations (R^2) between predicted and observed data points for each of the analogy item types in each of the three data sets.) Root-mean-square deviations (RMSDs) between predicted and observed data points (measuring absolute badness of fit) were .13, .26, and 1.68 seconds for schematic-picture, verbal, and geometric analogies, respectively. It was found that execution of the inference component was exhaustive (meaning that all encoded attributes were subjected to the inference process) but that execution of the mapping and application components was self-terminating (meaning that only a portion of the encoded attributes were subjected to the mapping and application components). It is worth noting that although the proposed theory did quite a reasonable job of accounting for variance in the latency data, the unexplained variance was statistically significant, meaning that the proposed theory is not equivalent to the "true theory." There is systematic variation that still remains unexplained.

External validation. Patterns of correlations between psychometric test scores and both the global scores (average response time over items for a given subject) and parameter scores (response latency for a particular processing component) of the analogies tasks were mixed in terms of their accord with prior predictions. The perceptual – motor psychometric tests had been included for purposes of discriminant validation, meaning that I had hoped that individuals' task scores would *not* be correlated with them. Significant correlations of this kind would suggest that the tachistoscopically administered analogies test was measuring perceptual—motor speed, a construct that was not of interest in the present studies. Happily, neither global task scores nor parameter scores showed any significant correlations with the perceptual—motor speed measures. But the psychometric reasoning tests were included for purposes of convergent validation, meaning that I had hoped that global task and appropriate parameter scores would be correlated with the reasoning measures. Although the correlations between the global task and test scores were adequate (ranging from about -.4 to -.6 across the three tasks, with negative correlations indicating that shorter task latencies were associated with greater numbers correct on the psychometric tests), attempts at localization of the source of these correlations were disappointing. Although there were some significant correlations of reasoning-type parameters (inference, mapping, application, justification) with the test scores, most of the global correlation turned out to be localized in the correlation of the response parameter with the reasoning score! Although I proposed at this time several possible explanations for this surprising phenomenon (Sternberg, 1977b), it remained for later research to show that the result was due to several factors, namely (a) unreliability of the reasoning component scores in contrast to the response component score (which depressed the possible correlations one could obtain with the former type of score), and (b) confounding of metacomponential latencies (which would be expected to correlate with psychometrically measured reasoning) and the response-component latency.

Why did this confounding occur? The response component score was estimated as a regression constant in the mathematical model, meaning that it was estimated as that portion of response time that was constant across item types within a given set (schematic-picture, verbal, or geometric) of analogies. The use of this (fairly standard) procedure for estimating response component time had the unfortunate result that any component latency that was constant across item types was confounded with the response constant. In subsequent studies, my colleagues and I attempted to obtain more reliable reasoning component scores and to increase the range of item difficulty and variety in order better to isolate the response component from any other component.

Extension of tests to series completions and classifications. The modeling data described above provided good support for the proposed theory of analogical reasoning processes. But the correlational results were perplexing. The data set as a whole raised two important theoretical questions.

First, could the theory of inductive reasoning processes actually account for performance on problems other than analogies? The theory would be of considerably greater psychological interest if it could be shown that it was, in fact, generalizable to problem types other than analogies. To the extent that the historical claim is correct that reasoning by analogy provides a paradigm for inductive thought (Reitman, 1965; Spearman, 1923), then the theory should indeed be generalizable.

Second, the patterns of correlation between parameters of inductive reasoning tasks and scores on psychometric tests needed to be clarified. If the proposed theory of reasoning were correct, then with sufficiently reliable task parameter estimates and psychometric test scores, and with sufficient variation in item types, parameters representing durations of reasoning components – inference, mapping, application, comparison, justification – should show statistically reliable correlations with psychometrically measured reasoning ability, and the response parameter should not show a significant correlation.

Twenty-four Yale undergraduates were confronted with three tasks – analogies, series completions, and classifications – presented via three kinds of contents – schematic pictures, words, and geometric forms (Sternberg & Gardner, 1982, 1983; see also Sternberg, 1983a). An example of each of the nine kinds of items used (3 tasks × 3 contents) is shown in Figure 5.6. A total of 2,880 items were administered to each subject. This large number of items was intended to insure highly reliable global-task scores and individual parameter estimates. In addition, subjects in the experiment received two forms of each of six psychometric tests of reasoning abilities and three of perceptual–motor speed abilities, again to insure reliability of scores. Total testing time was about 25 hours per subject, spread out over a number of separate sessions. As in the earlier analogy experiment, the primary dependent variable was response time (with error rate as a secondary dependent variable), and independent variables were formed by manipulations of various aspects of item difficulty. Also as in the earlier experiments, task items were presented tachistoscopically, with subjects timed in their latency of response to each item.

As in the analogies research, it was assumed that performance components were executed sequentially. Because the comparison component was being newly added to the theory, the ability of the theory to account for the latency data with the additional component was compared to the ability of the theory to account for the data without this additional component. The question of interest was whether the comparison component latency – as represented by an additional parameter in the mathematical model – accounted for statistically significant and practically substantial additional amounts of variance in the data. The answer to this question proved to be affirmative, and the data presented here are for the full set of parameters used

SHELL : NUT :: PEEL : (a) ORANGE (b) HOUSE

TREE : FOREST :: SOLDIER : (a) GENERAL (b) ARMY

SECOND : MINUTE : HOUR ::
DECADE : (a) TIME (b) CENTURY

RARELY : SOMETIMES : OFTEN ::
MANY : (a) FREQUENTLY (b) MOST

BABY CARRIAGE : TRICYCLE : BICYCLE ::
MEASLES : (a) ILLNESS (b) ACNE

(a) DICTIONARY ENCYCLOPEDIA (b) LEMONADE RUM
GASOLINE

(a) FURNACE STOVE (b) REFRIGERATOR AIR CONDITIONER
OVEN

(a) GERMANY FRANCE (b) VIETNAM KOREA
ITALY

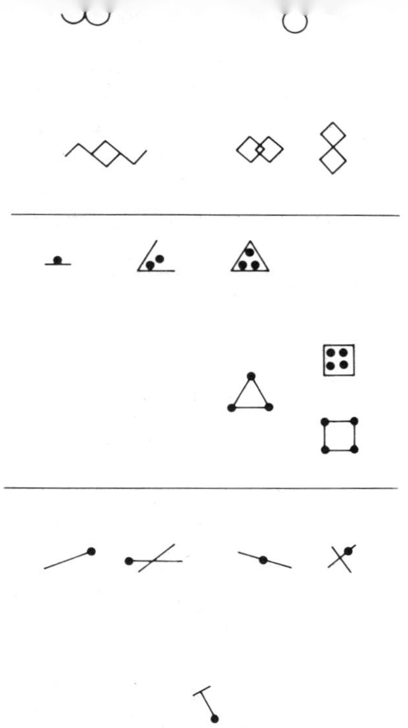

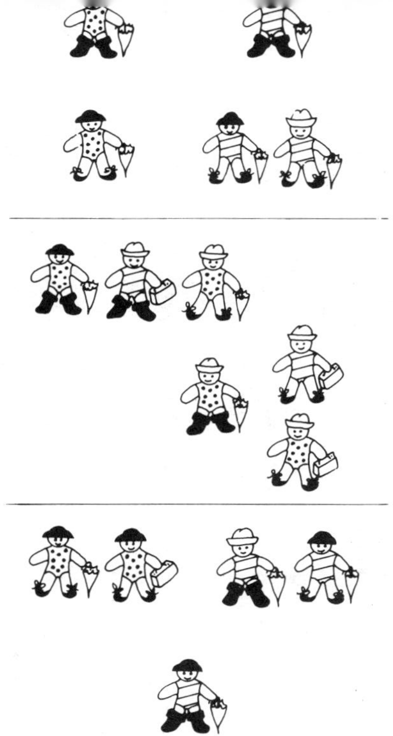

Figure 5.6. Examples of schematic-picture, verbal, and geometric analogies, series completions, and classifications. All items were forced-choice. In the analogies, subjects had to choose the final term that was related to the third term in the same way that the second term was related to the first term. In the series completions, subjects had to choose the final term that completed the series pattern set by the first three terms as projected to the fourth term. In the classifications, subjects had to decide in which of the two categories (each represented by two terms) a target stimulus fit better. Subjects solving schematic-picture items were told that four binary attributes – hat color (white, black), vest pattern (striped, polka-dotted), handgear (umbrella, briefcase), and footwear (boots, shoes) – were relevant to item solution. (From "Unities in inductive reasoning," by Robert J. Sternberg and Michael K. Gardner, 1983, *Journal of Experimental Psychology: General*, *112*, pp. 96–98. Copyright 1983 by the American Psychological Association. Reprinted by permission of the publisher.)

to model the full set of data points (with each group–mean item latency serving as a data point) for the nine tasks. Again, mathematical modeling was accomplished by linear multiple regression.

Internal validation. Mean response times across the nine tasks ranged from 2.92 to 5.87 seconds, with a median of 4.50 seconds. There was only a weak effect of type of reasoning task, but in terms of content, geometric items were clearly more difficult than the other two kinds of items. Error rates ranged from .002 to .055, with a median of .028 across the nine tasks.

Task latencies were highly intercorrelated. Averaged over contents, these intercorrelations were .97 between analogies and series completions, .97 between analogies and classifications, and .96 between series completions and classifications. Intercorrelations were also computed across tasks between correspondent parameters (e.g., "encoding" in analogies and "encoding" in series completions) and between noncorrespondent parameters (e.g., "encoding" in analogies and "response" in series completions). Collapsed over contents (and thus comparing tasks), the mean correlation for corresponding component scores was .32 and the mean for noncorresponding component scores was .24. Collapsed over tasks (and thus comparing contents), the mean correlation for corresponding component scores was .40 and the mean for noncorresponding component scores was .24. No significance test is appropriate for comparing pairs of mean correlations, but the results suggest at least some convergent and discriminant validity for the hypotheses regarding which components do and do not correspond across tasks.

Values of R^2 (proportion of variance accounted for in the group-mean latency data) ranged over the nine tasks from .49 to .94, with a median of .67. The major variable affecting R^2 was content rather than reasoning task. In particular, values of R^2 were lower for geometric items. Median values of R^2 were .76 for schematic-picture items, .67 for verbal items, and .58 for geometric items. As was the case in the previous experiments, the unaccounted-for variance was statistically significant. Values of RMSD ranged across the nine tasks from .18 second to 1.90 seconds, with a median of .71 second.

These results provide good support for the proposed theory. First, overall task scores were highly intercorrelated. Second, corresponding component scores were more highly intercorrelated than noncorresponding component scores. Third, the proposed models provided good fits to the data for each task.

External validation. We were particularly interested in these experiments in examining patterns of correlations between experimental task and psychometric test scores. Correlations for global task scores with averaged reasoning tests ranged from -.47 to -.72, with a median of -.64; correlations with the perceptual–motor speed tests, however, ranged only from .16 down to -.13, with a median of .00. The overall correlations thus demonstrated both convergent validity (the task scores correlated with reasoning test scores, as predicted) and discriminant validity (the task scores did not correlate with perceptual–motor test scores, as predicted). The correlational patterns for the component scores were also promising. A combined inference–mapping–application parameter (with the combination having been computed to increase reliability of the estimate) correlated with the combined reasoning score -.70 for analogies, -.50 for series completions, and -.64 for classifications (in each case, collapsed across the three types of contents). The comparison parameter also correlated significantly and substantially with psychometrically measured reasoning, with correlations of -.61, -.66, and -.67 for analogies, series completions, and classifications (collapsed over contents) respectively. The encoding and justification parameters showed mixed patterns of correlations (some statistically significant, others not). The response parameter did not correlate significantly with reasoning in any case: These correlations were -.39, -.01, and -.25 for analogies, series completions, and classifications, respectively. No parameters correlated significantly with the psychometric perceptual–motor speed scores.

These patterns of correlations were theoretically important for two reasons. First, they showed the desired pattern of convergent–discriminant validation with psychometrically measured reasoning and perceptual–motor speed: Substantial correlations were obtained with the former but not with the latter. Second, and even more importantly in view of the results of the earlier analogy experiments, convergent and discriminant validations were demonstrated in the particular pattern of correlations between the task parameters and psychometrically measured reasoning: The reasoning parameters showed substantial correlations with psychometrically measured reasoning, but the response parameter did not. The use of highly reliable parameters and psychometric test scores, and the use of a wide range of item difficulties, seemed to have paid off.

In a separate experiment, we tested the models of reasoning processes for analogies, series completions, and classification problems on items that used animal-name terms. Thirty-six college-age adults from the New Haven area each received 30 animal-name analogies, 30 animal-name series completions, and 30 animal-name classifications. Each item was presented in forced-choice format. Subjects were tested tachistoscopically on the animal-name items and via pencil and paper on the psychometric items (Sternberg & Gardner, 1983, Experiment 2). Although subjects received psychometric ability tests in this experiment, reliabilities of individual subject scores in this experiment were insufficient to permit external validation of task scores.

Mean solution latencies for analogies, series completions, and classifications were 8.51 seconds, 7.08 seconds, and 6.65 seconds, respectively. Corresponding respective error rates were .23, .26, and .26, quite a bit higher than in the previous experiments discussed earlier. Intercorrelations of latencies across tasks were high: .85 between analogies and series completions, .86 between analogies and classifications, and .88 between series completions and classifications. This suggests that it was indeed plausible to believe that a single model or very similar models accounted for performance in all three tasks.

The proposed models of information processing (as described earlier, with minor modifications to adjust for differences in item content and format) were fit to response latencies for the three kinds of items. Statistically reliable parameter estimates could be obtained for encoding, comparison, justification, and response. Only the justification parameter differed significantly in value across tasks. Values of R^2 for the analogies, series completions, and classifications were .77, .67, and .61 respectively. Corresponding respective values of RMSD were 1.10, .92, and 1.09 seconds. The task models – which employed Euclidean distances over three dimensions of size, ferocity, and humanness – were compared to alternative models each based only on a single one of these dimensions. The Euclidean models provided superior fits in every case. In every case, however, the unaccounted-for variance was statistically reliable.

These results provide further support for the notion of cross-task consistency in information processing. First, task latencies were highly intercorrelated. Second, only one of four corresponding parameter estimates differed significantly across tasks. Third, the proposed task models provided good fits to the data in each of the three tasks. Thus, the data further supported the notion of a single set of information-processing components underlying performance on each of the three tasks that were investigated.

Extension of theory to children's performance. The proposed information-processing theory seemed to provide a good account of adults' inductive reasoning performance. In a set of further experiments, my collaborators and I sought to test the theory developmentally (Sternberg & Nigro, 1980; Sternberg & Rifkin, 1979).

The theory to be tested was essentially the same as that described previously, with various alternative models pitted against each other that differed in which performance components were exhaustive (executed the maximum number of times possible) and which were self-terminating (executed the minimum number of times possible). Sequential information processing and an attribute–value representation for information were again assumed. An extension of interest was the introduction of a word association component into the theory for verbal analogies. Some children have been found to rely on word association in the solution of analogies (Achenbach, 1970). They look for associative rather than analogical relations among terms. For example, in the analogy TREE : ANIMATE :: PENCIL : (a) INANIMATE, (b) PAPER, the answer PAPER shows the greater associative relationship, although it is the poorer analogical completion. The association component seemed necessary to take account of a possible associative strategy in the solution of analogies by children.

Children ranging in educational level from grade 2 to college received either one of two kinds of schematic-picture analogies or verbal analogies. The primary dependent variable was again response time, and independent variables were formed by various manipulations of item difficulty designed to separate parameters of the information-processing theory. Schematic-picture analogies were presented in paper-and-pencil format; verbal analogies were presented tachistoscopically.

Mean response times for the schematic-picture analogies (Sternberg & Rifkin, 1979, Experiment 2) were 7.0, 5.7, 5.1, and 4.7 seconds for grades 2, 4, 6, and college students, respectively. Corresponding error rates were .15, .10, .07, and .02. For the verbal analogies (Sternberg & Nigro, 1980), mean response times were 7.6, 5.9, 4.6, and 3.7 seconds for grades 3, 6, 9, and college, respectively. Corresponding error rates were .30, .29, .22, and .09. Fits of theory to data (R^2) for the schematic-picture analogies ranged from .80 to .89 across the four grade levels, with a median of .84; for the verbal analogies, values of R^2 ranged from .72 to .85 across grade levels, with a median of .78. The proposed theory thus did a reasonable job of accounting for the latency data, although the unexplained variance was statistically significant.

In these experiments, the most interesting data were qualitative data illustrating the functioning of metacomponents. Consider a few of the main findings.

First, selection of lower-order performance components varied across age levels. In the schematic-picture analogies, the mapping component was apparently used by fourth-graders, sixth-graders, and college students, but not by second-graders. This finding makes sense developmentally: Mapping requires the recognition of a second-order relation between relations, not just a first-order relation between objects. One might therefore expect its use to develop later and for it to be either unavailable or inaccessible to young children. Indeed, Piaget's (1972) theory of the development of intelligence states that recognition of second-order relations does not occur until the "formal-operational" period, which usually begins around the age of 11 or 12. Of course, it is quite possible that a mapping component might be elicited in some task other than analogies. The present data do not address this issue.

We also found differential component selection across age levels in the verbal analogies. In particular, younger children tended to rely more heavily upon word association (a nonlogical component) and less heavily upon inference (a logical component). Older children showed the reverse pattern. By grade 9, there was little or no use of word association at all. In sum, the metacomponent for performance component selection seems to have played an important role in intellectual development in this task, resulting in the use of different performance components at different age levels.

Second, selection of a strategy for combining performance components also varied across age levels. The critical difference, shown by subjects in solving both the schematic-picture and the verbal analogies, was that older children tended to be more nearly exhaustive in their information processing than were younger children. In other words, the older the child, the more nearly completely he or she was apt to process the information contained in the problem. This tendency toward more exhaustive information processing, which has been found in other tasks as well (see Brown & DeLoache, 1978), had an important consequence in the analogies tasks. A consistent finding in this (and other) research is that error rates tend to decrease with age. Mathematical modeling of error rates reveals that errors in analogy solution are due almost entirely to premature termination, that is, incomplete information processing (Sternberg, 1977b). The set of results taken together strongly suggests that one source of the observed decline in error rates with age is the increased use of more nearly complete information processing. From an alternative point of view, one might view children as becoming more reflective and less impulsive in their cognitive style as they grow older (see Baron, 1982). In sum, the metacomponent of strategy selection appears to play an important role in intellectual development.

Third, children of different ages represented information about the schematic-picture analogies in different ways. In particular, the second-graders appear to have encoded the attributes of the schematic pictures separably, that is, attribute by attribute. The older children seem to have achieved a more integral or unitary encoding of the pictures (see Garner, 1974). This difference has important processing consequences, because separable encoding of stimulus attributes tends to require more memory storage capacity per unit of information than does integral encoding. As a result, the second-graders are probably obliged to seek a strategy that does not overtax the storage capacities of their working memories. In analogy solution, more self-terminating strategies, which are what these younger children in fact use, tend to place lesser requirements on memory at the cost of increased errors in information processing. This effect of mental representation upon strategy shows, I believe, the importance of considering representation and strategy in conjunction. Neither can be well understood independently of the other.

In short, the metacomponent of selection of a mental representation for information is important to an understanding of intellectual development.

Fourth and finally, children of different ages differ in their allocations of processing resources. The difference can be seen most clearly in the tradeoff between encoding time and time to operate upon information already encoded. Whereas performance components other than encoding decrease monotonically in duration with increasing age, encoding first shows a decrease in latency and then a subsequent increase (Sternberg & Rifkin, 1979). The initial decrease can presumably be attributed to straightforward intellectual development: Second-graders have not yet acquired full capacity to encode the analogy terms. By fourth grade, they have acquired this capacity. At this point, encoding times start to increase as the children realize that more careful and complete encoding of the terms of a given problem will facilitate operations upon these encodings, just as more careful cataloging of books in a library, after an initial time investment for the cataloging, will facilitate lending and borrowing of the books. This finding regarding encoding of analogy terms can be seen in other domains as well. Larkin, McDermott, Simon, and Simon (1980), for example, have found that expert solvers of physics problems spend relatively more time than novices encoding the terms of a given physics problem but relatively less time actually operating upon these encodings. In short, the metacomponent of allocation of processing resources appears to play an important role in intellectual development.

Testing the theory via componential training. The experiments described previously have focused upon the issue of what subjects do, but not upon the issue of why subjects do it. Why do people choose particular strategies, and how does strategy choice interact with task variables such as item content and people's knowledge about the strategies they select? We addressed these questions in the context of a study involving training of strategies for analogical reasoning (Sternberg & Ketron, 1982).

Some subjects were trained to use one of three different strategies that previous research had shown differed widely in terms of their frequency of spontaneous usage among untrained subjects; other subjects were not trained and were told to use a strategy of their own choice. Training was conducted and performance measured either with analogies having integral stimulus attributes or with analogies having separable stimulus attributes.

Untrained subjects were told simply to solve the analogies in "whatever way you think is best." Trained subjects were told to solve the analogies, of the form $A:B::C:(D_1, D_2)$, in a specific way. The specific way differed in whether all attribute value changes or just some attribute value changes were to be inferred from A to B (exhaustive versus self-terminating inference of relations) and in whether all attribute value changes or just some attribute value changes were to be applied from C to each of D_1 and D_2 (exhaustive versus self-terminating application of relations). In a fully exhaustive group, subjects were told to infer and to apply all possible relations. In a mixture-strategy group, subjects were told to infer all possible relations but to apply only the minimum possible number of relations. In a self-terminating group, subjects were told to infer and apply only the minimum possible number of relations. (Exact instructions are given in Sternberg & Ketron, 1982.) Previous research had shown that the fully exhaustive model was almost never spontaneously chosen, whereas the other two models were spontaneously chosen with roughly equal frequency.

Mean solution latencies for the integral stimuli were 7.97 seconds for the fully exhaustive group, 4.89 seconds for the mixture-strategy group, 3.00 seconds for the self-terminating group, and 2.75 seconds for the untrained group. Mean solution latencies for the separable stimuli were 7.20 seconds for the fully exhaustive group, 4.66 seconds for the mixture-strategy group, 3.06 seconds for the self-terminating group, and 2.84 seconds for the untrained group. Higher error rates were associated with higher latencies. The effect of strategy training on the latencies was significant, although the effect of content was not. The interaction was also nonsignificant. Further analysis revealed that the mean latency for the self-terminating group did not differ from the mean latency for the untrained group but that the latencies of the exhaustive and mixture groups did differ significantly from that for the untrained group. These data weakly suggest that subjects spontaneously and optimally use the fully self-terminating strategy. When they are trained in either of the other strategies, their performance is impeded and their latencies and error rates increase.

Correlations were computed between response latencies in the various conditions. Of greatest interest were the correlations of the trained conditions with the untrained condition. The correlations with the untrained group were, for integral stimuli, .59 for the exhaustive group, .85 for the mixture group, and .95 for the self-terminating group; for the separable stimuli, the correlations were .74 for the exhaustive group, .96 for the mixture group, and .99 for the self-terminating group. These results, like the means, suggest that subjects spontaneously use the self-terminating strategy.

Alternative models of analogical reasoning were fit to the latency data for each group. The goal of this analysis was to confirm whether subjects were doing what they were trained to do or, if not, to determine what they were in fact doing. The results can be summarized quite simply. Subjects in the integral-stimulus conditions did what they were told: The best-fitting mathematical model was that corresponding to the model that had been trained. But subjects in the separable-stimulus conditions did not do what they were told: The best-fitting mathematical model was always the fully self-terminating one. These results suggested an interaction between strategy options and item content: Subjects could adjust their strategies for the integral stimuli but not for the separable stimuli. Interestingly, earlier developmental results (Sternberg & Rifkin, 1979) had also found an interaction with stimulus content: Subjects became increasingly exhaustive in strategy over age with analogies involving integral stimuli (Experiment 2) but were fully self-terminating at all ages with analogies involving separable stimuli (Experiment 1). For reasons that are still unknown, then, separable attributes seem to resist strategy flexibility, whereas integral ones do not.

These results told us something about what subjects did but not about why they did it. After solving the analogies, subjects received a questionnaire that asked them to rate the strategy they used in terms of a number of attributes. The questionnaire results showed that the fully self-terminating strategy was viewed as faster, less difficult to use, less difficult to maintain, and better overall than were the other strategies. In the separable-attributes condition, the fully self-terminating strategy was also seen as requiring less demand on memory capacity than was required by the alternative strategies. An overall analysis of the questionnaire results clearly indicated that the fully self-terminating strategy was viewed as most expeditious and the full exhaustive strategy as least expeditious. Subjects thus could give us a pretty good idea of why they preferred self-terminating over exhaustive processing in these schematic-picture analogies.

An interesting sidelight to these data is that subjects in each of the two content conditions were equally likely to say that they used the strategy that they had been trained to use. What this means is that subjects were unaware of the difference in optionality between the two kinds of content. Subjects in the separable-content condition for the most part fully believed they were doing what they had been instructed to do, even though converging sources of direct data suggested that they were not in fact doing so.

In addition to the tachistoscopically administered analogies, subjects received a psychometric test of abstract reasoning ability. Scores on this test were correlated with subjects' solution latencies. It turned out that significant correlations obtained only for the two groups that used the preferred strategy – the untrained and self-terminating groups. For these subjects, the correlations between latencies and psychometric test scores were slightly over -.6 in the self-terminating group and slightly over -.4 in the untrained group. But training subjects to use either of the other two strategies (mixture or exhaustive) reduced the correlation with reasoning to statistical nonsignificance.

In sum, the spontaneous selection of the fully self-terminating strategy by untrained subjects as the preferred model for schematic-picture analogy solution makes sense in terms of overall efficacy and efficiency of the strategy. It appears to be the strategy that can be executed most rapidly (perhaps because it maximizes the number of self-terminating component processes); it results in error rates no higher than the other strategies; and it is the strategy perceived by subjects to be fastest, easiest to use, easiest to maintain, requiring the least memory load, and best overall. From a metacomponential point of view, then, subjects' strategy selections make good sense.

Tests of the theory of response choice

Michael Gardner and I sought to test our theory of response choice in inductive reasoning through the use of animal-name analogies, series completions, and classifications (Sternberg & Gardner, 1983, Experiment 1). Thirty college-age adults received 30 of each type of problem. Their task was to rank-order the 4 response options of each item from best (1) to worst (4).

Problems of all three types were composed of mammal names from the set multidimensionally scaled by Henley (1969). Analogies were taken from Experiment 1 of Rumelhart and Abrahamson's (1973) study. All 30 analogy problems were of the form $A:B::C:(D_1,D_2,D_3,D_4)$ – for example, TIGER : CHIMPANZEE :: WOLF : (a. RACCOON, b. CAMEL, c. MONKEY, d. LEOPARD). Series completions were of the form $A:B:(C_1 C_2,C_3,C_4)$ – for example, SQUIRREL : CHIPMUNK : (a. RACCOON, b. HORSE, c. DOG, d. CAMEL). Classification problems were of the form $A, B, C, (D_1, D_2, D_3, D_4)$ – for example, ZEBRA, GIRAFFE, GOAT, (a. DOG, b. COW, c. MOUSE, d. DEER). Details of item construction can be found in Sternberg & Gardner (1983).

The main dependent variable was proportion of subjects choosing each possible response as first, second, third, and fourth best. The independent variable used to predict these proportions was distance of each option from the ideal point. One parameter, α, was estimated for the predicted negative exponential function. All subjects received all items in counterbalanced order.

The main results were these:

First, the patterns of response choices for the 16 cells in the analogies data (4 possible answer options $\times$ 4 possible ranks for each option) closely replicated those in the 16 cells of Rumelhart and Abrahamson's data, $r = .99+$, RMSD = .02.

Second, the patterns of response choices across the three tasks in the present experiment were highly similar: for analogies and series completions, $r = .99$, RMSD = .03; for analogies and classifications, $r = .97$, RMSD = .05; for series completions and classifications, $r = .98$, RMSD = .04.

Third, the value of α was estimated as 2.52 for the analogies, 2.56 for the series completions, and 2.98 for the classifications. Although the difference among the three values was statistically significant, the difference was due to the somewhat discrepant value of α for the classifications task, where items were constructed in a way that diverged somewhat from the way items in the other two tasks were constructed. Moreover, the value of α for the classifications was quite close to Rumelhart and Abrahamson's analogy value of 2.91.

Fourth, the fit of the exponential model to the data from each type of inductive reasoning task was excellent. For analogies, $R^2 = .94$, RMSD = .05; for series completions, $R^2 = .96$, RMSD = .04; for classifications, $R^2 = .98$, RMSD = .03. Alternative models were also fit that employed only single dimensions (size, ferocity, or humanness) rather than overall Euclidean distance in distance computations. The alternative models provided worse prediction than the full Euclidean model in every case. However, residuals of predicted from observed values were statistically significant for each task.

To summarize, these results provided further support for the notion of commonalities in inductive reasoning across tasks. In particular, subjects seem to use very similar or identical means for selecting response choices in each of the analogies, series completions, and classifications tasks. The probability of selecting a given option as best is an exponentially decreasing function of its distance from the ideal point, and the algorithm appears to be iterated in successive response choices.

Higher-order inductive reasoning

Theory. In the preceding discussion, inductions involving mapping utilized mapping of *second-order* relations, that is, relations between relations. It is possible, however, to conceive of *third-order* relations between second-order relations. Such relations might even be construed as providing the basis for understanding intellectual development in post–formal-operational thought (Sternberg, 1984b). The notion would thus be that whereas the formal reasoning period postulated by Piaget (1972) is differentiated from the concrete-operational period by the development of a person's ability to perceive second-order relations, a post–formal-operational period could be differentiated from the formal-operational period by the development of a person's ability to perceive third-order relations (i.e., relations between second-order relations).

Consider a third-order analogy of the form, $(A_1 : B_1 :: C_1 : D_1) :: (A_2 : B_2 :: C_2 : D_2)$, such as (BENCH : JUDGE :: PULPIT : MINISTER) :: (HEAD : HAIR :: LAWN : GRASS). The subject's task is to evaluate the degree of (higher-order) analogy between the two analogies. In other words, the subject must rate how related the two analogies are. In this task, as in the standard second-order analogy task, there are no "right" or "wrong" answers: There never are right or wrong answers, strictly speaking, in inductive tasks. But whereas there is a set of generally accepted procedures for evaluating the goodness of a second-order analogy (how close is the C–D relation to the A–B one?), there is not, to my knowledge, a set of generally accepted procedures for evaluating the goodness of a third-order analogy. Hence, in proposing a set of procedures subjects might use in making such an evaluation, one must start from intuitions, which can then be tested empirically. As was the case for second-order analogies, two kinds of issues need to be faced, issues of representation and issues of processing.

With respect to representation, it is proposed that third-order analogies, like those of the second order, can be represented in a multidimensional semantic (or other conceptual) space. But whereas the representation of a second-order analogy is via a parallelogram, the representation of a third-order analogy is via a parallelepiped, which is a parallelogram extended to a third dimension (see Figure 5.7). Each planar surface of the parallelepiped represents an embedded analogy, with the $(A_1B_1C_1D_1)$ and $(A_2B_2C_2D_2)$ surfaces forming the main analogies of interest.

With respect to processing, it is proposed that each of the two main analogies constituting the third-order analogy are solved in essentially the same way as individual second-order analogies that occur in isolation. However, the evaluation of a third-order analogy requires the consideration of additional relations that are not considered (or relevant) in the evaluation of a second-order analogy. Consideration of these relations must follow solution of each of the two second-order analogies that constitutes the third-order analogy. Four relations are proposed to form "valid" bases for evaluation, and a fifth is proposed to form an "invalid" basis that is nevertheless sometimes used:

1. *Second-order relatedness of corresponding* inferences *across (second-order) analogies.* This relation is a function of the closeness of the second-order relations between $A_1–B_1$, on the one hand, and $A_2–B_2$, on the other. To the extent that these relations do not correspond, the three-dimensional object representing the third-order analogy will depart from being a parallelepiped. Either one of the AB bases will be longer than the other, or the two AB bases will depart from parallelism with each other. In the sample third-order analogy, BENCH : JUDGE is compared with HEAD : HAIR, much as these relations would be compared if they formed the two halves of a regular analogy. The more correspondent the two relations are, in terms of both the lengths and the directions of their correspondent vectors in semantic space, the more they contribute toward the formation of an acceptable higher-order analogy.

2. *Second-order relatedness of corresponding* mappings *across (second-order) analogies.* This relation is a function of the closeness of the second-

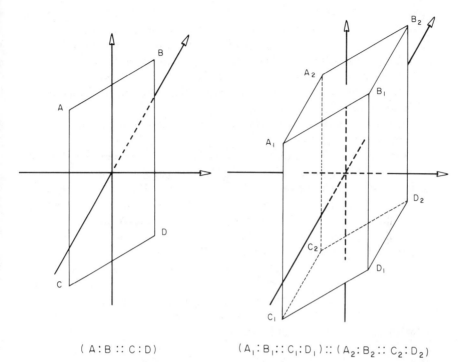

(A : B :: C : D) $(A_1 : B_1 :: C_1 : D_1) :: (A_2 : B_2 :: C_2 : D_2)$

Figure 5.7. Representations of second-order and third-order analogies in semantic space. (From "The development of higher-order reasoning in adolescence," by Robert J. Sternberg and Cathryn J. Downing, 1982, *Child Development, 53*, pp. 211–212. Copyright 1982 by the Society for Research in Child Development. Reprinted by permission of the publisher.)

order relations between $A_1 - C_1$, on the one hand, and $A_2 - C_2$, on the other. To the extent that these relations do not correspond, the three-dimensional object representing the third-order analogy will depart from being a parallelepiped. Either one of the AC bases will be longer than the other, or the two AC bases will depart from parallelism with each other. In the sample third-order analogy, BENCH : PULPIT is compared with HEAD : LAWN. The more correspondent the two relations are, in terms of both the lengths and the directions of their correspondent vectors in semantic space, the more they contribute toward the formation of an acceptable third-order analogy.

3. *Second-order relatedness of corresponding* applications *across (second-order) analogies.* This relation is a function of the closeness of the second-order relations between $C_1 - D_1$, on the one hand, and $C_2 - D_2$, on the other. To the extent that these relations do not correspond, the three-dimensional

object representing the third-order analogy will depart from being a parallelepiped. Either one of the CD bases will be longer than the other, or the two CD bases will depart from parallelism with each other. In the sample higher-order analogy, PULPIT : MINISTER is compared with LAWN : GRASS, much as these relations would be compared if they had formed the two halves of a second-order analogy. The more correspondent the two relations are, in terms of both lengths and the directions of their correspondent vectors in semantic space, the more they contribute toward the formation of an acceptable third-order analogy.

4. *Second-order relatedness of corresponding* inferences and applications *across (second-order) analogies.* This relation is a function of the closeness of the second-order relations between $A_1 - B_1$ and $C_2 - D_2$ and between $A_2 - B_2$ and $C_1 - D_1$. To the extent that these relations do not correspond, the three-dimensional object representing the third-order analogy will depart from being a parallelepiped. There will be a discrepancy in the lengths or directions of the two corresponding sets of AB and CD vectors. In the sample third-order analogy, BENCH : JUDGE is compared with LAWN : GRASS, and HEAD : HAIR is compared with PULPIT : MINISTER. The more correspondent the two relations are, in terms of both the lengths and directions of their correspondent vectors in semantic space, the more they contribute toward the formation of an acceptable third-order analogy.

The last relation that is sometimes used but that is irrelevant to the goodness of the structure of the parallelepiped is basically associative in nature:

5. *First-order* associative relatedness *of corresponding terms across (second-order) analogies.* This relation is a function of the closeness of associations between A_1 and A_2, B_1 and B_2, C_1 and C_2, and D_1 and D_2. Reference to these relations as "associative" underscores the belief that use of this variable in the evaluation is essentially "regressive": The closeness of corresponding terms across second-order analogies affects the volume of the parallelepiped but does not affect the goodness of the figure as a parallelepiped. Use of this criterion could possibly lead to a rather unfavorable evaluation of the sample third-order analogy, in that none of BENCH and HEAD, JUDGE and HAIR, PULPIT and LAWN, or MINISTER and GRASS is a highly related pair of words. According to this associative criterion, a better third-order analogy than the sample one would be (BENCH : JUDGE :: PULPIT : MINISTER) :: (CHAIR : COURTROOM :: PEW : CHURCH), because BENCH and CHAIR, JUDGE and COURTROOM, PULPIT and PEW, and MINISTER and CHURCH are all highly related pairs of words. Yet almost anyone would agree that the third-order analogy between these two second-order analogies is not as good as that between the two second-order analogies constituting the third-order analogy (BENCH : JUDGE :: PULPIT : MINISTER) :: (HEAD : HAIR :: LAWN : GRASS). The terms of the newly introduced third-order analogy are more highly associa-

tively related across the two second-order analogies, but the degree of analogical correspondence between the two second-order analogies is quite a bit worse.

There are certain parallels in the evaluation of second- and third-order analogies that are instructive to note. First, the third-order analogy requires a second-order inference in addition to the first-order inference required for second-order analogies. Second, the third-order analogy requires a second-order mapping in addition to the second-order mapping required for second-order analogies. Third, the third-order analogy requires a second-order application in addition to the first-order application required for second-order analogies. Finally, associative relations can play a role in the solution of third-order analogies, just as they can in the solution of second-order analogies; in each case, the associative relation is actually irrelevant to the true goodness of the analogy. These various informational inputs are combined to form a basis for the third-order analogical mapping between the two analogies that is used to rate the goodness of the third-order analogy.

The representational and process parallels between second-order and third-order analogies suggest at least the possibility that solution of the two kinds of analogies may undergo parallel courses of development, but at different time periods in the cognitive-developmental course. In particular, one might hypothesize that at least some of the processing changes in second-order analogical reasoning one observes in the transition from "concrete"- to "formal"-operational reasoning might be paralleled by processing changes in third-order analogical reasoning in a possible transition from formal- to post–formal-operational reasoning (see also Case, 1978). Consider some of the main developmental findings for the concrete- to formal-operational transition and possible parallels in a formal- to post–formal-operational transition:

1. Children tend to decrease their use of first-order associative relations with increasing age (see, e.g., Sternberg & Nigro, 1980). One might therefore expect decreased use of associative relations in third-order analogies with increasing age.
2. Children show a compensating increase in their use of first-order inference with increasing age (Sternberg & Nigro, 1980). One might therefore expect, with increasing age of subjects, increased use of second-order inference in third-order analogies.
3. Children seem to acquire the ability to map in second-order analogies with the onset of formal operations. One might therefore expect adolescents to acquire the ability to map in third-order analogies with the onset of post-formal operations.

In essence, then, the thrust of the predictions is that there will be, in the onset of post–formal operations, a recapitulation of developmental trends that appeared in the onset of formal operations. The recapitulation, however, will be at an order of analysis one level higher than was made possible at the onset of formal operations.

Data. Third-order analogies comprised the basis of an experiment on higher-order analogical reasoning (Sternberg & Downing, 1982). Subjects received 72 different items, which they were asked to rate on a scale from 1 (low) to 9 (high) indicating how closely related two second-order analogies were to each other, that is, how "analogous" they were. Examples of third-order analogies are (a) (SUN : DAY :: MOON : NIGHT) :: (SUNNY : SUMMER :: SNOWY : WINTER); (b) (SAND : BEACH :: STAR : GALAXY) :: (WATER : OCEAN :: AIR : SKY); and (c) (LETTER : MAILMAN :: NEWSPAPER : PAPERBOY) :: (EMPTY BOTTLES : MILKMAN :: GARBAGE : GARBAGE MAN). Subjects solving these third-order analogies were 20 eighth-graders, 20 eleventh-graders, and 20 college freshmen.

Performance on the third-order analogies was modeled by using ratings of third-order analogy goodness as the dependent variable and various ratings of distances between terms and relations as independent variables. The ratings were chosen so as to provide the appropriate measures of the psychological constructs of interest. For example, the independent variable for estimating the effect of second-order inference (relation 1 for third-order analogies) was the distance between the (A, B) relation for the first analogy in the third-order pair and the (A, B) relation for the second analogy in the third-order pair; the independent variable for estimating the effect of first-order associative relatedness (relation 5 for third-order analogies) was (X_1, X_2), where X_1 is a term of the first analogy in the third-order pair and X_2 a term of the second analogy in the third-order pair. In the first example in the preceding paragraph, SUN would be paired with SUNNY and rated for its degree of semantic relatedness. Subjects supplying these ratings were 140 students (in grades 8 through 11) who were nonoverlapping with the subjects providing the ratings of goodness of higher-order analogies.

The model of third-order analogical reasoning provided a very good account of the goodness ratings, accounting for 78% of the variance in the eighth-grade data, 81% of the variance in the eleventh-grade data, and 90% of the variance in the college data. All of these percentages differ significantly from zero. In contrast, a model based simply upon the basic model for *second*-order analogical reasoning (without augmentation by the higher-order variables) accounted for only trivial and nonsignificant percentages of variance in the data.

Of greatest importance, all three of our hypotheses were confirmed. Consider each hypothesis in turn:

1. *Associative relatedness:* First-order associative relatedness showed a decreasing standardized regression (beta) weight across the three grade

levels: .23, .10, and .09 for grade 8, grade 11, and college, respectively. Only the weight for grade 8 was statistically significant. Thus, adolescents did appear to show a declining use of associative relatedness with increasing age.

2. *Inference:* In contrast, second-order inference showed an increasing standardized regression weight across the three grade levels: .68, .81, and .82 for grade 8, grade 11, and college, respectively. All three weights were significant, indicating that second-order inference played at least some role in reasoning at each age level, although a diminished role at the grade 8 level relative to grade 11 and college.

3. *Mapping:* The standardized weight for second-order mapping across higher-order analogies did not show a monotonic trend across age levels: .13, .09, and .16 for grade 8, grade 11, and college, respectively. However, only the weight at the college level was significant (at the 1% level). Thus, there is at least some evidence of increased use of mapping at the oldest grade level.

In sum, there is at least some support for each of the developmental predictions, suggesting the possibility that patterns of development for third-order analogical reasoning recapitulate earlier patterns of development for second-order analogical reasoning. Moreover, the fact that a preliminary index of quality of performance on the third-order analogies correlated at the level of .52 with scores on Miller Analogies Test items for the college students (the only students for whom the Miller item scores were available) further suggests the likelihood that there are significant parallels (ontogenetic, structural, or otherwise) between the third-order analogies used in this study and the second-order analogies used in many previous studies and ability tests. Although the results of the experiment are not conclusive, they suggest the fruitfulness of further pursuing notions regarding third-order reasoning with analogies and possibly other types of induction problems as well.

One might wonder whether the theory of third-order reasoning applies beyond testlike items. I believe it does. Consider, for example, the third-order analogy (MACHINE LANGUAGE : HARDWARE :: PROGRAMMING LANGUAGE : SOFTWARE) :: (LANGUAGE OF THE BRAIN : NEURAL CONNECTIONS :: ORDINARY LANGUAGE : COGNITIVE STRUCTURES). This implicit analogy seems to underlie much of the current debate regarding the usefulness of computer programs as bases for understanding linguistic and other forms of information processing. Making the implicit analogy explicit facilitates understanding of the tacit assumptions underlying the debate, at least as put forward by researchers in artificial intelligence. Or consider the third-order analogy (U.S. ADVISERS : EL SALVADOREAN GOVERNMENT FORCES :: COMMUNIST ADVISERS : EL SALVADOREAN REBEL FORCES) :: (U.S. ADVISERS : SOUTH VIETNAMESE GOVERNMENT FORCES :: COMMUNIST FORCES : SOUTH VIETNAMESE REBEL FORCES). The validity (or invalidity) of this third-order analogy may be seen as underlying recent debates regarding the advisability of U.S. intervention in the El Salvadorean conflict. Those who accept the third-order analogy as valid are unlikely to support U.S. intervention through military advisers. Again, clarifying the implicit analogy underlying the conflict helps one understand just what the conflict (in this case, over the intervention in El Salvador) is about.

The theory of third-order analogical reasoning has actually been extended to series completion and classification problems (Sternberg, 1984b), but this augmented theory is not presented here due to considerations of space. At present, however, it seems safe to conclude that analogies of the third order do represent a psychologically interesting basis for assessing reasoning at levels beyond that of formal operations. Indeed, they provide a means for making analogies difficult that bypasses the usual route of very difficult or trivial vocabulary as possible bases for item difficulty.

Theory of induction for metaphors

In the previously described research, the theory of induction was applied to the three kinds of items that are probably most frequently used to measure fluid intelligence. The demonstrated commonalities in information processing and response choice have suggested that testlike induction, at least, can be understood in terms of a unified theory of induction. But one might well question whether the theory, or aspects of it, can be extended to stimuli that are less testlike and perhaps less highly formal in their stimulus properties. My collaborators and I have shown that the theory can be so extended in our research on metaphorical understanding and appreciation (Sternberg & Nigro, 1983; Sternberg, Tourangeau, & Nigro, 1979; Tourangeau & Sternberg, 1981, 1982). Our work has been divided into two subprograms, one seeking to test a theory of information processing, the other seeking to test a theory of mental representation.

Theory of metaphorical understanding and appreciation

In comprehending and appreciating a metaphor, we conceive of something new in terms of something old. In the metaphor "Man is a wolf," for example, the new term, or *tenor* of the metaphor, *man*, is seen in terms of the old term, or *vehicle* of the metaphor, *wolf*. The basis for the comparison between man and wolf, or *ground* of the metaphor, is left implicit.

Because the conception of something new in terms of something old forms the basis for analogical thinking as well as for metaphorical thinking, and because analogical thinking has generally been thought to comprise a broader range of mental phenomena than has metaphorical thinking, some students of metaphor have been inclined to view metaphorical understanding as a form of analogical thinking (e.g., Aristotle, 1927; Billow, 1977; Gentner, 1977, 1983; Miller, 1979). According to this view, the metaphor "Man is a wolf" can be viewed as an implicit analogy in which some properties of man are seen as analogous to some properties of a wolf; the metaphor "The lion is the king of beasts" can be understood as the incomplete analogy "LION : BEASTS :: KING : ?" (Miller, 1979).

Some theorists have proposed that to view metaphors as nothing more than abridged analogies is to miss the essence of metaphors. They propose that in metaphors there is an interaction between tenor and vehicle so that the resulting meaning of the metaphor involves a blending of the two terms (Black, 1962; Richards, 1936). Some recent studies by Malgady and Johnson (1976), Verbrugge and McCarrell (1977), and others have supported this view. Thus, one might theorize that metaphors are often built upon a foundation of analogy, but that they involve an interaction between terms that is either minimally present or entirely absent in the base analogies. We have proposed that this view – of metaphors as analogically based with the addition of some kind or kinds of elements of interaction – can give a good account of metaphorical comprehension and appreciation.

Theory of information processing. The proposed theory of metaphorical information processing is an augmented version of the previously presented theory of induction. Consider an analogy presented earlier as reexpressed in multiple-choice format: LION : BEASTS :: KING : (a) RULERS, (b) HUMANS. When the metaphor is presented in this form, the theory of inductive reasoning described earlier, as applied to analogies, can be directly applied to the understanding of the metaphor. The subject must *encode* the given terms, *infer* the relation of LION to BEASTS, *map* the higher-order relation that links the LION half of the metaphor to the KING half of the metaphor, *apply* the previously inferred relation as mapped to the new domain to generate an ideal answer, *compare* this answer to each of the alternatives, *justify* one of the given answers as better than the other, although possibly nonideal, and *respond*.

The theorized identity of performance components does not imply equivalence in the difficulty of the metaphor and its corresponding analogy. On the one hand, the additional verbal material contained in the metaphor increases the reading load of this presentation format; on the other hand, this additional mediating context may make the metaphor more readily comprehensible. Hence, the relative difficulties of the two presentation formats will depend upon the relative effects of increased reading load and increased mediating context.

Moreover, processing may be affected by the interaction between tenor and vehicle. In particular, more apt metaphors will tend to be those with more interactive and, we believe, more highly visually imaginable interactive terms. Increased visualizability of the interaction may also facilitate information processing.

Proportional metaphors are often presented in ways that leave at least some of the terms of the underlying analogy implicit. The "lion and king" metaphor, for example, could be presented in any of the following formats (among others), where either no terms or some terms are left implicit:

1. A lion among beasts is a king among people.
2. A lion among beasts is a king.
3. A lion is a king among people.
4. A lion is a king.
5. A lion is a king among beasts.

An important thing to notice in these various metaphorical forms is that different terms are left implicit in different forms of presentation. These different forms may differ in their comprehensibility, as well as in their aptness, as a function of the terms that are left implicit and, in the fifth form, as a function of the reordering of terms: "Beasts," the second term of the implicit analogy, is presented last. According to the present theory, the reason for these variations in comprehensibility and information-processing difficulty would be found in the fact that these metaphorical forms require not only *comprehension* of the explicit terms and of the relations that can be formed between these terms, but also the *generation* of terms that are left implicit and the comprehension of relations between these pairs of terms (as well as between implicit and explicit terms). Miller (1979) seems to take a similar view.

Theory of mental representation. The account presented above emphasizes real-time processing of metaphorical information. Consider now the issue of how metaphorical information is mentally represented (Sternberg, Tourangeau, & Nigro, 1979; Tourangeau & Sternberg, 1981, 1982).

Imagine an array of "local subspaces" comprising sets of terms, such as U.S. historical figures, modern world leaders, mammals, birds, fish, airplanes, land vehicles, and ships. Each local subspace represents the terms within it as points with coordinates on each of several dimensions. Each of these local subspaces might also be viewed as of roughly the same order (level of abstraction) and as of a lower order than a higher-order hyperspace that contains the lower-order subspaces as points embedded within it. Thus, the points of the higher-order hyperspace map into the lower-order subspaces and can be labeled by the names of these subspaces. This hyperspace can, in turn, be viewed as one of multiple subspaces of some still higher-order hyperspace, although such very-high-order subspaces will not be discussed here.

One needs some rule for restricting the subspaces that map into a single hyperspace and some way of establishing comparability across subspaces. Both of these goals can be accomplished by requiring all subspaces to have at least one corresponding dimension. Thus, for example, the subspaces of modern world leaders, bird names, and ships must have at least one corresponding dimension if they are to be local subspaces of the same order and of a common hyperspace.

Using the semantic-differential paradigm of Osgood, Suci, & Tannenbaum (1957), we asked subjects to rate each of 20 items within each domain on 21 scales, such as *warlike – peaceful, noble – ignoble*, and *strong – weak*, with a different group of 16 subjects supplying ratings for each of the 8 domains considered. We hoped in this way to obtain a corresponding set of dimensions for the 8 domains named above (U.S. historical figures, modern world leaders, mammals, birds, fish, airplanes, land vehicles, and ships). It seemed plausible to us that at least two such corresponding dimensions would be obtained: prestige (similar to Osgood and colleagues' "evaluative" dimension) and aggression (similar to Osgood and colleagues' "potency" or "activity" dimensions). The adjective pairs for each domain were then factor-analyzed.

Visual inspection of the results of the factor analyses supported our hypothesis: Two corresponding dimensions of prestige and aggression appeared for each domain, although the order in which the two dimensions appeared was variable across domains. In order to confirm our visual impression, statistical analyses were performed to ascertain degrees of dimensional interrelatedness. Corresponding dimensions according to the visual analysis were found to be highly statistically related as well, and noncorresponding dimensions to be only poorly statistically related.

This representational framework was used as a basis for constructing rules that would identify metaphors as more or less aesthetically pleasing. Two distances in the proposed spaces were deemed relevant: (1) "superimposed within-subspace distance" between the tenor (first term) of the metaphor and the vehicle (second term) of the metaphor and (2) "between-subspace distance" between these two terms.

Consider first the meaning of "superimposed within-subspace distance." Because at least two dimensions correspond (or, at least, are very similar) for each domain, one can imagine superimposing the dimensions of one local subspace onto the corresponding dimensions of another local subspace. Once this superimposition is accomplished it is also possible to imagine computing the superimposed within-subspace distance between two points that are actually in different subspaces. One simply computes the distance between points as though they were in the same subspace. Thus, if the coordinates of some point in one subspace were (x, y), then the superimposed within-subspace distance to some point in another subspace would be zero if that point also happened to occupy location (x, y), and would depart from zero as the Euclidean distance of that point from (x, y) increased.

An example may help clarify the concept. The superimposed within-subspace distance from *wildcat* to *hawk* is very small, because the coordinates of *hawk* in the bird subspace are very close to those of *wildcat* in the mammal subspace. The superimposed within-subspace distance from *wildcat* to *robin* is quite large, however, because the coordinates of *wildcat* and *robin* are quite disparate. Similarly, the superimposed within-subspace distance from *wildcat* to *ICBM* (intercontinental ballistic missile) is small, whereas the superimposed within-subspace distance from *wildcat* to *blimp* is large. The distance concept is further illustrated in Figure 5.8.

Consider next the meaning of "between-subspace distance." In order for the concept to have meaning, it must be possible somehow to compute the distance between a pair of subspaces. This computation is possible, in our representational formulation, because the distance between two subspaces is equal to the distance between the corresponding points within the appropriate hyperspace. Thus, if the coordinates of some local subspace in the hyperspace are (x, y), the distance from that subspace to another subspace increases as the Euclidean distance of that subspace from (x, y) increases.

Let us return to our earlier example to illustrate the concept of between-subspace distance. The between-subspace distance from *wildcat* to *hawk* is the same as that from *wildcat* to *robin*, because both *hawk* and *robin* are in the same local subspace. This distance is small, because mammal and bird names are viewed as relatively close to one another in the hyperspace. The between-subspace distances from *wildcat* to *ICBM* and *blimp* are also the same, because these latter two terms fall within the same local subspace; and this distance is relatively large, because mammal names and names of airplanes are viewed as relatively far from one another in the hyperspace. This distance concept is illustrated further in Figure 5.8.

Turning now to the theory of metaphorical aptness, we proposed that *a metaphor is aesthetically pleasing, or apt, to the extent that the superimposed within-subspace distance is small but the between-subspace distance is large.* Consider some examples of metaphors derived from the terms discussed above:

1. A wildcat is a hawk among mammals.
2. A wildcat is a robin among mammals.
3. A wildcat is an ICBM among mammals.
4. A wildcat is a blimp among mammals.

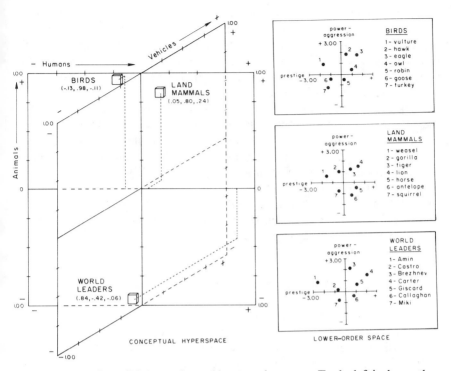

Figure 5.8. Relation of higher-order and lower-order spaces. To the left is shown the space of domains, or hyperspace. Each point in this space is itself a full space of a lower order, as shown to the right. For example, the point "Birds" in the hyperspace maps into the space of birds at the top right of the figure. (From "Aptness in metaphor," by Roger Tourangeau and Robert J. Sternberg, 1981, *Cognitive Psychology, 13*, pp. 32–33. Copyright 1981 by Academic Press, Inc. Reprinted by permission of the publisher.)

What empirical claims does the proposed theory make about each of these metaphors? According to the theory, metaphor 3 should be the metaphor of highest quality, because although *wildcat* and *ICBM* are quite close to one another in terms of superimposed within-subspace distance, they are from distant local subspaces. Metaphor 2 should be lowest in quality, because the tenor and vehicle occupy discrepant positions in their local subspaces and are from proximal subspaces. Metaphors 1 and 4 should be intermediate in quality. Because we expected superimposed within-subspace distance to carry more weight than between-subspace distance, we predicted that metaphor 1 would be perceived as more apt than metaphor 4. Thus, the ordering of metaphors in terms of aptness was, from greatest to least: 3, 1, 4, 2.

Although the theory has been applied only to items falling within semantic fields, its general principles can be applied to items outside such fields. For example, the theory predicts that Donne's famous conceit relating lovers to stiff twin compasses will be apt because the superimposed within-subspace distance, as shown by Donne, is low (i.e., lovers and stiff twin compasses can be shown to bear many similarities) but the between-subspace distance is high (i.e., lovers and stiff twin compasses are from very distant domains). At the opposite extreme, literal statements make for poor metaphors because their between-subspace distance is zero, regardless of what their superimposed within-subspace distance may be. For example, "An ICBM is an intercontinental missile" has zero superimposed within-subspace distance (which is good for metaphorical aptness), but zero between-subspace distance as well (which is bad for metaphorical aptness). Anomalous statements such as "An ICBM is a haystack" make for poor metaphors, because whatever may be their between-subspace distance, their superimposed within-subspace distance will generally be very high.

Tests of the theory of metaphorical understanding and appreciation

Information-processing theory. The proposed view of information processing led us (Sternberg & Nigro, 1983) to several predictions about metaphorical information processing. First, the information-processing components used in the understanding of metaphors, especially metaphors with relatively fewer implicit terms, should be highly overlapping with the components used in the understanding of analogies. Second, metaphors should become more comprehensible and be viewed as more apt as the number of terms of the underlying analogy that are made explicit is increased, thereby clarifying the meaning of the metaphor. Third, metaphors should become more comprehensible and be viewed as more apt as tenor – vehicle interaction is made more clear and vivid by the language in which the metaphor is presented. These hypotheses were tested in two experiments.

The first experiment investigated the first hypothesis. Base statements were presented in either metaphorical or analogical form with two forced-choice options for completion of the statements. All elements in the metaphors from the underlying analogy were made explicit. Thus, a subject might see either "Bees in a hive are a Roman mob in the (a) Coliseum, (b) streets" or "BEES : HIVE :: ROMAN MOB : (a) COLISEUM, (b) STREETS." Subjects were asked to complete the statements as quickly and as accurately as possible. Half of the 96 subjects saw the metaphorical format and half saw the analogical format. Each subject was presented with a set of 50 different test items.

Mean response latencies were 3.84 and 3.90 seconds for the metaphorical and analogical item formats, respectively. The difference between these two latencies was nonsignificant. Error rates were .06 in each condition, and these, too, obviously did not differ significantly. These mean data are thus consistent with the notion that similar or identical processing components are used in each task. The correlation between latencies (computed across item types) was .80; the correlation between error rates was not meaningful because of the very low error rates on individual item types. The correlation between latencies needs to be considered in conjunction with the internal-consistency reliabilities of the latency data, which were .90 for the metaphors and .93 for the analogies. The comparison between the task intercorrelation and the task reliabilities shows that although processing of metaphors and analogies was probably highly similar in nature, it was not identical, in that there was still some systematic variance left unaccounted for. As mentioned earlier, at least some difference would be expected, since the metaphors supplied mediating context that was absent in the analogies and may have increased tenor–vehicle interaction.

The data were mathematically modeled by predicting response latencies from the independent variables specified by the proposed theory of analogical and metaphorical reasoning. The overall fit of the model to each data set was quite good: Squared correlations (R^2) between predicted and observed latencies were .86 for the metaphors and .73 for the analogical format. RMSDs of observed from predicted values were .30 and .60 second in the metaphorical and analogical conditions, respectively. These model fits are based upon only the four strongest regression parameters of the proposed model. If all parameters allowed by the theory are entered in, the values of R^2 increase to .87 for metaphors and .83 for analogies. Clearly, the proposed model does a reasonable job of accounting for latency data, reflecting the comprehension of both the metaphors and the analogies.

A second experiment investigated the second and third hypotheses, as well as providing additional confirming evidence for the first hypothesis. In this experiment, base statements were presented in each of the five different metaphorical formats presented earlier, where the formats differed in the number and identities of the terms of the underlying analogy that were left implicit. Subjects were asked to rate either the aptness or the comprehensibility of each metaphorical statement. Half of the 48 subjects rated aptness, the other half comprehensibility, for each of the 50 metaphors of Experiment 1 presented in the five formats described earlier – e.g., (1) Bees in a hive are a Roman mob in the Coliseum; (2) Bees in a hive are a Roman mob; (3) Bees are a Roman mob in the Coliseum; (4) Bees are a Roman mob; and (5) Bees are a Roman mob in a hive.

For aptness, the effect of metaphorical form was highly significant. An examination of the pattern of ratings revealed that for forms 1–4, higher ratings were attained for metaphorical formats in which fewer terms were left implicit, as predicted. Thus, when terms are presented in the natural A – B – C – D order corresponding to the order of terms in the implicit analogy, the presentation of more terms is associated with higher aptness. But form 5, where the order of the second and third terms was reversed relative to the implicit underlying analogy ("Roman mob," in the example, precedes rather than follows "hive"), was rated as most apt. The high form 5 rating did not merely reflect its intermediate number of terms. We suggested that the form 5 metaphor was rated as most apt because the ordering of terms suggested something more than was suggested in the other metaphorical forms: In particular, it better suggested an *interaction* between tenor and vehicle than the interaction suggested by the other forms. In metaphors such as "A pear is a Buddha on a sill" or "Bees are a Roman mob in a hive" or "Tombstones are teeth in a graveyard," the tenor is more easily conceived in terms of the vehicle, and it is especially easy in many cases to create an image of tenor – vehicle interaction. One can easily imagine a Buddha transplanted to a window sill, a Roman mob scurrying mindlessly in a hive, or teeth sticking up from the ground in a graveyard. The fifth form thus provides an ordering of terms that facilitates one's understanding of tenor – vehicle interaction, and thus aptness is increased. In the other metaphorical forms, adherence to the order of terms in the underlying analogy reduces ease of perceived interaction of tenor and vehicle, and aptness is correspondingly reduced. In order to test our hypothesis that the fifth metaphorical form encouraged formation of interactive imagery more than did the second metaphorical form (which contained exactly the same terms in the standard analogical order) or than did any other form, we had a separate group of 20 subjects rate vividness of interactive imagery for each metaphor in each format. Mean ratings were highest for form 5. Most critically, the mean for form 5 was higher than for form 2, which differed only in order but not in content of terms. The same pattern of results obtained for aptness was obtained as well for comprehensibility.

We also mathematically modeled the ratings of aptness and comprehensibility on the basis of the independent variables in our theory. For the full model plus the effect of interactive imagery plus the effect of comprehensibility on aptness or the effect of aptness on comprehensibility, values of R^2 between predicted and observed data for the five respective metaphorical formats were .71, .77, .69, .78, and .71 for aptness, and .78, .80, .73, .86, and .82 for comprehensibility. These model fits were quite impressive in view of the fact that the theory was originally formulated to predict response latencies rather than ratings of aptness or of comprehensibility.

The results of the second experiment thus confirmed our second and third hypotheses, as well as providing additional confirming evidence for our first hypothesis. The componential theory of analogical reasoning seems to extend to metaphorical comprehension and aptness.

Tests of the theory of mental representation. The predictions of our "dual-distance" theory of metaphorical aptness were tested in two experiments.

In Experiment 1, the 37 subjects were asked to rate the aptness of metaphors such as "The owl is the horse among birds." Tenors and vehicles were taken from local subspaces described earlier. According to our theory, metaphorical aptness should be negatively correlated with the superimposed within-subspace distance between tenor and vehicle and positively correlated with the between-subspace distance. Both predictions were confirmed. Correlations were -.39 for superimposed within-subspace distance and .27 for between-subspace distance (both statistically significant, if small). When multiple regression was used to predict aptness from these two distances plus comprehensibility of the metaphor, the multiple correlation was .76. A fact of incidental interest is that the simple correlation of overall distance with metaphorical goodness was just -.01. This trivial correlation suggests why many previous investigations that have failed to make our distinction between the two kinds of distances have been inconclusive.

In Experiment 2, the 20 subjects were asked to rank-order the goodness of metaphorical completions in terms with the format exemplified by "A crab is a _____ among sea creatures. (1) TIGER, (2) MONGOOSE, (3) RAT, (4) HORSE." Half the items had options chosen from a single local subspace, as in the example, and half had options chosen from multiple local subspaces, for example, "A blue whale is a _____ among sea creatures. (1) KILLER WHALE, (2) GISCARD D'ESTAING, (3) SATELLITE, (4) LION." The rank-order correlation between superimposed within-subspace distance and option popularity (aptness) was -.46 for metaphors of the first kind (options from a single local subspace) and -.48 for metaphors of the second kind (options from multiple local subspaces). The correlation with between-subspace distance, which could be computed only for metaphors of the second kind, was a nonsignificant .06. An exponential model was also fit to the response-choice data, with choice proportions predicted on the basis of the two kinds of distances. The model was successful for the options of the first kind (correlation between predicted and observed values equal to .98) but not for the options of the second kind, where between- as well as superimposed within-subspace distance were manipulated.

To conclude, we have proposed theories of metaphorical information processing and representation that seem to capture major aspects of metaphorical comprehension and appreciation. The theories suggest that metaphorical processing can be related to other kinds of inductive information processing in terms of the representations and components used in metaphorical understanding, but that an additional element, that of interaction, applies uniquely to metaphorical (or possibly any figurative) format of verbal presentation.

Theory of judgment in causal inference

The accounts of induction described in the preceding sections of this chapter are all based on the componential theory presented early in the chapter. But as has been noted in the past (Pellegrino & Lyon, 1979), the components in the theory tend to be something like "black boxes." Labeling a mental act *inference*, for example, says little about the kinds of judgments that actually take place when an inference is made. The theory described here attempts to open up the black box for what many would call the most fundamental component of induction, namely, *inference*. It does so in the context of inferences about causal antecedents for observable events. Thus, the theory does not attempt to catalog all possible kinds of inferences (as do Collins, Warnock, Aiello, & Miller, 1975, for example).

Theory of causal inference

People frequently seek to infer the causal antecedent or antecedents of significant real-world events. Consider, for example, the response of the United States government to the Soviet invasion of Afghanistan. This response was predicated upon the motives U.S. government officials inferred to underlie the Soviet attack. Their response would almost certainly have been different if government policymakers had believed Soviet claims that the Soviets were merely responding to a request from the Afghan government for help in resolving domestic turmoil.

We have proposed that people use four basic kinds of evidence in evaluating the likelihood that a given event is a causal antecedent for a given consequent (Schustack & Sternberg, 1981; Sternberg & Schustack, 1980):

1. *Confirmation by joint presence of possibly causal event and outcome.* The potential cause and the given outcome tend to occur in conjunction. For example, because widespread increases in wages tend to be followed by widespread increases in prices, we tend to attribute the price increases at least in part to the increases in wages (the well-known "inflationary spiral"). This relation between the possibly causal event and the outcome event is evidence in favor of the sufficiency of the possibly causal event for the outcome; that is, if the possibly causal event occurs, so does the outcome.

2. *Confirmation by joint absence of possibly causal event and outcome.* The absence of the potential cause tends to be associated with the absence of the given outcome. For example, countries that are disarmed (or almost disarmed) tend not to start wars, so that one might reasonably conclude that

the starting of wars is at least in part attributable to the presence of armaments in a country's arsenal. This relation between the possibly causal event and the outcome event is evidence in favor of the necessity of the possibly causal event for the outcome; that is, the outcome event (here, starting wars) tends to occur only if the antecedent event is present (here, armaments in the country's arsenal).

3. *Disconfirmation by presence of possibly causal event but absence of outcome.* The presence of the potential cause tends to be associated with the absence of the given outcome. For example, the presence of large numbers of members of a given ethnic group in a country originally foreign to them does not (usually!) lead to overt action on the part of these ethnics to take over the country by force. This relation between the possibly causal event and the outcome event is evidence against the sufficiency of the possibly causal event for the outcome; that is, the occurrence of the possibly causal event does not always lead to the occurrence of the outcome. Thus, in the United States, there are large ethnic populations, but such populations have not been associated with attempts to overthrow the government.

4. *Disconfirmation by absence of possibly causal event but presence of outcome.* The absence of the potential cause tends to be associated with the presence of the given outcome. For example, a suspect's having been 100 miles away from the scene of a murder at the time the murder occurred would tend to disconfirm the inference that the suspect committed the crime. This relation is evidence against the necessity of the possibly causal event for the outcome; that is, the occurrence of the outcome (the crime in this example) was not preceded by the occurrence of the possibly causal event (the suspect's having been present).

A fifth kind of information can also be relevant to causal inference, namely, prior probability, by which is meant the probability of a given outcome occurring in the absence of any new information regarding the probability of occurrence in the particular situation. One simply uses one's world knowledge about concurrences of events. We theorized that such information would receive minimal usage.

It is important to note that the kinds of information considered above can be used to test one's preferred hypothesis and to test alternative hypotheses as well. Thus, the various kinds of evidence can be combined to give a causal likelihood for each of a set of potential causal antecedents.

Tests of the theory of causal inference

Unicausal inference. In our research on unicausal causal inference, subjects had to evaluate the likelihood that a given outcome event was the result of a particular hypothesized causal event. Individuals had to make these judg-

ments with incomplete information about complex problems varying simultaneously on many dimensions. In making the judgments, subjects had to
decide what kinds of evidence to consider, how to weigh each kind of evidence, how to combine the various kinds of evidence, and how to translate
their conclusions into a probability that the target hypothesis was responsible
for the target outcome.

The problems used in our research resembled in many respects problems
encountered in real-world settings that require causal inferences. We used
three basic kinds of problems that differed in the content domain in which
the causal inference was to be made: (a) an epidemiological domain, in
which the individual had to judge the likelihood that a particular hazard was
responsible for a given epidemic; (b) a securities domain, in which the
individual had to judge the likelihood that a particular circumstance was
responsible for a precipitous decline in the value of a company stock; and (c)
an abstract domain, in which the individual had to judge the likelihood that a
particular circumstance (labeled only by a letter) was responsible for some
other particular circumstance (also labeled only by a letter).

Consider a sample problem from the securities domain:

A market analyst noted that, among pharmaceutical manufacturers:
   In Company 1,
The office staff of the company organized and joined a union.
The company's major product was under suspicion as a carcinogen.
   There was a drastic drop in the value of the company's stock.

   In Company 2,
The office staff of the company did not organize or join a union.
The company's major product was under suspicion as a carcinogen.
   There was a drastic drop in the value of the company's stock.

   In Company 3,
Illegal campaign contributions were traced to the company's managers.
The company's major product was not under suspicion as a carcinogen.
   There was not a drastic drop in the value of the company's stock.

*What is the probability that, for some other pharmaceutical manufacturer, stock
values would drop drastically if the company's major product were under suspicion
as a carcinogen?*

In each problem of each kind, individuals were presented with the hypothesis that a particular event was responsible for some outcome. They
were asked to use a given body of evidence to estimate the probability (placed
on a 0–100 scale to eliminate decimal points) with which that event, by
itself, would produce that outcome. Individuals were explicitly warned that
they were being given incomplete information and that interactions between
potentially causal events were possible; these warnings were aimed at evok-

ing the same kinds of mental set as are evoked in real-life causal inference.

Within any situation in any kind of problem, each possible cause was in one of three states: observed to be present (e.g., "The office staff of the company organized and joined a union"), observed to be absent (e.g., "The office staff of the company did not organize or join a union"), or not observed (e.g., nothing is said about unionization). Over the sets of problems in three content domains, there were from two to five situations (cities, companies, or lines of problems) described in a single problem, as well as from two to five possibly causal events observed per situation independently of the number of situations. Within a single problem, each situation had the same number of observed possibly causal events.

Sixty-two subjects supplied probability ratings for each of the two concrete content domains, with order of domain counterbalanced. Forty subjects supplied probability ratings for the abstract content domain only. An additional 21 subjects supplied base-rate ratings for the concrete content domains. These subjects were asked the question without being given the prior information about the companies (or epidemics). Other experiments used similar designs (see Schustack & Sternberg, 1981, for a full description of the complete set of experiments, only one of which is described here), with similar results.

Mean response probabilities were .35 for epidemics, .37 for securities, and .35 for abstract items (with decimal points now inserted for ease of comprehension). The means did not differ significantly from each other. Values of R^2 between predicted and observed probabilities were .90, .88, and .90 for epidemics, securities, and abstract content, respectively. Deviations from the model were statistically significant, despite the high levels of fit. RMSDs of observed from predicted values were .07, .06, and .06 (with decimal points again inserted here) for the three respective content types. The proposed theory of causal inference was tested against a number of plausible alternative theories and was found to provide a superior account of the data. These alternatives included both linear and nonlinear models.

It is worth noting that parameter estimates for the four kinds of evidence considered by the theory were highly similar across the three content domains. Consistent with past evidence in research on causal inference (e.g., Wason, 1960), people weighed positive confirming evidence the most highly. Also consistent with past evidence, base rates were hardly used at all (see Nisbett & Ross, 1980). Evidence about hypotheses alternative to the one being considered was evaluated but was assigned much less weight than would have been optimal. On the whole, we found that people used a wide variety of types of evidence in making their judgments, but the weights they assigned these types of information were rather far from those that would be assigned if all types got equal weight. There were relatively small individual differences in these weights (making individual-difference analyses uninteresting).

In sum, the proposed theory of causal inference provided a good account of the unicausal probability-judgment data and seems to be generalizable across at least three content domains. The theory does seem to give a reasonable account of just what *inference* is in a unicausal judgment task.

Multicausal inference. The theory of unicausal inference has been extended to the multicausal case as well. Consider an instance requiring the need for multicausal inference and how it differs from the unicausal case:

In City 1,
Annual health inspection of food-service workers was stopped.
A new type of pesticide was tried by local vegetable farmers.
    An epidemic of Hammond's disease was reported.

In City 2,
A new type of pesticide was tried by local vegetable farmers.
A new type of hair dye was used in the area.
    An epidemic of Hammond's disease was reported.

In City 3,
A new type of pesticide was tried by local vegetable farmers.
There was a water-main break.
    An epidemic of Hammond's disease was reported.

In City 4,
Annual health inspection of food-service workers was not stopped.
A new type of hair dye was not used in the area.
    An epidemic of Hammond's disease was not reported.

In City 5:
There was a water-main break.
Annual health inspection of food-service workers was not stopped.
    An epidemic of Hammond's disease was not reported.

In another city,
Annual health inspection of food-service workers was stopped.
A new type of pesticide was tried by local vegetable farmers.
What is the likelihood that an epidemic of Hammond's disease would occur?

The critical difference between this multicausal problem type and the former unicausal type is that *more than one* antecedent is introduced in the final scenario for which a causal judgment has to be made. In other words, the possibility is allowed that there will be multiple pieces of information about the situation for which a causal estimate has to be made. Indeed, such an allowance seems more ecologically valid than the unicausal case, in which a judgment was to be made on the basis of only a single piece of information.

Downing, Sternberg, and Ross (1983) extended the theory of unicausal inference to account for the multicausal case and tested the augmented theory in two experiments using abstract content and concrete content (epidemics). Alternative models of the causal inference judgments were tested and compared to each other (see original article for details). One new variable was introduced into the final causal model: representativeness, or resemblance, of the events in the hypothetical situation (to be judged) to causal events in antecedent situations that led to the proposed outcome. If one of the antecedent situations (in the examples, citywide epidemics) evidenced both the proposed outcome (e.g., the epidemic) and an exact resemblance of possible causal conditions to the possible causal conditions in the situation to be judged, then subjects tended to raise their likelihood judgments beyond the ratings that would have been predicted on the basis of the original theory alone. Note that this new variable did not apply in the unicausal case, because only a single piece of causal evidence was presented for the last situation.

For abstract items (using letters), a proposed averaging model for causal information (i.e., averaging of the kinds of information in the proposed model) accounted for 95% and 93% of the variance in the judgment data in two experiments with two separate sets of subjects. Strength of alternative causes seemed not to be considered in these judgments, and hence this variable was not included in the final model. For concrete items (using epidemic information), the proposed averaging model accounted for only 84% of the variance in the data. However, it appeared that in this condition (and only in this condition) there were significant individual differences in strategy, with some subjects using a simplified model that only took into account limited information (namely, the causal event in a given situation that was judged most likely to lead to the outcome of interest). Thus, when situations become sufficiently complicated, at least some subjects seem to resort to strategies that simplify the given information in order to make it more manageable. Of course, the use of representativeness may itself be seen as a simplification that uses a holistic kind of correspondence between earlier events and events to be judged as a basis for causal inference.

To conclude, causal inferences, like all of the other kinds of inferences considered earlier, represent *inductive* thought. In the next chapter, attention is turned to the "other half" of reasoning, *deductive* thought.

6 Fluid abilities: deductive reasoning

Fluid abilities have most often been measured by tests of inductive reasoning, such as the analogies, series completions, and classifications problems considered in the previous chapter. Deductive reasoning tests have been used less frequently, although if one were to include in the domain of deductive reasoning mathematical reasoning problems as well as strictly logical reasoning problems, then the frequency with which deduction problems appear would be considered to be somewhat greater.

Deduction problems can be of many kinds. The three kinds of problems that seem to have played the greatest part in the literature on intelligence are probably the three major kinds of syllogisms: linear, categorical, and conditional. Each of these kinds of syllogisms will be considered in turn in the present chapter.

Linear syllogisms

In a linear syllogism, an individual is presented with two premises, each describing a relation between two items. At least one of the items overlaps between premises. The subject's task is to use this overlap to determine a relation between two (or more) items not occurring in the same premise. An example of such a problem is

Tom is trickier than Dick.
Dick is trickier than Harry.
Who is trickiest?

In general, the terms of a linear syllogism (or three-term series problem, as it is also called), form a linear array of items, say (A, B, C). Each of two premises describes a relation between one pair of adjacent items, say, $(A r_1 B), (B r_2 C)$. To solve the problem, an individual must combine information from the two premises in order to determine the relation between the two nonadjacent items, $(A r_3 C)$. Solution of the example problem above requires the individual to infer the relation between the two nonadjacent items, Tom and Harry.

Transitive inferences of the kind required by linear syllogisms are widely used in everyday life. In such inferences, one makes a decision about the relation between A and C on the basis of knowledge about the relations between A and B, on the one hand, and B and C, on the other. Comparisons and decisions of almost every kind that we make on a daily basis usually involve at least an implicit transitive inference. Consider, for example, the plight of a customer eating at a restaurant. The customer is faced with what may well be a bewildering choice of meals. The customer has neither the time nor the patience to compare every possible pair of meals and to order the meal that is preferred to every other. More typically, the customer will narrow down his or her preferences to a few possible choices, assuming that if the eliminated choices are less desirable than the minimally acceptable choice, they are less desirable than any other acceptable choice as well. In narrowing down the choices, the customer will probably assume transitivity of preferences at each step along the way. Without such an assumption, he or she would be faced with a bewildering number of choices, indeed. In general, without the use of transitive inference, many of even our simplest decisions would become unmanageably complex.

Although useful, it is important to note that transitivity is sometimes assumed when its application is questionable. For example, in selecting candidates for graduate school and for faculty positions, Yale (and many other universities) often make use of a rank-order list. But when it comes to the credentials of people who vary on many attributes, not all of which seem strictly comparable across persons, transitive inferences may break down. On many occasions, one finds that candidate A is preferable to candidate B, and candidate B is preferable to candidate C, but it is not at all clear that candidate A is preferable to candidate C. The point, then, is that part of the intelligence involved in transitive inference is knowing when such inferences apply.

Psychologists have long recognized the fundamental importance of transitive inferences in everyday cognition; as a result, transitive inference has played a key role in psychological theory. Research on transitive inference has appeared in diverse psychological literatures and under a number of different guises. Differential psychologists have recognized the linear syllogism form of transitive inference as a useful psychometric tool since Burt's (1919) use of the problem in a battery of mental tests, although our knowledge of the psychometric properties of the problem as a test item remains rudimentary (Burt, 1919; Shaver, Pierson, & Lang, 1974; Sternberg, 1980e; Sternberg & Weil, 1980). Developmental psychologists have investigated the transitive inference problem extensively, many of them in response to Piaget's (1921, 1928, 1955, 1970) claim that preoperational children (of roughly 2 to 6 years of age) are unable to perform the reasoning necessary to infer a transitive relation. Trabasso (Bryant & Trabasso, 1971; Riley & Trabasso, 1974), for example, has taken issue with Piaget's interpretation of the data and in a series of ingenious experiments has found evidence suggesting that memory rather than reasoning limitations are responsible for much of the difficulty young children encounter in attempting to solve transitive inference problems. Cognitive-experimental psychologists have also devoted a great deal of attention to the transitive inference problem, especially in its linear-syllogistic form. They have engaged in a vigorous debate regarding the representations and processes subjects use in solving such problems (Clark, 1969a, 1969b, 1971, 1972a, 1972b; DeSoto, London, & Handel, 1965; Egan & Grimes-Farrow, 1982; Handel, DeSoto, & London, 1968; Hunter, 1957; Huttenlocher, 1968; Huttenlocher & Higgins, 1971, 1972; Huttenlocher, Higgins, Milligan, & Kauffman, 1970; Johnson-Laird, 1972; Potts & Scholz, 1975; Sternberg, 1980b, 1980d, 1980e; Sternberg & Weil, 1980).

The primary issue in the cognitive-experimental literature has been that of whether information about transitive relations is mentally represented in a spatial format, a linguistic format, or both. Of the investigators noted above, the major proponent of the linguistic position has been Clark, the major proponent of the spatial position has been Huttenlocher, and the major proponents of mixture positions have been Johnson-Laird, Shaver, and myself. But whereas Johnson-Laird and Shaver have claimed that subjects switch representations and strategies (Johnson-Laird has argued for a spatial-to-linguistic switch, Shaver for a linguistic-to-spatial switch) over the course of trials of practice, I have claimed that most subjects use both kinds of representations on all problems. My proposed theory, then, is a spatial–linguistic mixture one. Individuals are theorized to use both kinds of representation in every problem, rather than to switch from one kind of representation to the other over the course of practice with the problems. This theory is considered below.

The linguistic–spatial mixture theory

Motivation

Two basic ideas motivate the proposed linguistic–spatial mixture theory of linear syllogistic reasoning.

The first basic idea is that in solving transitive inference problems, subjects seem likely to use both linguistic and spatial operations: First, they linguistically decode the verbal information presented in the premises; then they spatially recode the information into a form that permits the transitive inference to be made. This kind of mixture theory is consistent with the obvious need for subjects to interpret the verbal input presented to them and with their frequent reports of spatial imagery in combining information from the two premises. The position adopted here is similar to that adopted by Lawson (1977), who in studying linear ordering problems concluded that

whatever the nature of the representation, the results of this study indicate that two distinct types of information are available in memory: first, information about the holistic idea conveyed by the entire set of sentences, and second, information in propositional form about what sentences were presented. (P. 9)

Lawson suggests that holistic "knowledge of the ordering is represented in a form that is *analogical* to a visual depiction of the scene" (p. 8).

The second basic idea is that a major but previously unappreciated source of difficulty in solving linear syllogisms is the need for the subject at various points in the solution process to locate specific items in the spatial array, in particular, the pivot (that is, the middle, or B term) and the response. In solving a transitive inference problem, the subject's mind's eye traverses the spatial array as necessary. Every time it moves from one location to another, real time is consumed. This notion of visual scanning of a spatial representation is consistent with the sorts of visual scanning processes suggested by Shepard (Cooper & Shepard, 1973; Shepard & Metzler, 1971) and by Kosslyn (1975). The basic notion is that scanning of a visual array is analogous to scanning of a physical array and consumes measurable time.

Processing strategy

A flowchart for the proposed linguistic–spatial strategy is shown in Figure 6.1. The strategy will be illustrated with reference to the example "C is not as tall as B; A is not as short as B; who is shortest?" The correct answer is C, and by convention, A will always refer to the extreme item at the tall (and, in general, unmarked) end of the continuum, and C to the extreme item at the short (and, in general, marked) end of the continuum. The unmarked end of a continuum is that end that is used to name the scale. For example, one asks "how tall" an individual is, rather than "how short" that individual is. Similarly, *good* represents the unmarked end of the good–bad continuum, because one typically asks how good rather than how bad a thing (or person) is.

The subject begins solution by reading the first premise. In order for the premise to be understood, it must be formulated in terms of a kind of deep-structural proposition. Encoding a marked adjective into this deep-structural format takes longer than encoding an unmarked one. Also, the presence of a negation requires a reformulation of the deep-structural propo-

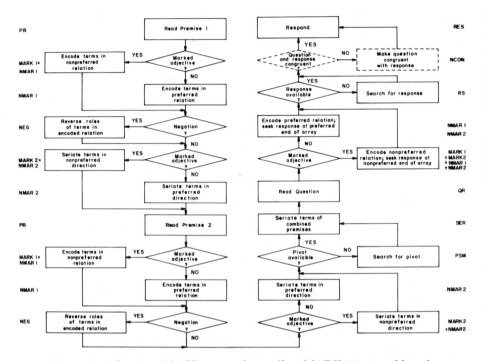

Figure 6.1. Mixed model. (PR = premise reading; MARK1+ = marking plus confounded operations (linguistic); NMAR1 = nonmarked (linguistic); NEG =
negation; MARK2+ = marking plus confounded operations (spatial); NMAR2 =
nonmarked (spatial); PSM = pivot search (mixed); SER = seriation; QR = question
reading; RS = response search; NCON = noncongruence; RES = response.) (From
"Representation and process in linear syllogistic reasoning," by Robert J. Sternberg,
1980, *Journal of Experimental Psychology: General, 109*, p. 127. Copyright 1980 by
the American Psychological Association. Reprinted by permission of the publisher.)

sition. Thus, "C is not as tall as B" is originally formulated as (C is tall +; B is
tall) and is then reformulated as (B is tall +; C is tall) (as would be true in
Clark's linguistic strategy). Once the deep-structural propositions for the
premise are in final linguistic form, the terms of the propositions are seriated
(i.e., arranged) spatially. If there is a marked adjective (such as *short*), the
subject takes additional time in seriating the relation spatially in the nonpreferred (usually bottom–up) direction. If the adjective is not marked, then the
premise is seriated in the preferred (usually top–down) direction. Note that
whereas a negation is processed linguistically, a marked adjective is processed first linguistically (in comprehension) and later spatially (in seriation). After seriating the first premise, the subject repeats the steps described
above for the second premise.

In order for the subject to combine the terms of the premises into a single spatial array, he needs the pivot (overlapping term). The pivot is either immediately available from the linguistic encoding of the premises or else it must be found spatially. According to the mixture theory, there are two ways in which the pivot can become available immediately: (a) It is the single repeated term from all previous linguistic encodings; or (b) it is the last term to have been linguistically encoded. These rules have different implications for affirmative and negative premises.

In problems with two affirmative premises, the pivot is always immediately available, since each premise has been linguistically encoded just once. One term, the pivot, is distinctive from the others in that more than one relational tag has been associated with it, one from its encoding in the first premise and one from its encoding in the second premise. The other two terms each have just a single relational tag associated with them.

The use of distinctiveness as a cue to the identity of the pivot fails in problems with at least one negative premise. In these problems, each premise containing a negation is encoded in two different ways – in its original encoding and in its reformulated encoding in which the roles of the terms have been reversed. The pivot is therefore no longer the only term with more than one relational tag associated with it, and it thus loses its distinctiveness. The subject must therefore search for the term with the largest number of relational tags, unless he or she can apply the second principle.

When the distinctiveness principle fails, the subject attempts to link the first premise to the last term to have been encoded in working memory. If this term of the second premise happens to be the pivot, the link is successful, and the subject can proceed with problem solution. Pivot search can thus be avoided if the last term to have been encoded is the pivot. But if this term is not the pivot, the link cannot be made, and the subject must search for the pivot – the term with the largest number of relational tags. This search for the pivot takes additional time.

Once the pivot has been located, the subject seriates the terms from the two spatial arrays into a single spatial array. In forming the array, the subject starts with the terms of the first premise and ends with those of the second premise. The subject's mental location after seriation, therefore, is in that half of the array described by the second premise. The subject next reads the question. If there is a marked adjective in the question, the subject will take longer to encode the adjective and to seek the response at the nonpreferred (usually bottom) end of the array. The response may or may not be immediately available. If the correct answer is in the half of the array where the subject just completed seriation (his or her active location in the array), then the response will be available immediately. If the question requires an answer from the other half of the array, however, the subject will have to search for the response, mentally traversing the array from one half to the other and thereby consuming additional time.

One final search operation is used optionally under special circumstances. If the subject has constructed a sharp spatial encoding, then he or she is now ready to respond with the correct answer. If the subject's encoding is fuzzy, however, the subject may find that he or she is unable to respond with a reasonable degree of certainty. The subject therefore checks his or her tentative response as determined by the spatial representation with the encoding of that reponse term in the linguistic representation. If the question and response are congruent, the check is successful, and the subject responds. If the question and response are not congruent, however, the subject reformulates the question to ascertain whether it can be made congruent with the response. Only then does he or she respond.

The notion of optional search for congruence depending upon quality of encoding makes a strong prediction: that the use of this additional operation should be associated with reduced encoding time. Indeed, subjects seek to establish congruence only because they did not take the time to create a sharply defined spatial encoding. Experimental manipulations can be controlled so that the subject is either encouraged to or discouraged from creating a sharp spatial encoding. The experimental manipulations that result in one or the other kind of encoding will be described later, as will the degree to which the data conform to the prediction made above.

Comparison of the mixture theory to other theories

Although the alternative theories to the proposed mixture theory have not been described in detail (see Sternberg, 1980e, for such a comparison), it would probably be helpful to point out some of the similarities and differences among the theories.

The theories all agree that marked adjectives and negations should increase solution latency. They disagree, however, as to why solution latency is increased. According to the spatial theory, solution latency is increased because processing of negations and marked adjectives requires a more complex encoding of information into a visualized spatial array. According to the linguistic theory, the additional time results from increased difficulty in a linguistic encoding process. According to the mixture theory, negations require a more complex linguistic encoding process, whereby marked adjectives require first more complex linguistic encoding and then more complex spatial encoding.

The theories also agree that some form of pivot search is needed under special circumstances. The theories disagree, however, as to what these circumstances are. In the spatial theory, pivot search is required for premises that are not end-anchored, that is, for premises in which the first term is the middle rather than an end of the spatial array. Absence of end-anchoring necessitates a search through the visualized spatial array. In the linguistic theory, pivot search results from compression of the first premise in the deep-structural encoding. If the term that was dropped from working memory in compression happens to be the pivot term, then the subject has to retrieve that term from long-term memory. In the mixture theory, pivot search is required if the reformulated deep-structural version of the negative second premise does not have the pivot in its latter (and hence most recently available) proposition.

The spatial and mixture theories agree that the terms of the two premises are combined into a single, unified representation. This combination is accomplished through a seriation operation in which each of the two partial spatial arrays is unified into a single array. The linguistic theory disagrees: Functional relations from the two premises are stored separately.

The linguistic and mixture theories agree in the need for an operation to establish congruence between question and answer, but only in the mixture theory is the establishment of congruence optional. It is used only when the spatial encoding of terms is of insufficient quality to permit the subject to respond to the problem with a reasonable degree of certainty. No operation for the establishment of congruence exists in the spatial theory.

In the spatial theory, subjects are hypothesized to prefer working in a certain direction (usually top–down) between, as well as within, premises. Generally, this preference means that extra time will be spent in seriation if the term at the preferred end of the array does not occur in the first premise. No corresponding "additional latency" exists in either the linguistic or mixture theory.

In the linguistic theory, subjects search the deep-structural propositions for the term that answers the question. In a spatial array, it is obvious which term corresponds to which question adjective. For example, the tallest term might be at the top, the shortest term at the bottom. In linguistic propositions, there is no such obvious correspondence, so that the subject must check both extreme terms relative to the pivot, seeking the correct answer.

In the mixture theory, subjects have to search for the response to the problem if their active location in their final spatial array is not in the half of the array containing the response. Subjects mentally traverse the array to the other half, looking for the response. No corresponding operation exists in either the spatial or linguistic theory.

Experimental tests of the mixture theory

Quantification. The proposed information-processing theory, as well as alternative spatial and linguistic ones, were quantified by assuming that (a) each operation represented by a box in the flowchart for that theory contributes toward the total real time consumed in the solution of a linear syllogism and that (b) these contributions toward solution time are additive.

Methods. Seven experiments have been conducted that were designed to distinguish among the mixture, spatial, and linguistic theories. The first six experiments involved college undergraduates; the last involved children in grades 3, 5, 7, 9, and 11. All of the experiments involved presentation of 32 basic types of linear syllogisms with three different adjective pairs (usually *taller – shorter, better – worse,* and *faster – slower*). Items were constructed by varying whether (a) the adjective in the first premise was marked or unmarked; (b) the adjective in the second premise was marked or unmarked; (c) the adjective in the question was marked or unmarked; (d) both premises were affirmative (for example, "John is taller than Bill") or negative equative (for example, "Bill is not as tall as John"); and (e) the correct answer was in the first premise or in the second premise. Terms in the problems were common first names, half of them male and half female, although male and female names were never mixed in the same problem. Consider some examples of the kinds of problems used:

Ken is taller than Sam.   Bill is not as good as Pete.
Sam is taller than Joe.   Pete is not as good as Jack.
Who is tallest?   Who is worst?
Sam Ken Joe   Bill Jack Pete

Jane is faster than Anne.   Sue is not as young as Lyn.
Jane is slower than Kate.   · Sue is not as old as Jan.
Who is slowest?   Who is youngest?
Anne Kate Jane   Jan Lyn Sue

The length of the experiments ranged from one to three sessions, and all experiments, except the last, included administration to each subject of tests of verbal reasoning, spatial visualization, and abstract reasoning abilities.

I will consider first the initial five experiments and then consider the last two separately and individually.

In the first experiment, 16 Stanford undergraduates received linear syllogisms such as "Sam is taller than Joe. Joe is taller than Bob. Who is tallest? Joe Bob Sam?" Items were presented to all subjects in both of two cueing conditions. In the first condition, subjects received a blank field in the first part of a trial. Subjects indicated readiness to see the item by pressing a foot pedal, and following this indication of readiness the entire item appeared on a tachistoscope screen. In the second condition, subjects received the two premises of the syllogism in the first part of the trial. Subjects processed the premises as fully as they could and then pressed the foot pedal, resulting in the appearance of the entire item on the screen. Adjective pairs were *taller–shorter, better–worse, older–younger,* and *faster–slower.*

In the second experiment, the linear syllogisms were presented to 18 Yale undergraduates with the question first: "Who is tallest? Sam is taller than Joe. Joe is taller than Bob. Joe Sam Bob?" In this experiment, there were three rather than two precueing conditions. Subjects received either a blank field, just the question, or the question and the two premises in the first part of the trial. They always received the whole item in the second part of the trial. Adjective pairs were the same as in Experiment 1, except for the deletion of *older–younger.*

In the third experiment, the linear syllogisms (with the question last) were presented to 18 Yale undergraduates without precueing. However, subjects also received eight basic types of two-term series problems – for example: "Jim is taller than Bob. Who is tallest? Jim Bob?" (The ungrammatical superlative is conventionally used in the question for this kind of problem.) These two-term series problems were used to separate parameters in the parameter estimation procedure, much as the precueing was used in the previous two experiments. Two-term and three-term series problems were each blocked into sets, so that subjects always knew what kind of problem to expect. Adjective pairs were the same as in the preceding experiment.

The fourth experiment was similar to the third experiment except that each of the 54 Yale undergraduates participating received two-term series problems and three-term series problems with just one of the adjective pairs, rather than with all three, as in the previous experiments.

The fifth experiment was similar to the third experiment except that the 18 Yale summer-session students were encouraged to solve items rapidly, and a bonus was paid to encourage more rapid (and hence less accurate) performance. The speed–accuracy tradeoff manipulation proved to be successful: Mean solution latencies decreased by about a second (from approximately 7 to approximately 6 seconds), and mean error rates increased from 1% in the previous experiments to 7% in this experiment.

Model fits. Mean response times were typically about 7 seconds per item. The median fits (R^2) were .84 for the mixture theory, .60 for the linguistic theory, and .58 for the spatial theory. The superiority of the mixture theory held up over all individual adjective pairs and over all individual sessions as well. More detailed results can be found in the original papers (Sternberg, 1980d, 1980e). Of greatest interest here are the model fits (in terms of R^2) for the latency data from each of the five experiments. In each experiment, the mixture theory was clearly superior to either the linguistic or the spatial theory: The differences in R^2 between the mixture theory and the second-best theory (the linguistic theory in four of the five experiments) were .213,

.148, .155, .240, and .237 in Experiments 1, 2, 3, 4, and 5, respectively. Patterns for other measures of fit, such as root-mean-square deviation (RMSD), were comparable. Thus, regardless of whether the question came before or after the premises, whether or not precueing was part of the experimental design, whether different adjectives were presented within or between subjects, and whether subjects emphasized speed or accuracy, the mixture theory best accounted for the data. The optional parameter for establishment of congruence was relevant to performance in Experiments 3, 4, and 5. With this parameter deleted, the values of R^2 for the mixture theory were .765, .832, and .761 in Experiments 3, 4, and 5, respectively. Thus, even without the optional parameter, the mixture theory was clearly superior to its competitors. Moreover, this superiority held up in every comparison for every adjective and session of testing and with precueing conditions included in this analysis. Thus, there was no evidence of a strategy change as a function of practice with the linear syllogisms. It should be noted, though, that the mixture theory could be rejected relative to the true theory in all but the first experiment: The unexplained variance was statistically significant in four of the five experiments. Thus, the mixture theory, although the best available approximation to the true theory, is not identical to it.

Parameter estimates. Parameter estimates were quite stable across experiments. For those (first four) experiments in which there was no particular speed pressure, typical estimates were about 4.6 seconds for encoding, .3 second for negation, .4 second for marking, 1.1 seconds for pivot search, .6 second for response search, .5 second for noncongruence, .4 second for question answering, and .5 second for response plus other constant operations. Not all of these operations could be separated in each of the five experiments.

Correlations with ability tests. Correlations between parameter estimates for the mixture theory and composite verbal and spatial ability test scores were, respectively, -.25 and -.51 for encoding, -.10 and -.56 for negation, -.26 and -.65 for marking, -.18 and -.38 for pivot search, -.28 and -.58 for response search, -.41 and -.38 for noncongruence, and -.30 and -.09 for response. (These correlations are based only upon subjects for whom significant parameter estimates were obtained. Hence, the number of subjects contributing to each correlation differs somewhat from one correlation to another. The original report contains both these correlations and those for all subjects.) The encoding parameter (ENC+) was significantly correlated with scores on both types of ability tests. This pattern is consistent with the mixture theory, according to which the ENC+ parameter includes both linguistic and spatial–abstract processes. A strictly linguistic or spatial theory would have difficulty accounting for this pattern. Although ENC+ contains a mixture of operations, the predominant operation – according to the mixture theory – is spatial seriation between premises. This mixture theory therefore predicted that the spatial – abstract correlations would be higher than the verbal correlations, and this was in fact the case.

The negation parameter (NEG) showed significant correlations with the spatial but not with the verbal composite. This pattern of correlations was inconsistent with the prediction of the mixture theory, according to which negation was supposed to be a linguistic operation. It now appears that negation is accomplished spatially by reversing the positions of the two relevant terms in a within-premise spatial array.

The marking parameter (MARK) showed some relationship to both composite ability scores, as predicted by the mixture theory but not by the spatial or linguistic theories. It thus appears that marked adjectives are both linguistically more difficult to encode and spatially more difficult to seriate in an array.

Pivot search (PSM) was significantly correlated with the spatial but not with the verbal composite. This pattern of correlations is consistent with the mixture theory, according to which pivot search is a spatial – abstract operation.

Response search (RS) was significantly correlated with both composite scores. The significant correlation with verbal ability came as a surprise, because response search is postulated by the mixture theory to be a spatial operation. A possible explanation of the correlation with the verbal composite is that subjects may differ in the rates at which they read off names from a spatial array, resulting in individual differences along a verbal dimension.

Search for congruence (NCON) was significantly correlated with the verbal composite but not with the spatial composite. This correlational pattern is as predicted by the mixture theory, which – like the linguistic theory – postulates that the search for congruence is a linguistic operation.

Finally, response (RES+) was significantly correlated with the verbal composite but not with the spatial composite. Response was a confounded parameter containing mostly linguistic operations, and hence this pattern of correlations was consistent with the theory.

Generally speaking, the results of the individual-differences analysis were consistent with the predictions of the mixture theory, according to which particular operations should show patterns of individual differences along either verbal, spatial – abstract, or both lines. The two exceptions to the predictions suggest a need for slight reconceptualization.

Extension of the theory to indeterminate linear syllogisms. The linear syllogisms considered in the experiments described above were all determinate, which is to say that there was always a unique, correct answer to each of the problems. Such an answer is not always available for all problems, however. Consider, for example, the problem "Len is taller than Bob. Len is taller than Sam. Who is shortest?" The question is not uniquely answerable, because the premises do not contain sufficient information to infer a unique answer. Although one can infer that Len is tallest, one cannot distinguish between the relative heights of Bob and Sam. Linear syllogisms such as this one, which do not permit inference of the relation between each possible pair of terms, are referred to as *indeterminate*.

The mixture theory of linear-syllogistic reasoning has been extended to account for performance on indeterminate as well as determinate linear syllogisms (Sternberg, 1981i). In the extended theory, indeterminate linear syllogisms are assumed to be easier to solve, on the average, than determinate ones, because in constructing a single three-item array from the two two-item arrays one initially forms, one needs to construct a determinate relation between only two of the three possible pairs of relations; in contrast, a determinate linear syllogism requires construction of a three-item array showing determinate relations between all three possible pairs. Processing of indeterminate linear syllogisms can be facilitated only if subjects recognize such syllogisms as indeterminate. In this theory, recognition is assumed to occur once the individual premises are each linguistically and spatially encoded. These encodings will be needed regardless of whether the problem is determinate or indeterminate. First, the subject is theorized to question whether the adjectives in the premises are the same and the positions of the repeated terms the same in each premise. If so, the problem is indeterminate; if not, the problem may still be indeterminate. The subject next questions whether the adjectives in the premises are different and the positions of the repeated terms different in each premise. If so, the problem is indeterminate; if not, the problem is determinate. If the problem is indeterminate, the positions of the overlapping term in the two spatial arrays representing the two premises are the same, and the two arrays can be essentially superimposed at the pivot point rather than joined end to end at the pivot point. Superimposition is assumed to be faster than end-to-end joining. Finally, the subject responds.

The extended theory was tested in an experiment with 18 undergraduates attending the Yale summer term. Stimuli were two-term series problems and three-term series problems. Half of the three-term series problems were determinate and half were indeterminate. Subjects were instructed to respond "I" to problems without a unique answer. Determinate and indeterminate problems were randomly intermixed.

The fit of the quantified model to the latency data was quite good. R^2 for the total data set was .93. For indeterminate three-term series problems only,

R^2 also happened to be .93. Parameter estimates were .46 second for marking, .76 second for negation, .68 second for response search, 2.75 seconds for construction of the full determinate array, 4.49 seconds for detection of a mismatch of the premise adjectives or position of repeated terms, and 4.28 seconds for the response constant. Correlations with reference ability tests were similar to those in the previously described experiments. Of some interest is that the new parameter, mismatch of premise adjectives or position of repeated term, correlated -.61 with an abstract reasoning test score but did not correlate significantly with either verbal or spatial test scores.

This study provided the first quantitative test of the ability of any of the primary current theories of linear-syllogistic reasoning to account for performance on indeterminate linear syllogisms. In particular, mathematical modeling of the latency data showed the success of the proposed mixture theory in accounting for performance on indeterminate as well as determinate linear syllogisms, and the correlations with ability tests showed the predicted pattern. Because no other theories have been explicitly extended to indeterminate linear syllogisms, no competitive theories were tested. But the proposed theory seems to provide a reasonable account of what subjects do when confronted with such syllogisms.

Initial summation. In sum, the results of the five experiments provide strong support for the mixture theory, considered either by itself or in comparison to alternative theories of linear-syllogistic reasoning. Parameter estimates for the mixture theory were sensible and generally consistent across experiments, and patterns of individual differences generally supported the predictions as to which operations were spatial and which linguistic. But a finer-grained analysis reveals the existence of individual differences in strategies that were not the object of study in these five experiments.

What, exactly, does it mean for one theory to be "better" than the rest? A possible interpretation of this result is that more people use the indicated strategy than use other strategies, but that the differences in quantitative fits reflect individual differences in strategy as a function of the proportion of people who use each of the various strategies. Data collected by Sternberg and Weil (1980) seem consistent with this interpretation of differences in fits.

Individual differences in strategies and the effects of strategy training. In the Sternberg–Weil experiment, particular attention was paid to the strategies used by individual subjects. Mathematical modeling of latency data revealed that in a standard linear-syllogisms paradigm, there was in fact variation in strategies used by individual subjects. Of 48 subjects given standard instructions, 30 yielded latency data best fit by the mixture theory, but 18 yielded data best fit by other theories: 7 by a linguistic theory, 5 by a spatial theory, and 6 by an algorithmic theory (which is based upon a subject strategy that uses a shortcut for solving linear syllogisms that bypasses transitive inference). Group fits again indicated the superiority of the mixture theory, but clearly this superiority indicated that the mixture strategy was the most widely used strategy, not that it was the only one used.

The main experimental manipulation in this experiment was one of instructions for solving the linear syllogisms. The group noted above that received standard instructions was a control group. A second group received instructions in how to use a strategy involving spatial visualization; and a third group received instructions in how to use a strategy involving a shortcut algorithm that practically bypassed altogether the need for deductive reasoning of any kind. It was originally expected that the groups would yield different regression patterns when solution latencies were correlated with scores on verbal and spatial ability tests. In particular, it was expected that the uninstructed group would show significant correlations with both kinds of psychometric tests (because the mixture strategy that they would presumably use involves both verbal and spatial elements), that the spatially instructed group would show significant correlations only with the spatial tests, and that the algorithmically instructed group would show only minimal or trivial correlations with the two kinds of tests, in that standard verbal and spatial patterns of reasoning would be bypassed by these subjects. The results that emerged, however, were a "mishmash." There was no clear pattern at all.

Analyses of individual subject data revealed the reason for the lack of clearly differentiable correlational patterns: Not everyone followed the strategy they were told to follow. For example, in the algorithmically instructed group, the number of subjects using the instructed strategy was more than three times as great as the number in the untrained group (21 as opposed to 6), but there were still substantial numbers of people using other strategies. In particular, about as many people (22) used the standard mixture strategy (which most subjects use spontaneously) as used the instructed algorithmic strategy. Subjects were therefore re-sorted into new groups on the basis of the strategy the mathematical modeling showed they actually used, as opposed to the strategy that we, the experimenters, had hoped they would use on the basis of the instructions. The number of subjects in each group thus differed, reflecting the number of subjects using the particular strategy characterizing the performance of that group. When subjects were re-sorted, the correlations showed the kind of aptitude–strategy interactional pattern we had hoped for. Correlations in the mixture-strategy group were significant with both verbal (-.45) and spatial (-.27) tests. Correlations in the linguistic-strategy group were significant only with the verbal (-.76) but not spatial (-.28) tests. Correlations in the spatial-strategy group were significant only with the spatial (-.61) but not the verbal (-.08) tests. And correlations in the algorithmic-strategy group were significant, but reduced, with verbal (-.32) and marginal with spatial (-.28) tests. Thus, it is important to consider individual differences in strategy, even in the face of instructional manipulations designed to eliminate such differences.

Clearly, the mixture strategy is the strategy of choice for most adult subjects. But does this preference extend to lower age levels? Might it be, for example, that the mixture strategy arises developmentally through some kind of progression that first involves a spatial strategy, then a linguistic strategy (or vice versa), and only finally a mixture strategy?

Development of strategies for linear-syllogistic reasoning. This question was addressed in a study investigating linear-syllogistic reasoning in children from grades 3 to 11 (with an age range of roughly 8 to 17 years) (Sternberg, 1980b). With one exception, the results of model fitting were straightforward. The mixture theory performed better than three alternative theories (linguistic, spatial, algorithmic) at each of the grade 3, grade 5, grade 7, and grade 11 levels. This superiority held up overall and in each of three sessions of testing. The linguistic theory was better at the grade 9 level. An examination of the data revealed that the superiority of the linguistic theory at this level was time-bound: The linguistic theory performed better than the mixture theory in the first session, but worse in the second session. Because the superiority of the linguistic theory in the first session was greater than the superiority of the mixture theory in the second session, the linguistic theory performed better overall. But because there was no evidence of this or any other strategy shift at any other grade level, it seems wise to interpret the strategy shift with caution, pending replication of the result. The result seems as likely to be due to chance as to systematic variation. At the present time, it appears that the mixture strategy is probably preferred by most subjects at each of the grade levels; at the grade 9 level, it is possible that this strategy is not used until some practice with the items is attained.

Conclusions

Consider now how the mixture theory answers three important theoretical questions regarding representation and processing of information in linear syllogistic reasoning.

Representation of information. The available evidence suggests strongly that both linguistic and spatial representations for information are used during the course of solution of linear syllogisms. Subjects first decode the linguistic surface structure of the premises into a linguistic deep structure and then recode the linguistic deep structure into a spatial array. Both the linguistic deep structure and the spatial array are available for search and retrieval processes that occur after recoding has taken place. Noncongruence, when used, operates upon the linguistic representation, whereas response search operates upon the spatial representation (primarily).

Processing of information. The preferred mixture theory accounts for linear syllogistic reasoning in terms of 12 elementary information-processing components, not all of which are used in every type of problem and not all of which have been estimated as separate parameters in the experiments described here. Of the 12 processes, 6 were hypothesized to be linguistic (premise reading, linguistic encoding of unmarked adjectives, linguistic encoding of marked adjectives, noncongruence, question reading, negation), 5 were hypothesized to be spatial (seriation, spatial encoding of unmarked adjectives, spatial encoding of marked adjectives, pivot search, response search), and 1 was hypothesized to be neutral (response). Negation turned out to be spatial. The operations were found to differ widely in their latencies and in their contributions to individual differences in overall performance. Moreover, not all subjects did, in fact, use exactly the same operations. At best, it can be said that the mixture theory was used by most subjects most of the time.

Generality of representations and processes. Consider the major kinds of generality that are at issue here.

Across adjectives. Four different adjective pairs – *taller–shorter, older–younger, better–worse, faster–slower* – were used in the course of the various experiments. Essentially the same results were obtained with each. These results seem to support the generality of the representations and processes of the mixture theory across adjectives. Of course, this generality is consistent with the earlier findings of DeSoto et al. (1965) and of Handel et al. (1968) that subjects may differ in the directions they use between and within adjective pairs for representing spatial arrays.

Across sessions. The numbers of sessions in the experiments ranged from one to three. The evidence supported the generality of the representations and processes of the mixture theory across all sessions. There was no evidence of the kinds of strategy shifts suggested by Johnson-Laird (1972) (see also Wood, Shotter, & Godden, 1974) or by Shaver et al. (1974). As would be expected, there was evidence that subjects speed up with increasing practice.

Across subjects. Analyses of individual data revealed a striking consistency in the superiority of the mixture theory. As noted above, however, the mixture strategy was not used universally. At least some subjects use the spatial, linguistic, or algorithmic strategies spontaneously.

Across tasks. The experiments described here have tested the generalizability of the representations and processes of the mixture theory across a variety of experimental paradigms using linear syllogisms. The presence or absence of a particular operation in the linear syllogisms task obviously does not guarantee the presence or absence of that operation in other tasks. How generalizable are the operations identified in the mixture theory? This question can be answered in two different ways.

First, at least some generalizability has been shown by the significant correlations of each component latency with at least one of the reference ability composites. The correlations show that the patterns of individual differences generated by the component processes are not specific to the linear syllogisms task but are common to reference tests that have been shown to measure abilities called upon in a wide variety of psychometric and other tests. In particular, the correlation of each component latency with the type of ability it is hypothesized to represent demonstrates the convergent validity of the information-processing component. The lack of correlation of each component latency with a type of ability it is hypothesized not to represent demonstrates the discriminant validity of the information-processing component. Only two mispredictions arose. Negation showed a clear convergent – discriminant pattern, but it was spatial rather than linguistic. In addition to strong correlations with the spatial – abstract tests, response search also showed weak but significant correlations with the verbal tests, and these latter correlations were interpreted in terms of individual differences in times for reading names from the spatial arrays.

Second, the generalizability of encoding, negation, marking, and noncongruence operations to a wide variety of comprehension and reasoning tasks has been amply demonstrated in past research. (For a comprehensive review of relevant literature see Carpenter & Just, 1975; Clark, 1973; Clark & Chase, 1972; Trabasso, 1972.) It should be noted that although this past research has repeatedly identified these information-processing components as contributors to solution latency in a variety of tasks, the research has not adequately distinguished which of the identified operations are linguistic and which are spatial, although some progress has been made by MacLeod, Hunt, and Mathews (1978) and Mathews, Hunt, and MacLeod (1980).

The pivot search and response search operations as formulated here have not appeared previously in others' work, and so their generalizability has yet to be demonstrated fully. However, there is some evidence that provides further support for the plausibility of these operations. If pivot search as formulated by the mixture theory is used, then negative equative problems should show end-anchoring effects for their linguistically converted (recoded) form. Huttenlocher et al. (1970) have found such a result in their task requiring manipulation of physical objects rather than just abstract terms. Findings such as these and those of Shepard and Metzler (1971) and Kosslyn (1975) suggest that in scanning visualized arrays, subjects proceed in much the same way as they do in scanning physical arrays.

In sum, then, the mixture theory appears to give a good account of linear syllogistic reasoning. This account is generalizable across modes of problem presentation, adjectives, sessions, many subjects, and some tasks. It does not account, however, for all deductive reasoning. A distinct but related theory is required to deal with other kinds of deductive reasoning. One such theory is the transitive-chain theory proposed below.

Categorical syllogisms

The nature of categorical syllogisms

A categorical syllogism comprises three declarative statements, each of which describes a relation between two sets of items. The first two statements, called the major premise and minor premise, respectively, are given. The third statement, called the conclusion, follows with logical necessity from the premises. Categorical syllogisms are of two basic types. In the first type, both the major and minor premises express relations between two sets of objects, one of which overlaps between premises. The conclusion expresses a relation between the nonoverlapping sets of objects. An example of such a syllogism is "All B are C. All A are B. Therefore, all A are C." In the second type of syllogism, the major premise expresses a relation between two sets of objects, and the minor premise expresses a relation between a particular item and one of the two sets of objects. The conclusion expresses a relation between that member and the other set. An example of such a syllogism is "All A are B. X is an A. Therefore, X is a B." We have proposed a theory that accounts for performance in both kinds of syllogisms (Guyote & Sternberg, 1981; Sternberg, Guyote, & Turner, 1980; Sternberg & Turner, 1981).

The transitive-chain theory of categorical-syllogistic reasoning

I present in this section the transitive-chain theory as it applies to the first type of categorical syllogism noted above, namely, the type in which both the major and minor premises express relations between two sets of objects. The application of the theory to the second type of categorical syllogism will be

Set Relation	Symbolic Representation	Euler Diagram Representation
Equivalence	$a_1 \rightarrow B \mid b_1 \rightarrow A$ $a_2 \rightarrow B \mid b_2 \rightarrow A$	
Subset-Set	$a_1 \rightarrow B \mid b_1 \rightarrow A$ $a_2 \rightarrow B \mid b_2 \rightarrow -A$	
Set-Subset	$a_1 \rightarrow B \mid b_1 \rightarrow A$ $a_2 \rightarrow -B \mid b_2 \rightarrow A$	
Overlap	$a_1 \rightarrow B \mid b_1 \rightarrow A$ $a_2 \rightarrow -B \mid b_2 \rightarrow -A$	
Disjoint	$a_1 \rightarrow -B \mid b_1 \rightarrow -A$ $a_2 \rightarrow -B \mid b_2 \rightarrow -A$	

Figure 6.2. Five possible set relations and their corresponding symbolic representations. (From "A transitive-chain theory of syllogistic reasoning," by Martin J. Guyote and Robert J. Sternberg, 1981, *Cognitive Psychology*, *13*, p. 468. Copyright 1981 by Academic Press, Inc. Reprinted by permission of the publisher.)

considered in the next section, together with a consideration of the application of the theory to conditional syllogisms.

Representation of information. Figure 6.2 shows the five possible set relations and shows how these relations are represented in both conventional Euler diagram format and in the symbolic format proposed by Guyote and Sternberg (1981). Each symbolic representation consists of two distinct components – one (at the left) indicating how many members of set A are also members of set B, the other (at the right) indicating how many members of set B are also members of set A. In this notation, lowercase letters stand for disjoint, exhaustive partitions of a set. Thus, for example, lowercase a_1 and a_2 are mutually exclusive and exhaustive with respect to set A. Uppercase letters refer to whole sets, and the arrow relation indicates that the partition to the left of the arrow is a proper subset of the set to the right. Components can be referred to by the order of the terms within them. Thus, all left-hand components in the figure are AB components, and all right-hand components are BA components.

Consider a couple of examples to see how the notation works. Consider, for example, set equivalence (identity). Note that both partitions of A, a_1 and a_2, are proper subsets of B, and both partitions of B, b_1 and b_2, are proper subsets of A. Thus, all a's are B's, and all b's are A's, as is the case for set

INTERPRETIVE STAGE:

No C ARE B   (1)   C → -B | B → -C

ALL B ARE A   (2)   B → A | A → B

                     (3)   B → A | a_1 → B

                                  | a_2 → -B

COMBINATION STAGE:

P_1 ONLY (1) AND (2) ARE COMBINED, YIELDING

                     A → -C | C → -A

P_2 BOTH (1) AND (2) & (1) AND (3) ARE COMBINED, YIELDING

    A → -C | C → -A a_1 → C | c_1 → A a_1 → C | C → A

              , a_2 → -C | c_2 → -A, AND a_2 → -C |

COMPARISON STAGE:

   IF ONLY (1) AND (2) ARE COMBINED, THE RESULTING REPRESENTATION
   IS LABELLED "NO A ARE C" WITH $p = \beta_2$ AND IS LABELLED
   "SOME A ARE NOT C" WITH $p = 1 - \beta_2$.

   IF BOTH PAIRS OF REPRESENTATIONS ARE COMBINED, THE SUBJECT
   LABELS THE COMPOSITE REPRESENTATION INDETERMINATE WITH
   $p = c$, AND LABELS IT "SOME A ARE NOT C" WITH $p = 1 - c$.

Figure 6.3. Solution of a sample problem in the transitive-chain model. (From "A transitive-chain theory of syllogistic reasoning," by Martin J. Guyote and Robert J. Sternberg, 1980, *Cognitive Psychology, 13*, p. 478. Copyright 1981 by Academic Press, Inc. Reprinted by permission of the publisher.)

equivalence. Consider now the second set relation, subset – set. Notice at the right that although all a's are B's, only some b's are A's: In the component at the right, b_2 is a proper subset of not-A rather than of A. This relation, then, indicates that B is a superset of A. To summarize, the basic idea is that each set relation can be represented by a notation indicating the relative numbers of a's that are B's and of b's that are A's.

Combination of representations. Figures 6.3 and 6.4 show how two simple rules can be applied to the symbolic representations of set relations to effect the combination of any two representations. The proposed representation has the advantage of permitting combination to occur via the two rules.

   The first rule states that if a partition x_i is a proper subset of Y and a partition y_j (where j may but need not equal i) is a proper subset of Z, then x_i is a proper subset of Z. This rule applies when the two middle terms match in polarity – that is, are both affirmative. It is from this rule that the transitive-

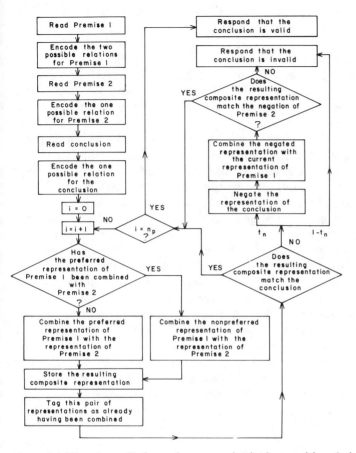

Figure 6.4. Flowchart of information processing in the transitive-chain model. (From "A transitive-chain theory of syllogistic reasoning," by Martin J. Guyote and Robert J. Sternberg, 1980, *Cognitive Psychology*, *13*, p. 481. Copyright 1981 by Academic Press, Inc. Reprinted by permission of the publisher.)

chain theory derives its name, because elements are combined by forming simple transitive chains.

The second rule states that if a partition x_i is a proper subset of not Y and a partition y_j (where j may but need not equal i) is a proper subset of Z, then x_i may be a proper subset of either Z or not-Z; one can't tell for sure. This rule applies when the two middle terms do not match in polarity – that is, when the first is negative and the second affirmative. In this case, one cannot form a transitive chain.

Further examples of how the transitive-chain combination process works and further details of the combination process can be found in the original papers (Guyote & Sternberg, 1981; Sternberg & Turner, 1981).

Information-processing model. The description of the transitive-chain theory up to now has been for the ideal subject – one who can process information without making errors. Subjects do make errors, of course, and the transitive-chain theory specifies the processes that give rise to these errors.

In the transitive-chain theory, as in other theories of categorical-syllogistic reasoning, there are four basic stages of information processing: encoding, during which the premises are read and interpreted; combination, during which the information from the premises is integrated; comparison, during which the combined representation is compared to possible labels for the representation (such as "All A are C" and "Some A are C"); and response, during which the subject communicates a response. According to the transitive-chain theory, encoding and response are error-free. Erroneous responses result from errors made in combination and comparison.

Errors during the combination stage arise from limitations in the ability of working memory to hold all possible combinations. A standard classical syllogism can require as few as 1 or as many as 16 pairs of set relations to be combined. For example, in the syllogism "No B are C. No A are B," each premise can be represented by only one set relation, meaning that only one combination need be performed. In the syllogism "Some B are C. Some A are B," however, each premise can be represented by four set relations, meaning that 16 (4×4) combinations need to be performed.

According to the theory, subjects combine a maximum of four set relations. Moreover, there is a three-tier preference hierarchy that places some constraints on the order in which set relations are combined. In particular, equivalence relations are combined before nonequivalent symmetrical ones (overlap and disjoint sets), which in turn are combined before asymmetrical ones (set–superset and set–subset). This ordering reflects the ease with which relations of each kind are stored and manipulated in working memory. Symmetrical relations are those for which the polarities of the elements of the left-hand side of each component match the polarities of the elements of the right-hand side of each component. A quick glance back at Figure 6.2 will reveal symmetry of polarities only for equivalence, overlap, and disjoint relations. Four parameters of information processing arise from the combination stage – p_1, p_2, p_3, and p_4 – representing the respective probabilities that exactly 1, 2, 3, or 4 pairs of set relations are combined.

Errors during the comparison stage arise from simplifying heuristics that subjects use to facilitate selection of a label for combined pairs of representations. If no label is consistent with all of the combined relations generated during combination, the subject labels the relationship between A and C indeterminate, choosing "None of the above" as an answer. If only one label is correct, then the subject chooses that one. But sometimes two labels are consistent with the representation generated during the combination stage. For example, the final set relation A-subset-of-C can be represented as "All A are C" or as "Some A are C." In this case, some basis is needed for choosing between labels.

Whenever two labels are consistent with all set relations generated during the combination stage, one of these labels will be stronger than the other, and one of the labels (but not the other) will match the atmosphere of the premises. The stronger of the two labels is the label with fewer possible set relations in its representation. For example, "All A are C" is stronger than "Some A are C," because the universal statement can be represented by only two set relations (equivalence and subset – set), whereas the particular statement can be represented by four set relations (equivalence, subset – set, set – subset, set overlap). The atmosphere of two premises is determined by the standard rules: It is particular (leading to the choice of a particular conclusion) if at least one premise is particular, and negative (leading to the choice of a negative conclusion) if at least one premise is negative.

The bases for choosing a label when two labels are possible take into account strength and atmosphere of the premises. It may be that each of the two possible labels meets one of the two criteria or that one of the two labels meets both. Suppose the former is true: Each label meets one criterion. When one label is weaker than the other label but matches the atmosphere of the premises, it is chosen with probability β_1, and the stronger label is chosen with probability $(1 - \beta_1)$. Suppose the latter is true: One of the two labels meets both criteria. When one label is both the stronger label and matches the atmosphere of the premises, it is chosen with probability β_2, and the other label is chosen with probability $(1 - \beta_2)$.

There is one more source of error in the comparison stage. This arises when the final set relations generated during the combination stage have different initial components. Consider the example described in Figure 6.3. Two of the pairs of components have a_1 and a_2 both linked to C, and two have a_1 linked to C but a_2 linked to not C. In such cases, subjects are hypothesized occasionally to mistake this discrepancy as indicating the indeterminacy of the conclusion. When this happens, the subject mistakenly labels the relationship between A and C indeterminate with probability c.

Alternative theories of categorical-syllogistic reasoning. Only the briefest description of the alternative information-processing theories to which we compared the transitive-chain theory will be given here. Details can be found in the original papers and in our own papers.

In the transitive-chain theory, errors occur during combination and comparison but not during encoding. In the complete-combination theory of Erickson (1974, 1978), errors occur during encoding and comparison but not during combination. In the random-combination theory of Erickson (1974, 1978), errors occur during encoding, combination, and comparison. The atmosphere theory of Woodworth and Sells (1935) is essentially one of alogical information processing. Subjects encode, combine, and compare only the quantification (universal or particular) and polarity (affirmative or negative) of the premises. In the conversion theory of Chapman and Chapman (1959), errors in syllogistic reasoning, due to conversion of premises, occur during the encoding and comparison stages of processing.

The numbers of parameters estimated differed widely across quantified models, an inevitable consequence of the different information-processing assumptions the theories make. Thus, the transitive-chain theory involved estimation of 7 free parameters; the complete- and random-combination theories involved estimation of 13 free parameters apiece; and the atmosphere and conversion theories each involved estimation of 1 free parameter. We were not particularly concerned with differing numbers of parameters, however, for three reasons. First, our major concern was with comparing the historically important theories in a way that did full justice to the initial conceptualizations, and these conceptualizations differ widely in their complexity and completeness. Second, we always estimated large numbers of data points (at least 100) in comparing theories, thus minimizing the opportunity for capitalization upon chance variation in the data. Third, the fits of the quantified models showed little correspondence to the numbers of parameters in the theories, suggesting that number of parameters was not an important determinant of fit.

Empirical tests of the theories

Method. Three experiments were conducted that are relevant to distinguishing between the theories already noted. All experiments were conducted with Yale undergraduates.

In a first experiment, subjects received pairs of premises with abstract content and had to choose one of five possible conclusions – for example: "All B are C. All A are B. (a) All A are C. (b) No A are C. (c) Some A are C. (d) Some A are not C. (e) None of the above." Half of 38 syllogisms had at least one valid conclusion from among options a through d; the other half did not. Each of 49 subjects received all of the syllogisms.

In a second experiment, subjects received pairs of premises with concrete content and again had to choose one of five possible conclusions. The idea of the experiment was to examine the effects of different kinds of concrete content on syllogistic reasoning performance. Content could be either factual – for example, "No cottages are skyscrapers. All skyscrapers are buildings"; counterfactual – for example, "No milk cartons are containers. All containers are trash cans"; or anomalous – for example, "No headphones are planets. All planets are frying pans." Note that anomalous premises could be either factually correct (as was the major premise of the example) or incorrect (as was the minor premise of the example): In either case, though, the subject and predicate of the premise were semantically unrelated (or close to it). Each of 20 syllogism types was presented to each of 50 subjects once with each type of content. Items were not blocked by content type. Subjects in this experiment were given the verbal reasoning, spatial visualization, and abstract reasoning subtests of the Differential Aptitude Test. The tests were subjected to a principal components analysis, yielding two orthogonal components, a verbal one, and a spatial–abstract one.

In a third experiment, premises were again presented with abstract content. This experiment differed from the first experiment, however, in that (a) the subject's task was to indicate whether a single presented conclusion was definitely, possibly, or never true; and (b) subjects might receive either a single premise or a pair of premises. Sixteen subjects received each of four premises, such as "All A are B," with each of four possible conclusions, such as "Some A are not B," and had to determine the truth value of each conclusion; 16 other subjects received 15 pairs of premises, such as "All B are C. All A are B," and had to determine the truth value of the conclusion. Eleven premise pairs had at least one valid conclusion; four did not. This decomposition of the task permitted us to test assumptions of the theories regarding encoding of single premises separately from assumptions of the theories regarding combination of pairs of premises.

Results. Three sets of results are of primary interest: fits of the quantified models to the data, parameter estimates for the preferred model, and relationships of parameter estimates to ability test scores. All parameter estimation was done by nonlinear regression.

Fits of the alternative models of categorical syllogistic reasoning to the response-choice data were quite variable across models. For those conditions in which all models could be fit to the data, median fits (R^2) were .92 for the transitive-chain model, .68 for the complete-combination model, .54 for the random-combination model, and .50 for an "ideal-subject" model predicting no errors in reasoning. Values of root-mean-square deviation (RMSD) showed comparable patterns. The results of these experiments, considered either singly or as a whole, are unequivocal: The transitive-chain theory gave a better account of the response-choice data than did any competing theory. And the results of the third experiment showed that the assumptions of the transitive-chain theory are plausible both for encoding considered alone and for encoding and combination considered jointly. Viewed by itself without regard to the other theories, the transitive-chain theory also did very well: R^2 was greater than .9 for all but one data set (in which it was .89). Of course, these are not the only alternative theories that have been proposed (see, e.g., Johnson-Laird & Steedman, 1978; Revlin, 1975; Revlis & Leirer, 1978), but they are the alternatives that we were able to quantify.

Although the fits of the transitive-chain theory to the data are most respectable, it is important to note that the theory could be rejected at the .05 level or better in every case. Thus, although the transitive-chain theory is the best of the competing theories we considered and shows respectable fits when considered just on its own, it is not the true theory. The most likely source of inadequacy seemed to us to be the assumption that encoding is always complete and correct (see, e.g., Ceraso & Provitera, 1971; Sternberg, 1979a). We therefore tried relaxing this assumption, estimating parameters for errors in encoding. Generally, this bought us about .02 or .03 point of R^2, and in about half of the data sets it resulted in nonrejection of the quantified model. But the small increases in R^2 did not seem to justify the increase by over 50% in the number of parameters, and so we did not modify the theory.

The value of the p_1 parameter (probability of combining just one pair of encoded representations) varied across experiments and conditions. It was .54 for abstract content, .29 for factual content, .49 for counterfactual content, and .47 for anomalous content. Parameters p_2, p_3, and p_4 were highly correlated and were therefore combined. Their combined value was thus equal to $1 - p_1$. The value of the β_1 parameter ranged from about .7 to .8 across conditions, and the value of β_2 ranged from .92 to .95. The value of c ranged from .37 to .48 across the four conditions. In general, the parameter estimates make good sense.

Consider first the p parameters. The value of p_1 is particularly low for syllogisms with factual content, suggesting that the working memory or other processing limitations that restrict the number of set relations a subject can combine are lessened when the subject is dealing with concrete, factual content. The value of β_1 is always considerably greater than .5, indicating that given a choice between a stronger label and a label that matches the atmosphere of the premises, subjects prefer the label that matches the atmosphere of the premises. One would expect β_2 to be quite close to 1, because it represents subjects' preferences for conclusions that both are stronger and match the atmosphere of the premises. In fact, β_2 is quite close to 1 in each data set. Finally, we can see that when the representation for combined premises contained nonidentical first components, subjects did show pronounced tendencies (indicated by nontrivial values of the c parameter) to label the final representation as indeterminate.

Next consider the relationship between the parameters of the transitive-chain theory and scores on the orthogonal verbal and spatial – abstract principal components. Means of parameter estimates in Experiment 2 were calculated for subjects high (that is, above the median) and low (that is, below the median) on the two components. High- and low-verbal subjects did not differ significantly on any of the parameters. High- and low-spatial – abstract subjects, however, did differ significantly on the p_1 parameter. Thus, subjects higher in spatial – abstract ability were better able to combine more set relations, presumably because of their ability to visualize more representations or the same representations more clearly than did the lower spatial – abstract subjects. There was no a priori theoretical reason to expect any differences in the parameters of the comparison stage, and none occurred.

It is obviously not possible to describe here all the data analyses we performed and presented in the original reports of our results. Worth noting, however, is the fact that we formulated a response latency model from the assumptions of the transitive-chain theory and tested it in Experiment 1, the only one of the three experiments in which latency data were collected. The model accounted for 80% of the variance in the latency data, indicating that even with response latencies as long (mean = 43.59 seconds) and as variable (standard deviation = 5.34 seconds) as those obtained for categorical-syllogism data, it is possible to obtain good fits of observed to predicted latencies.

Conditional syllogisms

The nature of conditional syllogisms

A conditional syllogism comprises three declarative statements. The first statement, called the major premise, expresses a relation between two events – for example, "If A, then B." The second statement, called the minor premise, asserts the truth or falsity of either the antecedent (first term) or consequent (second term) of the major premise – for example, "Not B." The third statement, or conclusion, is either the affirmation or negation of the term not appearing in the minor premise – for example, "Not A."

An interesting parallel exists between conditional syllogisms and categorical syllogisms of the second type, which were mentioned earlier but not further discussed. Consider the syllogism "All A are B. X is not a B. (Therefore) X is not an A." If A is taken to be the sets of states of the world in which event A is true, B is taken to be the set of states of the world in which event B is true, and X is taken to be a particular state of the world, then the conditional and categorical syllogisms become structurally isomorphic. Indeed, the transitive-chain theory assumes that categorical syllogisms of the second type are represented and processed in the same way as conditional syllogisms.

The transitive-chain theory of conditional-syllogistic reasoning

The transitive-chain theory applied to conditional syllogisms (and categorical syllogisms of the second type) is very similar to the theory applied to standard categorical syllogisms. First, the subject encodes both premises completely, using the same format for storing information as was described earlier. Then the subject attempts to construct a transitive chain involving the representations of the second premise and one of the components in the first premise. Because all major premises are universal in problems of these types, there is a maximum of two possible representations of the first premise (see Figure 6.2) and hence two sets of components. If the first rule for constructing transitive chains that was described earlier permits formation of a transitive chain, then the subject forms it and completes solution. If the first rule does not apply, the subject has two choices. He or she can apply the second rule, reason that no definite conclusion exists, and respond that the given conclusion is logically invalid. Or the subject can use indirect proof, trying to form a transitive chain integrating the negation of the conclusion with one of the components in the representation of the major premise. If such a transitive chain can be formed, and if the result contradicts the representation of the second premise, the subject can respond that the conclusion is valid. Otherwise, the conclusion is deemed invalid. The probability of a subject's using indirect proof and thus being able to form a second transitive chain (given that the first rule does not apply in the subject's initial attempt to combine the two premises) depends on the number of negations in the first premise. Parameter t_0 applies when there are no negations in the first premise, t_1 applies when there is one negation, and t_2 applies when there are two negations. Further details about the theory as it applies to conditional syllogisms can be found in Guyote and Sternberg (1981).

Empirical tests of the theory

Method. An experiment was conducted with 50 adults from the New Haven area. The stimuli were 64 syllogisms – half of which presented conditional relations and half of which presented categorical relations isomorphic to the conditional relations. The 32 syllogisms of each type were constructed according to a 2^5 design that was exhaustive with respect to the possible item types. In these syllogisms, it was possible to have as affirmative or negative (a) the first term of the major premise, (b) the second term of the major premise, (c) the single term of the minor premise, and (d) the conclusion; moreover, (e) the single term of the minor premise was the same (disregarding polarity) as either the first or second term of the major premise. The subject's task was to label each syllogism as having either a valid or an invalid conclusion. The content of each syllogism was abstract (with the letters *A* and *B* used as terms). All subjects received all syllogisms blocked by syllogism type and also the verbal reasoning, spatial visualization, and abstract reasoning sections of the Differential Aptitude Test.

Results. Three sets of results are again of primary interest: fits of the quantified model to the data, parameter estimates for the model, and relationships of parameter estimates to ability test scores. It is also of interest to note that the correlation across the 32 item types for the two kinds of syllogisms was .97, suggesting that the processes used to solve the two types of syllogisms were probably quite similar, if not essentially identical.

The transitive-chain theory provided an excellent fit to the response-choice data for both conditional and categorical syllogisms. For the conditional problems, R^2 was .95 and RMSD was .10; for the categorical problems, R^2 was .97 and RMSD was .07. As in the earlier experiments, however, the fit of the theory to each set of data could be rejected at the .05 level, indicating that the transitive-chain theory, although a close approximation to the true theory, is not identical to the true theory.

Parameter estimates for the conditional syllogisms were .36 for p_1, .64 for p_2, .52 for t_0, .48 for t_1, and .15 for t_2. (Parameters p_3 and p_4 are irrelevant in this type of syllogism, because there are never more than two possible set relations to combine; parameters β_1, β_2, and c are irrelevant, because the presentation of only a single conclusion in this experiment obviates the need for a comparison stage.) Parameter estimates for the structually isomorphic categorical syllogisms were .43 for p_1, .57 for p_2, .60 for t_0, .61 for t_1, and .16 for t_2.

Comparison of the value of p_1 in this experiment with that of p_1 in the first experiment with categorical syllogisms of the first kind reveals that with content type held constant, subjects combine more representations for problems of the types used in this experiment than for problems of the type used in that experiment. This result is a sensible one, because the representation of the minor premise in problems of the present type is simpler than the representation of the minor premise in problems of the previous type. In the present problems, the minor premise consists merely of a single term (conditionals) or indication of set membership (categoricals), whereas in the previous problems the minor premise consisted of a quantified relation between two sets.

We assumed that subjects have a fixed amount of processing capacity that they can devote to each problem and that increased consumption of processing capacity for one kind of operation results in decreased processing capacity left over for other kinds of operations. Using this reasoning, we expected the values of t_0, t_1, and t_2 to be successively smaller: The increased processing capacity allocated to comprehension of negations in the major premise was expected to leave decreased processing capacity to allocate to forming a second transitive chain from the negation of the conclusion. Instead, the values of t_0 and t_1 were approximately equal, whereas the value of t_2 was indeed considerably lower. Apparently, double negations cause considerably more difficulty for subjects relative to single negations than do single negations relative to straightforward affirmations.

Next, consider the comparison of orthogonal verbal and spatial–abstract principal component scores for high- and low-verbal subjects and for high and low spatial–abstract subjects. Our general expectation was that parameters reflecting processing capacity (those relevant to the combination stage) would differ in value across ability groups, whereas those parameters merely reflecting biases in response choice (those relevant to the comparison stage) would not differ in value across ability groups. Because the representation of information combined is assumed to be symbolic, our particular expectation was that larger differences would be obtained between the two spatial–abstract groupings than between the two verbal groupings. The results of the studies with categorical syllogisms described earlier confirmed both the general and specific expectations, and the results of the present experiment do as well. As in the previously described experiment, the values of p_1 for high- and low-verbal subjects, .38 and .43, did not differ significantly from each other; the values of p_1 for high and low spatial–abstract groups, .35 and .52, did differ significantly from each other. Similarly, the values of the t parameters (which are combination-stage parameters) did not differ significantly across high- and low-verbal subjects: .54 and .55 for t_0, .50 and .55 for t_1, and .16 and .17 for t_2. They did differ significantly across high- and low-spatial–abstract subjects: .66 and .43 for t_0, .63 and .42 for t_1, and .22 and .11 for t_2. The results of both experiments thus confirm that (a) parameters measuring processing capacity vary with spatial–abstract ability, whereas parameters not measuring processing capacity do not vary with this ability; and (b) no parameters vary with verbal ability. These results provide further support for the kind of symbolic representation and for the identification of processes proposed by the transitive-chain theory.

As in Experiment 1 for categorical syllogisms of the first type, a response latency model was formulated on the basis of the transitive-chain theory. The values of R^2 for this model were .91 for conditional syllogisms and .84 for categorical syllogisms of the second type. The model thus provides a good fit to the latency data.

Conclusions

The conclusions of the research on categorical and conditional syllogisms will be presented in terms of the theoretical questions addressed and the tentative answers provided by the transitive-chain theory.

Representation of premise information. The transitive-chain theory assumes that the categorical information contained in a premise is represented by one or more symbolic representations. Each representation corresponds to a possible relationship between two sets and includes two distinct pieces of information, called components. These components may be combined with each other in various ways to yield different relationships between the two sets.

The patterns of individual differences in four separate experiments provided some evidence for the use of a spatial–abstract representation (although not necessarily the one described) in syllogistic reasoning, as spatial–abstract reasoning ability correlated significantly with the mean number of correct responses in these experiments. Specifically, the ability to combine pairs of representations varied significantly with spatial–abstract reasoning ability but not with verbal reasoning ability.

Combination of premise information. The structure of the symbolic representations in the transitive-chain theory makes it possible to specify a performance algorithm for combining premise information. This algorithm includes two important processes. The first process is the formation of transitive chains; this process involves the rearrangement of components in the original representations. The second process is the application of two simple inferential rules to the transitive chains thus formed.

Sources of difficulty in syllogistic reasoning. The present research identified three major sources of difficulty in the solution of categorical- and conditional-syllogistic reasoning problems. The most important of these is the processing capacity required to combine two symbolic representations. The high level of p_1 for almost all of the data sets attests to subjects' difficulty in combining representations. In almost every case, subjects were as likely to combine just one pair of representations as they were to combine more than one pair. The probability of combining more than one pair of representations seemed to be affected by two problem variables: the content of the premises and the total number of pairs of representations to be combined. It should be noted that one important source of differential item difficulty in syllogistic reasoning – figure effects – is not dealt with by the present theory.

(See Johnson-Laird & Steedman, 1978, for a theoretical account of figure effects.)

Another source of error is the subjects' preferences for working with simpler representations (that is, symmetrical representations and represen- tations with no negatives). Since the values of the p parameters indicate that usually few pairs of representations are combined, we can conclude that pairs of complex representations are rarely combined. As a result, there are many errors in problems where the results of combining complex represen- tations are different from the results of combining simple representations.

A third source of error is found in biases subjects have in how they label the composite representations generated during the combination process. Three specific biases are identified by the theory. The first of these is a bias for strong labels, the second is a bias for labels that match the atmosphere of the premises, and the third a tendency to label a composite representation inde- terminate if it contains nonidentical initial components.

Generality of the processes used in syllogistic reasoning. We found, as did Osherson (1975), that a single theory could account for problems with var- ious types of abstract and concrete content. However, we also found, as did Wilkins (1928), a substantial difference in performance between problems with concrete, factual content and problems with abstract, anomalous, or counterfactual content. This difference was due to a higher probability of combining more than one pair of representations when dealing with factual problems.

The results of the experiments showed that a single theory could account for both categorical and conditional syllogisms, as proposed by Revlis (1975). The symbolic representations in the transitive-chain theory are capa- ble of representing both kinds of information, and the same combination process can be applied to each set of representations. Moreover, the sources of difficulty in categorical and conditional syllogistic reasoning are highly similar. Finally, the pattern of individual differences suggests that spatial– abstract processes are used to solve both types of syllogisms.

The present work replicates the findings of Thurstone (1938) and Frand- sen and Holder (1969) of a relationship between performance on syllogistic reasoning tasks and performance on tests of spatial ability. The present interpretation of this relationship is in terms of both the representations and processes used in syllogistic reasoning. In particular, the proposed represen- tation is an abstract, symbolic one: Combination of information about set relations requires visualization of relationships between pairs of informa- tional components expressed in this representation.

The transitive-chain theory successfully predicted subjects' performance on a wide variety of syllogistic reasoning problems and provided some preliminary answers to some of the major theoretical questions in the literature. It thus seems like a good first step toward understanding the representations and processes subjects used in syllogistic reasoning in particular and in deductive reasoning in general.

7 Crystallized intelligence: acquisition of verbal comprehension

Verbal comprehension refers to a person's ability to understand linguistic materials, such as newspapers, magazines, textbooks, lectures, and the like. Verbal comprehension has been recognized as an integral part of intelligence in both psychometric theories (e.g., Guilford, 1967; Thurstone, 1938; Vernon, 1971) and information-processing theories (e.g., Carroll, 1976; Hunt, 1978; Sternberg, 1980f) and has, under a variety of aliases, been an important topic of research in both differential and experimental psychology.

The theoretical construct of verbal comprehension can be and has been operationalized in a number of different ways. Most often, it is directly measured by tests of vocabulary, reading comprehension, and general information. Indeed, vocabulary has been recognized not only as an excellent measure of verbal comprehension, but also as one of the best single indicators of a person's overall level of intelligence (e.g., Jensen, 1980; Matarazzo, 1972). The importance of verbal comprehension in general and of vocabulary in particular to the measurement of verbal intelligence is shown by the fact that both of the two major individual scales of intelligence – the Stanford – Binet and the Wechsler – contain vocabulary items and by the fact that many group tests also contain vocabulary items (which may be presented in any of a number of forms, e.g., synonyms, antonyms, verbal analogies with very-low-frequency terms, and so on). Because of its importance both in the theory and measurement of intelligence and in everyday interactions with the environment, it seems important to understand the antecedents of observable individual differences in vocabulary levels.

Our theory of verbal comprehension comprises two parts. The first part is a theory of how verbal comprehension develops, in other words, how one acquires one's current level of verbal skills. The second part is a theory of information processing in verbal comprehension, that is, of the skills one uses in one's current verbal functioning. Thus, the first theory accounts for how "crystallized" ability becomes crystallized; the second theory accounts for how crystallized ability is utilized in information processing. Each of

214

these two subtheories of verbal comprehension as a whole will be considered in turn, with acquisition considered in this chapter and real-time processing considered in the next chapter.

In order for my presentation of the theory of the acquisition of verbal comprehension skills to be fully meaningful, it must first be placed in the context of other efforts toward the same or similar goals. There have been three major approaches to understanding the origins and development of verbal comprehension. These three major approaches are considered briefly below.

Alternative cognitive approaches to the acquisition of verbal comprehension skills

The three major approaches to the acquisition of verbal comprehension skills are a "knowledge-based" approach, a "bottom–up" approach, and a "top–down" approach. The knowledge-based approach deals with the role of prior information in the acquisition of new information. The bottom–up approach deals with speed of execution of certain very basic mechanistic cognitive processes. The top–down approach deals with higher-order utilization of cues in complex verbal materials. Consider each of these three approaches and some of the research that has been done under each.

The knowledge-based approach

The knowledge-based approach assigns a central role to old knowledge in the acquisition of new knowledge. Although "knowledge" is often referred to in the sense of domain-specific information, the knowledge-based approach can also encompass research focusing on general world knowledge, knowledge of structures or classes of text (as in story grammars), and knowledge about strategies for knowledge acquisition and application (see, e.g., Bisanz & Voss, 1981). Proponents of this approach differ in the respective roles they assign to knowledge and process in the acquisition of new knowledge. A fairly strong version of the approach is taken by Keil (1984), who argues for the primacy of knowledge over process in cognitive development.

Proponents of the knowledge-based approach usually cite instances of differences between expert and novice performance – in verbal and other domains – that seem to derive more from knowledge differences than from processing differences. For example, Keil (1984) suggests that development in the use of metaphor and in the use of defining features of words seems to be due more to differential knowledge states than to differential use of processes or speed of process execution. Chi (1978) has shown that whether children's recall performance is better than that of adults depends upon the knowledge domain in which the recall takes place and particularly upon the relative expertise of the children and adults in the respective domains. In related research, Chase and Simon (1973) found that differences between expert and novice performance in chess seemed largely to be due to differential knowledge structures rather than to processes (but see Charness, 1981).

I have no argument with the position that the knowledge base is highly important in understanding differences in current performance between experts and novices in both verbal and nonverbal domains. But accounts that slight the role of information processing in the development of expertise seem to beg an important question, namely, that of how the differences in knowledge states came about in the first place. For example, why did some people acquire better vocabularies than others? Or in the well-studied domain of chess, why is it that of two individuals given equally intensive and extensive exposure to the game, one will acquire the knowledge structures needed for expertise and the other will not? In sum, I accept the importance of old knowledge in the acquisition of new knowledge (indeed, this is what the "selective comparison" knowledge-acquisition component discussed in Chapter 4 is all about). But I do not believe the overemphasis on process that characterized some previous research should be replaced by an overemphasis on knowledge in present research. Rather, it should be recognized that knowledge and process work interactively in complex ways. What is needed is to understand what these ways are.

Bottom – up approach

Bottom – up research has emerged from the tradition of investigation initiated by Earl Hunt (e.g., Hunt, 1978, 1980; Hunt, Lunneborg, & Lewis, 1975) and has been followed up by a number of other investigators (e.g., Jackson & McClelland, 1979; Keating & Bobbitt, 1978; see also Perfetti & Lesgold, 1977, for a related approach). According to Hunt (1978), two types of processes underlie verbal comprehension ability – knowledge-based processes and mechanistic (information-free) processes; Hunt's approach has emphasized the latter kind of process. Hunt et al. (1975) studied three aspects of what they called "current information processing" that they believed to be key determinants of individual differences in developed verbal ability. These were:

(a) sensitivity of overlearned codes to arousal by incoming stimulus information, (b) the accuracy with which temporal tags can be assigned, and hence order information can be processed, and (c) the speed with which the internal representations in STM [short term memory] and intermediate term memory (ITM, memory for events occurring over minutes) can be created, integrated, and altered. (P. 197)

The basic hypothesis motivating this work is that individuals varying in verbal ability differ even in these low-level mechanistic skills – skills that are free from any contribution of disparate knowledge or experience. Intelligence tests are hypothesized to measure indirectly these basic information-processing skills by measuring directly the products of these skills, both in terms of their past contribution to the acquisition and storage of knowledge (such as vocabulary) and their present contribution in the current processing of information.

For example, in a typical experiment, subjects are presented with the Posner and Mitchell (1967) letter-matching task. The task comprises two experimental conditions, a physical-match condition and a name-match condition. In the physical-match condition, subjects are presented with pairs of letters that either are or are not physical matches (e.g., "AA" or "bb" versus "Aa" or "Ba"). In the name-match condition, subjects are presented with pairs of letters that either are or are not name matches (e.g., "Aa," "BB," or "bB" versus "Ab," "ba," or "bA"). Subjects must identify the letter pair either as a physical match (or mismatch) or as a name match (or mismatch) as rapidly as possible. The typical finding in these experiments is that the difference between mean name-match and physical-match times within a group of subjects correlates about -.3 with scores on a test of verbal ability.

The finding described above seems to be widely replicable, but its interpretation is a matter of dispute (Carroll, 1981; Hogaboam & Pellegrino, 1978; Sternberg, 1981g, 1981j). I have been and remain concerned that .3-level correlations are abundant in both the abilities and personality literatures (indeed, they are rather low as ability correlations go) and provide a relatively weak basis for causal inference. A further concern is that most of the studies that have been done on the name- minus physical-match difference have not used adequate discriminant validation procedures. When such procedures are used and perceptual speed is considered as well as verbal ability, this difference seems to be much more strongly related to perceptual speed than it is to verbal ability (Lansman, Donaldson, Hunt, & Yantis, 1982; Cornelius, Willis, Blow, & Baltes, 1983), although these findings are subject to alternative interpretations. Thus, the obtained correlation with verbal ability may reflect, at least in part, variance shared with perceptual abilities of the kind that the letter-matching task would seem more likely to measure. But whatever may be the case here, it seems likely that speed of lexical access plays *some* role in verbal comprehension, and what remains to be clarified is just what this role is.

Top–down approach

Top–down processing refers to expectation- or inference-driven processing, or to "knowledge-based" processing, to use Hunt's (1978) terminology.

Top–down processing has been an extremely popular focus for research in the past decade, with many researchers attempting to identify and predict the sorts of inferences a person is likely to draw from a text and how these inferences (or lack thereof) will affect text comprehension (see, e.g., Kintsch & van Dijk, 1978; Rieger, 1975; Rumelhart, 1980; Schank & Abelson, 1977). Usually, top–down researchers look at how people combine information actually present in the text with their own store of world knowledge to create a new whole representing the meaning of the text (e.g., Bransford, Barclay, & Franks, 1972).

The first of a small handful of investigators who looked at the use of inference in the acquisition of word meanings from context were Werner and Kaplan (1952), who proposed that learning from context provides a major source of vocabulary development. They devised a task in which subjects were presented with an imaginary word followed by six sentences using that word. The subjects' task was to guess the meaning of the word on the basis of the contextual cues they were given. They found that performance improves gradually with age, although the various processes underlying performance did not necessarily change gradually. They did not, however, provide an explicit model of what these processes are.

Daalen-Kapteijns and Elshout-Mohr (1981) pursued the Werner–Kaplan approach by having subjects think aloud while solving Werner–Kaplan-type problems. They found, among other things, that high- and low-verbal subjects learn word meanings differently, with high verbals performing a deeper analysis of the possibilities for a new word's meaning than was performed by low-verbal subjects. In particular, the high-verbal subjects used a well-formulated strategy for figuring out word meaning, whereas the low-verbal subjects seemed not to.

Keil (1981) presented children in grades kindergarten, 2, and 4 with simple stories in which an unfamiliar word was described by a single paragraph. An example of such a story is "*Throstles* are great, except when they have to be fixed. And they have to be fixed very often. But it's usually very easy to fix throstles." Subjects were asked what else they knew about the new word (here, *throstle*), and what sorts of things the new word described. Keil found that even the youngest children could make sensible inferences about the general categories denoted by the new terms and about the properties the terms might reasonably have (see also Keil, 1979, 1981).

Jensen (1980) has suggested that vocabulary is an excellent measure of intelligence "because the acquisition of word meanings is highly dependent on the deduction of meaning from the contexts in which the words are encountered" (p. 146). Marshalek (1981) has tested this hypothesis using a faceted vocabulary test, although he did not directly measure learning from context. He found that subjects with low reasoning ability did, in fact, have major difficulties inferring meanings of words. Moreover, reasoning was related to vocabulary measures at the lower end of the vocabulary difficulty distribution but not at the higher end. Together, these findings suggest that a certain level of reasoning ability may be prerequisite for extraction of word meaning. Above this level, the importance of reasoning begins to decrease rapidly.

Summary

To summarize, I have described three basic approaches to understanding the cognitive bases of verbal comprehension. These approaches – a knowledge-based one, a bottom—up one, and a top–down one – are complementary, and ultimately they would all have to be incorporated to understand fully the nature and development of verbal comprehension. In the next section, I present our own approach to understanding the antecedents and development of verbal comprehension skills.

Theory of learning from context

Our theory of the development of verbal skills emphasizes learning from context (see Sternberg, 1984e; Sternberg & Powell, 1983; Sternberg, Powell, & Kaye, 1983). We believe that the ability to infer the meanings of unfamiliar words from context deserves a prominent place within a discussion of verbal comprehension for three reasons. First, a theory describing how people use context to infer the meanings of words could tell us much about vocabulary-building skills. Identifying what types of information people of different ability levels use to construct a tentative definition of a word and how additional information influences a working definition of a word could also tell us about how to train vocabulary-acquisition skills. Second, a theory of learning from context can help explain why vocabulary is the single best predictor of verbal intelligence. Our hypothesis is that learning from context reflects important vocabulary-acquisition skills, the net products of which are measured by the extent of one's vocabulary. Thus, according to our view, vocabulary tests are such good predictors of one's overall verbal intelligence because they reflect one's ability to acquire new information. Third, a theory of learning from context is useful in illuminating the relationship between the more fluid, inferential aspects of verbal intelligence, usually measured by tests of verbal analogies, and the more crystallized, knowledge-based aspects of verbal intelligence, usually measured by vocabulary tests (see Horn & Cattell, 1966). Learning from context thus provides a way of integrating the two aspects of verbal ability – comprehension and vocabulary – and of placing vocabulary acquisition within the framework of general cognitive theories of language comprehension.

Two basic ideas underlie our theory of learning from context. The first idea pertains to why some verbal concepts are easier to learn than others: The difficulty of learning a new verbal concept is in large part a function of the degree of facilitation (or inhibition) of learning provided by the context in which the new verbal concept is embedded; the same or very similar contextual elements that facilitate (or inhibit) learning of the concept are hypothesized also to facilitate (or inhibit) later retrieval of the concept and also its transfer to new situations. The second idea pertains to why some individuals are better at learning verbal concepts than are others: Individual differences in verbal comprehension can be traced in large part to differences in people's abilities to exploit contextual elements that facilitate learning and to be wary of contextual elements that inhibit learning; the same or very similar sources of individual differences are hypothesized to be involved in people's differential abilities later to retrieve verbal concepts and to transfer these concepts appropriately to new situations.

The theory distinguishes between those aspects of vocabulary acquisition that lie strictly outside the individual, that is, contextual cues present in the verbal context that convey various types of information about the word, and those aspects of vocabulary acquisition that lie at least partially within the individual, that is, mediating variables that affect the perceived usefulness of the contextual cues. The contextual cues determine the quality of a definition that theoretically can be inferred for a word from a given context. The mediating variables specify those constraints imposed by the relationship between the previously unknown word and the context in which the word occurs that affect how well a given set of cues will be actually utilized, by an individual, in a particular task and situation. Moreover, the theory specifies the processes by which the cues and mediating variables are utilized. These various aspects of the theory will now be explained in turn.

Theory of decoding of external context

During the course of one's reading (or other encounters with words), one commonly comes upon words whose meanings are unfamiliar. When such words are encountered, one may attempt to utilize the external context in which the words occur in order to figure out the meanings of the words. Our theory specifies external cues, mediating variables, and processes that influence the likelihood that these meanings will be correctly inferred.

Context cues. Context cues are hints contained in a passage that facilitate (or, in theory and sometimes in practice, impede) deciphering the meaning of an unknown word. We propose that context cues can be classified into eight categories, depending upon the kind of information they provide. These context cues include the following:

1. *Temporal cues.* Cues regarding the duration or frequency of X (the unknown word) or regarding when X can occur; alternatively, cues describing X as a temporal property (such as duration or frequency) of some Y (usually a known word in the passage).

2. *Spatial cues.* Cues regarding the general or specific location of X or possible locations in which X can sometimes be found; alternatively, cues describing X as a spatial property (such as general or specific location) of some Y.

3. *Value cues.* Cues regarding the worth or desirability of X or regarding the kinds of affects X arouses; alternatively, cues describing X as a value (such as worth or desirability) of some Y.

4. *Stative descriptive cues.* Cues regarding properties of X (such as size, shape, color, odor, feel, etc.); alternatively, cues describing X as a stative descriptive property (such as shape or color) of some Y.

5. *Functional descriptive cues.* Cues regarding possible purposes of X, actions X can perform, or potential uses of X; alternatively, cues describing X as a possible purpose, action, or use of Y.

6. *Causal/enablement cues.* Cues regarding possible causes of or enabling conditions for X; alternatively, cues describing X as a possible cause or enabling condition for Y.

7. *Class membership cues.* Cues regarding one or more classes to which X belongs or other members of one or more classes of which X is a member; alternatively, cues describing X as a class of which Y is a member.

8. *Equivalence cues.* Cues regarding the meaning of X or contrasts (such as antonymy) to the meaning of X; alternatively, cues describing X as the meaning (or a contrast in meaning) of some Y.

Alternative and related classification schemes have been proposed in the past by Ames (1966), McCullough (1958), Miller and Johnson-Laird (1976), and Sternberg (1974), among others.

An example of the use of some of these cues in textual analysis might help concretize our descriptive framework. Consider the sentence "At dawn, the *blen* arose on the horizon and shone brightly." This sentence contains several external contextual cues that could facilitate one's inferring that *blen* probably means *sun.* "At dawn" provides a temporal cue, describing when the arising of the *blen* occurred; "arose" provides a functional descriptive cue, describing an action that a *blen* could perform; "on the horizon" provides a spatial cue, describing where the arising of the *blen* took place; "shone" provides another functional descriptive cue, describing a second action a *blen* could do; finally, "brightly" provides a stative descriptive cue, describing a property (brightness) of the shining of the *blen.* With all these different cues, it is no wonder that most people would find it very easy to figure out that the neologism *blen* is a synonym for the familiar word *sun*.

We make no claim that the categories we have suggested are mutually exclusive, exhaustive, or independent in their functioning. Nor do we claim that they in any sense represent a "true" categorization scheme of context cues. We have found, however, that this classification scheme is useful in understanding subjects' strategies in deriving meanings of words from context. Not every type of cue will be present in every context, and even when a given cue is present, our theory proposes that the usefulness of the cue will be mediated by the sorts of variables to be described in the next section.

Mediating variables. Whereas the contextual cues describe the types of information that might be used to infer the meaning of a word from a given verbal context, they do not at all address the problems of recognition of the applicability of a description to a given concept, weaning out irrelevant information, or integration of the information gleaned into a coherent model of the word's meaning. For this reason, a set of mediating variables is also proposed that specifies relations between a previously unknown word and the passage in which it occurs and that mediates the usefulness of the contextual cues. Thus, whereas the contextual cues specify the particular kinds of information that might be available for an individual to use to figure out the meanings of unfamiliar words, the mediating variables listed below specify those variables that can affect, either positively or negatively, the application of the contextual cues present in a given situation.

1. *Number of occurrences of the unknown word.* A given kind of cue may be absent or of little use in a given occurrence of a previously unknown word but may be present or of considerable use in another occurrence. Multiple occurrences of an unknown word increase the number of available cues and can actually increase the usefulness of individual cues if readers integrate information obtained from cues surrounding the multiple occurrences of the word. For example, the meaning of a given temporal cue may be enhanced by a spatial cue associated with a subsequent appearance of the unknown word, or the temporal cue may gain in usefulness if it appears more than once in conjunction with the unknown word. On the other hand, multiple occurrences of an unfamiliar word can also be detrimental if the reader has difficulty integrating the information gained from cues surrounding separate appearances of the word or if only peripheral features of the word are reinforced and are therefore incorrectly interpreted as being of central importance to the meaning of the unfamiliar word.

2. *Variability of contexts in which multiple occurrences of the unknown word appear.* Different types of contexts – for example, different kinds of subject matter or different writing styles, and even just different contexts of a

given type, such as two different illustrations within a given text of how a word can be used – are likely to supply different types of information about the unknown word. Variability of contexts increases the likelihood that a wide range of types of cues will be supplied about a given word and thus increases the probability that a reader will get a full picture of the scope of a given word's meaning. In contrast, mere repetition of a given unknown word in essentially the same context as that in which it previously appeared is unlikely to be as helpful as a variable-context repetition, because few or no really new cues are provided regarding the word's meaning. Variability can also present a problem in some situations and for some individuals: If the information is presented in a way that makes it difficult to integrate across appearances of the word, or if a given individual has difficulties in making such integrations, then the variable repetitions may actually obfuscate rather than clarify the word's meaning. In some situations and for some individuals, a stimulus overload may occur, resulting in reduced rather than increased understanding.

3. *Importance of the unknown word to understanding the context in which it is embedded.* If a given unknown word is judged to be necessary for understanding the surrounding material in which it is embedded, the reader's incentive for figuring out the word's meaning is increased. If the word is judged to be unimportant to understanding what one is reading (or hearing), one is unlikely to invest any great effort in figuring out what the word means. Whereas in explicit vocabulary-training situations the individual may always be motivated to infer a word's meanings, in real-world situations this will not be the case. Thus, a question of interest from the perspective of our model is the extent to which an individual reader can recognize which words are important to a passage and which are not. In some cases, it really may not be worth the individual's time to figure out a given word's meaning. It is possible to distinguish between importance at different levels of text organization. We distinguish between the sentence and paragraph levels, that is, the importance of a given word to understanding the meaning of the sentence in which it occurs and to understanding the meaning of the paragraph in which it occurs. The ability to recognize the importance of a word to understanding context may be seen as one form of comprehension monitoring of the form studied by Markman (1977, 1979, 1981), Flavell (1981), Collins and Smith (1982), and others.

4. *Helpfulness of surrounding context in understanding the meaning of the unknown word.* A given cue can be differentially helpful depending upon the nature of the word whose meaning is to be inferred and upon the location of the cue in the text relative to the word whose meaning is to be inferred. Consider first an example of how the nature of the word can affect cue helpfulness. A temporal cue describing when a *diurnal* event occurs would

probably be more helpful than a spatial cue describing where the event occurs in aiding an individual to figure out that *diurnal* means *daily*. In contrast, a spatial cue would probably be more helpful than a temporal cue in figuring out that *ing* is a low-lying pasture. It is unrealistic to expect a given kind of cue to be equally helpful in figuring out the meanings of all kinds of words. Consider now an example of how the location of the cue in the text relative to the word whose meaning is to be inferred can affect cue helpfulness. If a given cue occurs in close proximity to the word whose meaning is unknown, then there is probably a relatively high likelihood that the cue will be recognized as relevant to inferring the unknown word's meaning. If the cue is separated from the known word by a substantial portion of text, the relevance of the cue may never be recognized; indeed, the cue may be misinterpreted as relevant to an unknown word to which it is more proximal. The helpfulness of context cues may also be mediated by whether the cue comes before or after the unknown word. Rubin (1976), for example, found that context occurring before the placement of a blank in a cloze test was more helpful to figuring out what word should go in the blank than was context occurring after the placement of the blank.

5. *Density of unknown words.* If a reader is confronted with a high density of previously unknown words, he or she may be overwhelmed and be unwilling or unable to use available cues to best advantage. When the density of unknown words is high, relatively more text is occupied by unknown and therefore unhelpful words (for figuring out meanings of other words), and it can be difficult to discern which of the cues that are available apply to which of the words that are unknown. In such a situation, utilization of a given cue may depend upon figuring out the meaning of some other unknown word, in which case the usefulness of that cue (and very likely of other cues as well) is decreased.

6. *Concreteness of the unknown word and the surrounding context.* Concrete concepts are generally easier to apprehend, in part because they have a simpler meaning structure. Familiar concrete concepts such as *tree, chair,* and *pencil* are relatively easy to define in ways that would satisfy most people; familiar abstract concepts such as *truth, love,* and *justice,* however, are extremely difficult to define in ways that would satisfy large numbers of people. Indeed, each of these abstract concepts has been the subject of multiple books, none of which has provided "definitive" definitions. Moreover, the ease of inferring the meaning of the word will depend upon the concreteness of the surrounding description. A concrete concept such as *ing* might appear more opaque embedded in a passage about the nature of reality than it would embedded in a passage about the nature of food sources; similarly, an abstract concept such as *pulchritude* (beauty) might be more easily appre-

hended in a passage about fashion models than in one about eternal versus ephemeral qualities.

7. *Usefulness of previously known information in cue utilization.* Inevitably, the usefulness of a cue will depend upon the extent to which past knowledge can be brought to bear upon the cue and its relation to the unknown word. The usefulness of prior information will depend in large part upon a given individual's ability to retrieve the information, to recognize its relevance, and then to apply it appropriately.

Knowledge-acquisition components and representation of information. The theory of external decontextualization also relies upon three knowledge-acquisition components. These are the same ones discussed in more general terms earlier in the book.

1. *Selective encoding.* Selective encoding involves sifting out relevant from irrelevant information. When new words are presented in actual contexts, cues relevant to decontextualization are embedded within large amounts of irrelevant information. A critical task facing the individual is that of sifting out the "wheat from the chaff": recognizing just what information in the passage is relevant for word decontextualization.

2. *Selective combination.* Selective combination involves combining selectively encoded information in such a way as to form an integrated, plausible definition of the previously unknown word. Simply sifting out the relevant cues is not enough to arrive at a tentative definition of the word: One must know how to combine the cues into an integrated knowledge representation.

3. *Selective comparison.* Selective comparison involves relating newly acquired information to information acquired in the past. Deciding what information to encode and how to combine it does not occur in a vacuum. Rather, encoding and combination of new knowledge is guided by retrieval of old information. A cue will be all but useless if it cannot somehow be related to past knowledge.

Verbal information is theorized to be represented in terms of a network-type model that is similar in some respects to the node models found in Rumelhart and Norman's (1975) and Collins and Loftus's (1975) models of semantic memory. A given concept is represented as the "center" of a network describing the concept. Nodes emanate from the concept describing its properties. Nodes for different concepts are connected via the concept names, which serve as the origin for nodes with descriptive attributes. Unlike in other network models, the kinds of nodes extending from the concept, and from other nodes, correspond to the properties of cues used to understand word meanings, as specified by the proposed theory of cue utilization. For

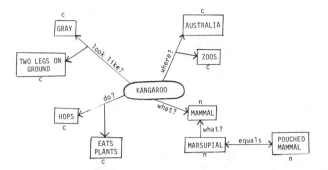

Figure 7.1. A hypothetical individual's mental representation of information according to the proposed theory. Attributes with the letter *n* adjacent to them are believed by the individual to be necessary or defining attributes. Attributes with the letter *c* are believed by the individual to be characteristic, or nonnecessary attributes of the word. (From "A theory of knowledge acquisition in the development of verbal concepts," by Robert J. Sternberg, 1984, *Developmental Review, 4,* p. 123. Copyright by Academic Press. Reprinted by permission of the publisher.)

example, spatial cues are fed into (where?) nodes, functional-descriptive cues are fed into (do?) nodes, stative descriptive cues are fed into (look like?) nodes, class membership cues are fed into (what?) nodes, equality cues are fed into (equals?) nodes, and so on. Each node has associated with it both an attribute (e.g., an attribute for (look like?) might be "gray") and an identification of the attribute as being necessary, sufficient, or characteristic of the concept. An example of this form of representation for "kangaroo" is shown in Figure 7.1.

How is the proposed representation developed during the course of acquisition of a verbal concept? This question is addressable in terms of the processes, cues, and moderating variables in the proposed theory. A general description of the development of representations will be presented first, followed by a specific example of how this development occurs. It is assumed that initial processing is done sentence by sentence, although further processing may follow if a subject reviews a passage and uses higher-order units (e.g., pairs of sentences) as a basis for further understanding. A person begins building up a representation of text as soon as he or she starts reading the text.

The subject begins selective encoding of information about the to-be-defined (target) word from the first sentence in which the word appears. The target word at this point becomes the center point of a new network; characteristic and defining attributes can "grow" into appropriate nodes in this network, which is constructed in working memory. This information also activates matching information stored in long-term memory networks. This activated knowledge then influences what further facts in the passage will be selectively encoded and fed into the nodes in the newly forming network. As more information about the new word is selectively encoded and incorporated into the new network, the subject's activated knowledge base in long-term memory is reduced: Concepts that might have helped define the word are now found to be excluded by the additional information and hence can be dropped from active consideration. When the subject has finished processing all of the information in the passage, he or she will select concepts from the long-term memory knowledge base whose nodes are still activated. The full network structure for these concepts is then compared to the newly formed network structure. If no such concepts exist (e.g., all concepts in long-term memory have been excluded as possible meanings of the word), the subject will either reprocess the passage or else view the new network structure as corresponding to a new concept nonidentical to any already in long-term memory. If one or more such concepts exist, the subject will compare defining attributes of the target word's network to defining attributes of the networks for each of the possible meanings. The subject will then select the activated concept that has the most defining attributes in common with the target concept, create a new concept, or else seek further information. A new concept will be based on an agglomeration of the new concept with that concept in long-term memory that is closest to the new one, appropriately modified so as to take into account those nodes in the new representation that do not match the nodes of the old representation. So, for example, if *ing* is found to be closest in its representation to *pasture* but to differ from *pasture* in having nodes describing the *ing* as low-lying, then *ing* will be defined as "a pasture that is low-lying." In some instances, the given information may allow the individual to propose a definition that he or she knows is at a more general level than the meaning of the word: There was simply insufficient information fully to restrict the meaning of the new concept.

Errors in understanding the meaning of a new word can occur in at least three ways. First, information about the new word's meaning as provided in the text will inevitably be incomplete. Thus, one may not have sufficient basis for choosing among alternative possible meanings stored in long-term memory, or one may provide a new but incomplete definition. Second, information about the new word's meaning may be misencoded. A cue in the passage may be misconstrued, so that the representation one builds up is simply wrong. Third, information in the passage may be properly encoded but lead to an incorrect representation of the new word because the information is misleading. In such a case, cues may actually serve to lead a subject astray.

The ideas expressed above can be made more explicit and concrete by considering an example of how the representation of a word is constructed. An illustration of the development of a representation of a word is shown in

Figure 7.2. It is important to note that the buildup shown is for a given hypothetical individual: There will be individual differences, and probably major ones, in the representational buildups of various people as a function of their decontextualization skills and prior knowledge. The subject is shown the following brief story about a *blumen* and is asked to figure out what a *blumen* is.

He first saw a *blumen* during his trip to Australia. He had just arrived from a business trip to India and felt very tired. Looking out at the plain, he saw the *blumen* hop across it. It was a typical marsupial, getting its food by chewing on the surrounding plants. Squinting because of the bright sunlight and an impending headache, he noticed a young *blumen* securely fastened in an opening in front of its mother.

In step 1 (see Figure 7.2), the subject considers the first sentence in the passage and *selectively encodes* two facts: that the individual saw a *blumen* and that he first saw it on a trip to Australia. The first cue, a stative – descriptive cue, indicates that the *blumen* is visible; the second cue, a spatial – locative cue, indicates that *blumens* can be found in Australia. In *selective combination*, the representation of *blumen* grows two nodes, a (look like?) node for the stative – descriptive cue and a (where?) node for the spatial cue. In *selective comparison*, the subject's knowledge about things that can be seen in Australia is activated in long-term memory. The names (network central entries) of these concepts are placed into working memory and the subject constructs a list corresponding to possible meanings of *blumen*. This list will be reduced in successive steps as entries in long-term memory and even classes of entries are found to be irrelevant to the new word's meaning. As each entry is deleted from the list of possible meanings in working memory, the nodes in long-term memory corresponding to that entry are deactivated.

In step 2, the subject considers the second sentence. Because the subject is now using his or her activated knowledge to guide what should be selectively encoded, none of the information in this sentence is perceived as relevant to the task at hand (figuring out the meaning of *blumen*). The reason for this is that the new information is uninformative (again, for *this* individual) with respect to *blumens* and their visibility in Australia. No further encoding, combination, or comparison is done.

In step 3, the subject considers the third sentence, *selectively encoding* that *blumens* can be found on plains (a spatial cue related to the subject's knowledge that plains exist in Australia) and that *blumens* hop (a functional – descriptive cue related to the subject's knowledge about what some animals do in Australia). The subject now *selectively combines* the new information with the information already in the *blumen* network, adding two new nodes. The subject grows "on plains" out of "Australia," so that, according to the modified network, *blumens* are now found on plains in Australia. "Hops" is fed into the (do?) node. Because of this newly encoded and combined information, the subject can eliminate some of the names of concepts that he or she is holding in working memory. In particular, by *selectively comparing* the new information with the activated information in long-term memory corresponding to the names of concepts being considered as possible word meanings in working memory, the subject can eliminate all names that do not represent objects that hop or that are found on plains.

In step 4, the subject *selectively encodes* the facts that a *blumen* is a marsupial and that it chews plants. (For someone who didn't know what a marsupial is, the information might be ignored, or an attempt might be made to infer the meaning of *marsupial* from context.) In *selective combination*, two further nodes are grown, a further (do?) node and a (what?) node. The two new attributes that have been added to the network can be used by the subject to reduce further the number of concept names he or she is holding in working memory. In particular, the subject can now eliminate names of objects whose network representations in long-term memory (which are still activated) do not represent marsupials that chew plants. Thus, *selective comparison* continues to reduce the relevant prior knowledge base at the same time that selective encoding and combination are increasing the relevant new knowledge base.

In step 5, the subject fails to selectively encode any of the information in the sentence as relevant to the meaning of *blumen*. This failure may derive either from his or her not realizing that there is relevant information or from his or her not knowing how to use the given information. This failure illustrates how some of the moderating variables specified by the proposed theory can affect the buildup of a word representation. With successive presentations of the word, the chances are improved that the representation will be more nearly complete; one presentation often will not be enough to achieve anything approaching a complete representation.

The subject now checks whether there are any concept names left in working memory that meet all of the constraints of the representation that he or she has built up. If there is only one such concept, the subject compares defining attributes of the network representation corresponding to the already stored word. If the attributes match or pass a criterion for being close enough, the subject defines the new word in terms of the old, in this case, *kangaroo*. If the attributes do not match or are not close enough to accept the old name as a definition, the subject either offers a definition that represents a new concept different from any already stored in long-term memory or else goes back to the passage and tries to obtain further information. If multiple old concept names are left in working memory, the subject compares the defining attributes of the new concept to the defining attributes of all of the

1. He first saw a BLUMEN during his trip to Australia.

   a. Selectively encode

        BLUMEN (saw,   Australia)
                 ↑   ↑
             stative   spatial
          descriptive   locative
             ↓   ↓
            visible   in Australia
              n   c

   b. Selectively combine

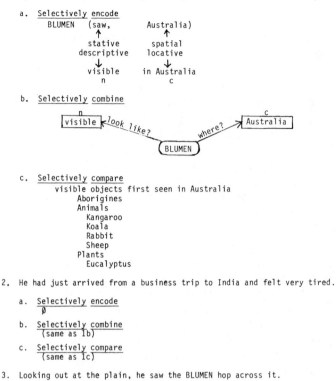

   c. Selectively compare
         visible objects first seen in Australia
             Aborigines
             Animals
               Kangaroo
               Koala
               Rabbit
               Sheep
             Plants
               Eucalyptus

2. He had just arrived from a business trip to India and felt very tired.

   a. Selectively encode
      Ø

   b. Selectively combine
      (same as 1b)

   c. Selectively compare
      (same as 1c)

3. Looking out at the plain, he saw the BLUMEN hop across it.

   a. Selectively encode

        BLUMEN (at the plain,   hop)
                 ↑   ↑
             spatial   functional
              ↓   descriptive
          on plains   ↓
             c   hops
                        c

   b. Selectively combine

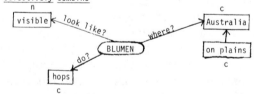

   c. Selectively compare
         visible objects first seen in Australia, that hop across plains
             ~~Aborigines~~
             Animals
               Kangaroo
               ~~Koala~~
               Rabbit
               ~~Sheep~~
             ~~Plants~~
               ~~Eucalyptus~~

4. It was a typical marsupial, getting its food by chewing on the surrounding plants.

a. Selectively encode

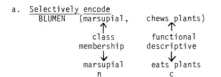

BLUMEN (marsupial, chews plants)
↑   ↑
class   functional
membership   descriptive
↓   ↓
marsupial   eats plants
n   c

b. Selectively combine

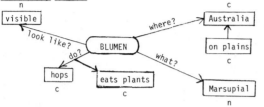

c. Selectively compare
   visible objects first seen in Australia, that hop across plains, are
   marsupials, and chew plants
        Animals
        Kangaroo
        ~~Rabbit~~

5. Squinting because of the bright sunlight and an impending headache, he noticed
   a young BLUMEN securely fastened in an opening in front of its mother.

   a. Selectively encode
      Ø

   b. Selectively combine
      (same as 4b)

   c. Selectively compare

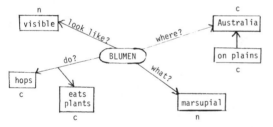

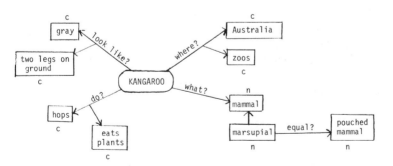

Figure 7.2. A hypothetical individual's buildup of a mental representation for a story
about a *blumen* (kangaroo). Attributes with the letter *n* adjacent to them are believed
to be necessary by the individual; attributes with the letter *c* adjacent to them are
believed by the individual to be characteristic ones. (From "A theory of knowledge
acquisition in the development of verbal concepts," by Robert J. Sternberg, 1984,
Developmental Review, 4, pp. 126–127. Copyright by Academic Press. Reprinted by
permission of the publisher.)

remaining old concepts and selects the best of the options if it is good enough (over criterion); if it is not good enough (i.e., if it is under criterion), the subject either defines a wholly new concept or else goes back to the passage for further information. Again, this new concept will be a modification of the best old-fitting concept, with the modification reflecting the mismatch between the new concept and the old one.

In conclusion, definitions of new words are constructed by adding defining and characteristic attributes onto new network representations at the same time that one reduces in size a list of possible meanings for the new word. The reduction is accomplished by comparing attributes of the new word to attributes of the listed words (as stored in long-term memory) and removing from the list words whose attributes do not match the attributes of the new word. Eventually, one is left with a built-up representation of the new word and a usually reduced list of possible meanings. One then compares in working memory attributes of the new word to attributes of each of the words on the reduced list and either (a) chooses one as the correct meaning if the match is close enough, (b) comes to view the new word as a new concept because it does not match any old concepts in memory, or (c) returns to the passage for more information. Should one see the word again in another context, one can return to the building-up process and use the new information to refine and elaborate the network representation of the new word. This refinement and elaboration is more likely to lead to a correct definition in the final comparison process whereby defining attributes of new and old words are compared.

Data testing the theory of external decontextualization

As of the present, we have some preliminary data regarding the validity of the proposed theory. In particular, we have only tested the cue-utilization and moderating-variable subtheories (Sternberg & Neuse, 1983; Sternberg & Powell, 1983).

The theory was first tested (Sternberg & Powell, 1983) by asking 123 high school students to read 32 passages each of roughly 125 words in length that contained embedded within them from 1 to 4 extremely-low-frequency words. Thirty-seven such words (all nouns) were used in the passages; each target word could appear from 1 to 4 times, resulting in 71 presentations altogether. Passages were equally divided among four different writing styles: literary, newspaper, scientific, and historical. An additional sample passage was written in the literary style. Consider it here as an example of the kinds of passages used:

Two ill-dressed people – the one a tired woman of middle years and the other a tense young man – sat around a fire where the common meal was almost ready. The mother, Tanith, peered at her son through the *oam* of the bubbling stew. It had been a long time since his last *ceilidh* and Tobar had changed greatly; where once he had seemed all legs and clumsy joints, he now was well-formed and in control of his hard, young body. As they ate, Tobar told of his past year, re-creating for Tanith how he had wandered long and far in his quest to gain the skills he would need to be permitted to rejoin the company. Then all too soon, their brief *ceilidh* over, Tobar walked over to touch his mother's arm and quickly left.

The students' task was to define, as best they could, each of the low-frequency words within each passage (except for multiple occurrences of a single word within a given passage, which required only a single definition). Students were not permitted to look back to earlier passages and definitions in making their current responses.

Qualities of definitions were rated independently by three trained raters. Because mean inter-rater reliability was .92, an average of the three ratings was used as a goodness-of-definition score for each word for each subject. These averages were then averaged over subjects to obtain a mean goodness-of-definition rating for each word. The main independent variables were ratings of the number or strength of the occurrences of our contextual cues and moderating variables (with the exact nature of the rating depending upon the independent variable) with respect to their roles in helping in the deciphering of the meaning of each low-frequency word in the passages.

Theory testing was done via multiple regression. We used a stepwise multiple-regression procedure in which we allowed only three variables plus a regression intercept to enter into our final models. The decision to limit the number of variables was made on the basis of our judgment of the degree of refinement of our data and in the hope of minimizing the risks of capitalization upon chance that inhere in stepwise regression. Because of multicollinearity (correlation) among independent variables, it was not possible to make strong inferences regarding the "true" subsets of variables that were differentially relevant from one passage style to the next. Variables that entered into at least one of four regressions were enablement, stative – descriptive, functional – descriptive, and equivalence cues, plus moderating variables of helpfulness and importance. The correlations between predicted and observed goodness ratings were .92 for literary passages, .74 for newspaper passages, .85 for science passages, and .77 for history passages. All of these values were statistically significant.

We concluded on the basis of these data that the contextual cues and moderating variables proposed by our subtheories provided good prediction of the goodness-of-definition data, although we certainly do not believe that our model accounted for all of the reliable variance. Indeed, the square roots of the internal-consistency reliability coefficients (based on all possible split halves of subjects) for our four data sets, which place upper limits on the values of R, were all .98 or above, showing that there was a considerable amount of reliable variance not accounted for by the fitted model. Nevertheless, the fits of the model subsets seemed sufficiently high to merit some optimism regarding our initial attempts to understand differential word difficulty in learning from context. Moreover, performance on the task was successful in distinguishing high- from low-verbal subjects: Goodness-of-definition ratings for individual subjects correlated .62 with IQ, .56 with vocabulary, and .65 with reading comprehension scores. The data, although extremely limited, are consistent with the notion that the proposed theory of cognitive competence is on the right track, at least in the domain of verbal declarative knowledge.

This first study had some clear limitations. Independent variables were nonorthogonal (multicollinear), resulting in difficulties isolating the effects of each variable; the possibility of interactions among model variables was not examined; and the population was limited to upper-middle-class high school students. A second study was designed to expand upon the first by removing these limitations.

In this experiment (Sternberg & Neuse, 1983), we tested 81 sophomores and juniors in an inner-city high school. The subjects were divided into two basic groups, a training group (59 subjects) and a control (no-training) group (22 subjects). The mean IQ of the subjects was 97, with a standard deviation of 11.

The experimental design involved seven independent variables: (a) training group (experimental, control); (b) testing time (pretest, posttest); (c) test format (blank, nonword); (d) clue type (stative–descriptive, functional–descriptive, class membership); (e) unknown word type (abstract, concrete); (f) restrictiveness of context with respect to the meaning of the unknown word (low, high); and (g) sentence function of the unknown word (subject, predicate). These variables were completely crossed with respect to each other. Treatment group was a between-subjects variable; all other variables were within-subject and were manipulated via a faceted testing arrangement. Two different test forms were used, and half the subjects received the first form as a pretest and the second form as a posttest; the other half of the subjects received the reverse arrangement. Test items, involving either neologisms or blanks (cloze procedure), were each presented in the context of a single sentence. There were 48 items on each test. Scores on the pretest were correlated .74 with an IQ test (Henmon–Nelson) given before training and .71 with an alternative form of the test given after training. Scores on the posttest were correlated .65 and .64, respectively, with the two administrations of the IQ test.

The training sequence was spread out over six sessions. The topics covered were (a) What is context? (b) Using sentence context; (c) 20 questions (spotting clue types); (d) Cues I (temporal, spatial, stative–descriptive, equivalence); (e) Using paraphrase to figure out word meanings; (f) Cues II (functional – descriptive, causal); and (g) Mystery words (neologisms presented in sentences or paragraphs). The six class periods proved ample to cover this range of theory-based material.

In the experimental group, significant main effects were obtained for testing time (posttest higher than pretest), clue type (stative – descriptive hardest, functional – descriptive in between, category membership easiest), context restrictiveness (higher restrictive more difficult than lower restrictive), and sentence function (predicates harder than subjects). In the control group, significant main effects were obtained for clue type (same ordering of means as above) and restrictiveness of context (same ordering of means as above). Thus, there was a significant pre- to posttest gain in the trained group, but not the untrained group. However, the interaction between group and training effect was not statistically significant. In addition, there were a number of statistically significant interactions between independent variables, suggesting that model effects were not wholly independent and additive but rather were interactive with each other.

Taken as a whole, these results suggest that (a) subsets of the cues and moderating variables do have additive effects that can be quantified and isolated, (b) the additive effects are supplemented by interactive ones, and (c) at least some training of decontextualization skills is possible. The set of results is thus supportive of the ideas in the theory of verbal decontextualization but emphasizes the need to consider interactions as well as main effects in analyses of model fits.

Theory of decoding of internal context

By internal context, I refer to the morphemes within a word constituted of multiple morphemes that combine to give the word its meaning. People attempting to figure out meanings of words will often use not only external context of the kinds discussed above, but also internal context deriving from their prior knowledge of a new word's constituent morphemes.

Context cues. Because internal context is much more impoverished than is external context, the diversity of kinds of cues is much more restricted (see, e.g., Johnson & Pearson, 1978; O'Rourke, 1974). The four kinds of cues constituting our scheme (Sternberg, Powell, & Kaye, 1983) are:

1. *Prefix cues.* Prefix cues generally facilitate decoding of a word's meaning. Occasionally, the prefix has a special meaning (e.g., *pre-* usually means *before*) or what appears to be a prefix really is not (e.g., *pre-* in *predation*); in these cases, the perceived cue may be deceptive.

2. *Stem cues.* Stem cues are present in every word, in the sense that every

word has a stem. Again, such cues may be deceptive if a given stem has multiple meanings and the wrong one is assigned.

3. *Suffix cues.* Suffix cues, too, generally facilitate decoding of a word's meaning; in unusual cases where the suffix takes on an atypical meaning, or in cases where what appears to be a suffix really isn't, the perceived cue may be deceptive.

4. *Interactive cues.* Interactive cues are formed when two or even three of the word parts described above convey information in combination that is not conveyed by a given cue considered in isolation from the rest of the word.

The usefulness of these kinds of cues in decoding meanings can be shown by an example. Suppose one's task is to infer the meaning of the word *thermoluminescence* (see Just & Carpenter, 1980). The word is probably unfamiliar to most people. But many people know that the prefix *thermo-* refers to heat, that the root *luminesce* is a verb meaning "to give off light," and that the suffix *-ence* is often used to form abstract nouns. Moreover, a reasonable interpretation of a possible relation between *thermo-* and *luminesce* would draw on one's knowledge that heat typically results in some degree of light. Note that this cue derives from an interaction between the prefix and stem: Neither element in itself would suggest that the light emitted from heat would be a relevant property for inferring word meaning. These cues might be combined to infer (correctly) that *thermoluminescence* refers to the property of light emission from heated objects.

Again, we make no claims that this simple (and unoriginal) parsing of internal contextual cues represents the only possible classification scheme, although we think it probably represents one, but not the only, plausible parsing. Collectively, these kinds of cues provide a basis for a person to exercise his or her competence in inferring word meanings.

Mediating variables. Again, there exists a set of variables that mediate the usefulness of cues. Our model includes five variables that affect cue usefulness. These variables are similar but not identical to those considered for external context:

1. *Number of occurrences of the unknown word.* In the case of internal contextual analysis, the context cues are the same on every presentation of a given unknown word. However, one's incentive to try to figure out the word's meaning is likely to be increased for a word that keeps reappearing relative to one's incentive to try to figure out the meaning of a word that appears just once or a very few times.

2. *Importance of the unknown word to understanding the context in which it is embedded.* Again, a word that is important for understanding the context in which it occurs is more likely to be worth the attention it needs for decontextualization. One can skip unimportant words, and often does. As

before, importance can be subdivided into the importance of the unknown word to the sentence in which it is embedded and the importance of the word to the paragraph in which it is embedded.

3. *Density of unknown words.* If unknown words occur at high density, one may be overwhelmed at the magnitude of the task of figuring out the meanings of the words and give up this task. Yet it is possible that the greater the density of unfamiliar words in a passage, the more difficulty the reader will have in applying the external context cues, and hence the more important will be the internal context cues. A high density of unfamiliar words may encourage word-by-word processing and a greater focus on cues internal to unfamiliar words. This mediating variable interacts with the next one to be considered.

4. *Density of decomposable unknown words.* Because internal decontextualization may not be a regularly used skill in many individuals' repertoires, individuals may need to be primed for its use. The presence of multiple decomposable unknown words can serve this function, helping the individual become aware that internal decontextualization is possible and feasible. In this case, the strategy is primed by repeated cues regarding its applicability.

5. *Usefulness of previously known information in cue utilization.* Again, one's knowledge of words, word cognates, and word parts will play an important part in internal decontextualization. The sparsity of information provided by such cues (in contrast to external cues) almost guarantees an important role for prior information.

Knowledge-acquisition components. The knowledge-acquisition components relevant to decontextualization of internal context are the same as those for decontextualization of external context and hence will not be repeated here, other than by name: selective encoding, selective combination, and selective comparison.

Data testing the theory of internal decontextualization

Our goal in our study of internal decontextualization (Kaye & Sternberg, 1983) was to determine the extent to which secondary school and college students could derive the correct definitions of very-low-frequency words on the basis of their knowledge of frequently used prefixes and stems. We sought to determine whether these students were attending to either of the words' constituents (prefix or stem) while attempting to define the words. We also examined relationships between students' metacognitive knowledge of such words and their actual performance in defining them. Given the present state of research in this area, we felt there is a need to know *whether* individuals use internal context before examining in detail *how* individuals use such context. Thus, our study tested a prerequisite for our theory to be applicable, rather than the theory itself, which we plan to test in subsequent research.

We tested 108 students, of whom 58 were in secondary school (approximately equally balanced among grades 8, 10, and 11) and of whom 50 were undergraduates at a state university. Each subject was exposed to 58 prefixed words that were selected each to contain 1 of 15 commonly used Latin prefixes and 1 of 15 commonly used Latin stems. Because there were 15 different prefixes and 15 different stems, there were a total of 30 different individual word parts. Each prefix and each stem appeared in from 2 to 6 different words. All words were of very low frequency and of 2 to 3 syllables in length. Each subject received half of the words in a multiple-choice word-definitions task and the other half of the words in a word-rating task. Words presented in each of the two tasks were counterbalanced across subjects.

In the word-definitions task, each word was paired with four possible definitions, one of which was correct and three of which were incorrect. One of the incorrect definitions retained the meaning of the prefix only, one retained the meaning of the stem only, and one retained the meaning of neither the prefix nor the stem. An example of such a problem is

Exsect:
(a) to cut out (totally correct)
(b) to throw out (prefix only correct)
(c) to cut against (stem only correct)
(d) to throw against (totally incorrect)

In the (metacognitive) word-rating task, each word was paired with four questions: (a) How familiar is the word? (b) How easily can you define the word? (c) How similar is the word to another word you have seen or heard? (d) How similar is the word to another word you can define? Subjects responded by circling numbers arrayed on a 7-point scale, with more positive responses to the questions answered in terms of higher-numbered values on the scale.

All subjects were also asked to rate the 30 word parts for their meaningfulness (i.e., familiarity of meaning). This task, which occurred at the end of the experiment, also involved a 7-point rating scale.

A hierarchical multiple-regression procedure was used to predict scores both on the learning-from-context cognitive task and on the metacognitive ratings of words and word parts. In such a procedure, sets of independent variables are entered into the regression in a fixed order and in successive steps. The variables entered at the first level of the hierarchy were always "dummy variables" for age, test form (i.e., which set of test words was received in which task), and age × test form. This level was used to control for the effects of those variables that might be expected to affect test performance but that were not directly relevant to the question of how subjects answered the test items or made their ratings. The particular independent variables entered at the second level of the hierarchy were the theoretically relevant ones and varied from one regression to the next. Consider, for example, the question of whether subjects are using prefixes in order to figure out word meanings. If they are, then performance on a word with a given prefix, such as *ex-* in the above example, should be better predicted by performance on other words sharing this prefix than by performance on words not sharing this prefix. If subjects are not using prefixes, then performance on words sharing the same prefix should be no better a predictor of performance on the given word than should performance on words not sharing the same prefix. The same logic applies for word stems. Thus, a typical independent variable at the second level of analysis would be performance on other words sharing the same prefix (for determining whether subjects use prefixes in figuring out word meanings) or sharing the same stem (for determining whether subjects use stems in figuring out word meanings). The variable entered at the third level of the hierarchical regression was an interaction term between the variables at the first and second levels of analysis.

The results suggested that college students, but not high school students, were able to use internal context to help infer word meanings. Values of R (the correlation between predicted and observed scores on each of the test items) were generally statistically significant for college students but not for high school students. However, both high school and college students had accurate metacognitive knowledge; that is, their metacognitive knowledge was predictive of their cognitive performance (and vice versa). Significant values of R for the various regressions ranged from .53 to .78, with a median of .63. The pattern of results suggested that the word stem was the central focus for determining what each of the various words meant, with the prefix modifying this stem meaning. Interestingly, knowledge of prefixes was better than knowledge of stems, at least for our word sample. This result may be attributable to the much larger number of stems than of prefixes in the language.

In conclusion, the data collected to date indicate the usefulness of the theory of verbal decontextualization for understanding something of how individuals acquire their vocabularies. The theory can explain, at some level, both differences in difficulty of learning individual words (stimulus variance) and differences in individuals' abilities to learn words (subject variance). Differences in word difficulty are understood in terms of differences in cue availability, applicability of mediating variables, and interactions between different cues and mediating variables. Differences between subjects are understood in terms of their differential ability to use selective encoding, selective combination, and selective comparison upon the cues and in terms of differences in susceptibility to the mediating variables. In the next chapter, I will present a theory of how verbal skills are used to understand words and texts in real time.

8 Crystallized intelligence: theory of information processing in real-time verbal comprehension

I have presented in the preceding chapter a theory of how verbal comprehension skills evolve. Consider now how these skills are executed in real time. I will first describe two general alternative approaches to this issue and then consider in more detail our own approach.

Alternative approaches to understanding real-time verbal comprehension

Approaches emphasizing current functioning seem divisible into two subapproaches – those that are essentially molar, dealing with information processing at the level of the word, and those that are essentially molecular, dealing with information processing at the level of word attributes. I shall consider each subapproach in turn.

A molar subapproach

The molar subapproach examines comprehension and understanding of individual words or groupings of words. A proponent of this approach, Marshalek (1981), administered a faceted vocabulary test along with a battery of standard reasoning and other tests. The facets of the vocabulary test were word abstractness (concrete, medium, abstract), word frequency (low, medium, high), item type (vague recognition – easy distractors in a multiple-choice recognition task; accurate recognition – difficult distractors in a multiple-choice recognition task; definition – subjects have to provide word definition rather than being given multiple-choice), and blocks (two parallel blocks of words). Marshalek found that vocabulary item difficulty increased with word abstractness, word infrequency, item formats requiring more precise discrimination of word meaning, and task requirement (such that word definition was harder than word recognition). He also found that partial concepts are prevalent in young adults and that word acquisition is a gradual process. Vocabulary level seemed to be related to reasoning performance at the lower but not the higher end of the vocabulary difficulty distribution. These results led Marshalek to conclude that a certain level of reasoning ability may be prerequisite for extraction of word meaning (see also Anderson & Freebody, 1979). Above this level, the importance of reasoning begins rapidly to decrease.

Marshalek's approach to understanding verbal comprehension is of particular interest because it breaks down global task performance into more specific facets. It is possible, in his research, to score each subject for the various facets of performance as well as for the overall level of performance. I believe this to be an important step toward understanding current verbal functioning. One concern I have, though, is with whether the experimenter-defined facets correspond to important psychological (subject-defined) aspects of performance. Although these facets may differentiate more and less difficult items and better and poorer performers, it is not clear that they do so in a way that bears any resemblance to the psychology of verbal comprehension. In other words, it is not clear how understanding these facets of performance gives us what could in any sense be construed as a causal – explanatory account of verbal comprehension and individual differences in it. The causal inferences that can be made are, at best, highly indirect.

A molecular subapproach

The molecular subapproach is the kind that we have taken in our work on the real-time representation and processing of information during verbal comprehension. The idea is to understand verbal comprehension in terms of how attributes of words are encoded and compared as well as to understand decision making in real-time reading through the specific decisions that are made about allocating time. For example, one would seek to understand performance on a synonyms test in terms of actual comparisons between the attributes of a given target word and the attributes of the potential synonyms given in a multiple-choice list. At minimum, one would have to know what kinds of attributes are stored, how these attributes are stored, how these attributes are accessed during verbal comprehension performance, and how these attributes are compared between the target and the options. Our theory of these phenomena (McNamara & Sternberg, 1983; Sternberg & McNamara, in press) and some data testing the theory, are presented next.

Theory of real-time representation and information processing

Performance components

In work investigating the performance components of real-time information processing, Timothy McNamara and I have sought to understand the mental representations and processes people use in understanding and comparing word meanings.

Alternative models of word representation. Several alternative models have been proposed for how word meaning is represented mentally. I consider below some of the major models that have been proposed.

Defining attribute (nonadditive) models. Traditional models of word meaning make use of necessary and sufficient – that is, defining – attributes of words (Frege, 1952; Russell, 1956). The idea is that the meaning of a word is decomposed into a set of attributes such that the possession of these attributes is necessary and sufficient for a word to refer to a given object or concept. For example, a bachelor might be represented in terms of the attributes *unmarried, male,* and *adult.* Being an unmarried male adult is then viewed as necessary and sufficient for being labeled as a bachelor. (Some might add *never-before-married* as an additional required attribute.) Traditional models can be viewed as "nonadditive," in the sense that either a given word has the attributes necessary and sufficient to refer to a given object or concept or it does not; there are no gradations built into this model of representation.

Characteristic attribute (additive) models. A second class of models, and one that has been more in favor in recent times, might be referred to as "characteristic attribute" models. In these models, word meaning is conceptualized in terms of attributes that tend to be characteristic of a given object or concept but neither necessary nor sufficient for reference to that concept. A well-known example of the usefulness of this kind of model stems from Wittgenstein's analysis of the concept of *game.* It is extremely difficult to speak of necessary attributes of a game. Similarly, it is difficult to speak of any attributes that guarantee something's being a game: Hence, it is difficult to find any sufficient attributes of a game. Yet games bear a "family resemblance" to each other. In today's parlance, various games cluster around a "prototype" for the concept of a game (Rosch, 1978). Games are either closer or further from this prototype depending upon the number of characteristic attributes of a game they have. A game such as chess might be viewed as quite close to the hypothetical prototype, whereas a game such as solitaire might be viewed as further away from the prototype.

The class of additive models can be divided into at least three submodels according to how the attributes are used to refer to a concept: (a) The reference of a word might be determined by the *number of attributes* possessed by an object that match attributes in the word's definition (Hampton, 1979; Wittgenstein, 1953). If the number of matching attributes exceeds some criterion, then the object is identified as an example of the word; otherwise, the object is not so identified. (b) The referent of a word might be determined by a *weighted sum of attributes*. This model is like the first one, except that some attributes are viewed as more critical than are others and hence are weighed more heavily (Hampton, 1979). For purposes of our analyses, the first model will be viewed as a special case of the second (the weighted case) and will not be treated as qualitatively distinct. (c) The referent of a word might be determined by a *weighted average of attributes*, in which case the sum of the weights of the attributes is divided by the number of attributes. The second and third models are distinguished by whether or not a given sum of weights counts equally without respect to the number of weights entered into the sum. To our knowledge, the difference between summing and averaging models has not been addressed in the literature on word meaning and reference, although it has certainly been considered in other contexts, such as information integration in people's formation of impressions about each other (e.g., Anderson, 1979).

Mixture models. A third class of models specifies words as being decomposable into both defining and characteristic attributes. An example of such a model would be that of Smith, Shoben, and Rips (1974), which proposes that words can be viewed as comprising both defining and characteristic attributes. Consider, for example, the concept of a *mammal*. Being warm-blooded would be a defining attribute of a mammal, whereas being a land animal would be a characteristic attribute, in that most, but not all, mammals are land animals.

In the mixture model (or at least the proposed variant of it), not all words need be composed of both defining and characteristic attributes (Clark & Clark, 1977; Schwartz, 1977). For example, one might view some words, such as *game*, as comprising only characteristic attributes. Intuitively, it seems much easier to find defining attributes for some kinds of concepts than for others, and this class of models capitalizes upon this intuition. It seems less likely that any words comprise only defining attributes. At least, we are unable to think of any words that do not have at least some characteristic attributes that are neither necessary nor sufficient for referring to a concept.

Tests of alternative models of representation. We conducted four initial experiments to test the alternative models of word-meaning representation (McNamara & Sternberg, 1983). Our concern in these experiments was with how word meaning is represented psychologically. The psychological issues of interest to us are not, of course, necessarily the same as those issues concerning philosophers of meaning and linguists.

The first experiment was intended to (a) determine whether people identify necessary and/or sufficient attributes of concepts and objects and (b) collect rating data needed for a second experiment that tested the various models of representation. Ten Yale students participated in the study. The study involved three kinds of nouns: (a) natural-kind terms (e.g., *eagle, banana, potato*); (b) defined-kind terms (e.g., *scientist, wisdom*); and (c) proper names (e.g., *Queen Elizabeth II, Aristotle, Paul Newman*). Proper names were included because they have been heavily used in the philosophical literature, often serving as the basis for generalization to all nouns. The main independent variables in the experiment were the type of term about which a rating was to be made (natural-kind, defined-kind, proper-name) and the type of rating to be made (necessary attributes, sufficient attributes, importance of attributes – see below). The main dependent variable was the value of the assigned ratings. Subjects were first asked to list as many properties as they could think of for the various objects of the three kinds noted above. Then they were asked to provide three kinds of ratings (with the order of the kinds of ratings counterbalanced across subjects). The first kind of rating was one of necessity: Subjects were asked to check off those attributes, if any, that they believed to be necessary attributes for each given word. The second kind of rating was one of sufficiency: Subjects were asked to check off those attributes, if any, that were sufficient attributes for each given word. They were also asked to indicate minimally sufficient subsets of attributes (such that the subset in combination was sufficient to define a word). In both of these kinds of ratings, it was emphasized that there might well be *no* necessary or sufficient properties (or subsets of properties) at all. The third kind of rating was one of importance: Subjects were asked to rate how important each attribute was to defining each of the given words. These ratings were used to determine how characteristic each attribute is of the concept it helps describe.

The major results were these:

First, all subjects found at least one necessary attribute for each of the eight natural-kind and proper-name terms. All but one subject found at least one necessary attribute for each of the defined kinds. One could therefore conclude that individuals conceive of words of these three kinds as having at least some necessary attributes. Examples of some of these attributes are, for a diamond, that it scratches glass, is the hardest substance known, and is made of carbon; and for Albert Einstein, that he is dead, was a scientist, was male, and that he formulated the equation $E = mc^2$.

Second, all subjects found at least one sufficient attribute or subset of attributes for all natural-kind terms. Almost all subjects found at least one sufficient attribute or subset of attributes for defined kinds and proper names. One could therefore conclude that most individuals conceive of most words as having at least some sufficient attributes or subsets of attributes. Examples are, for an eagle, that it is a bird that appears on quarters, and for a lamp, that it is a light source that has a shade.

Third, roughly half of the natural-kind and defined-kind terms were conceived as having attributes that were both necessary and sufficient. More than three-fourths of the proper names were conceived as having such attributes. Examples are, for sandals, that they are shoes that are held on with straps and that do not cover the whole foot, and for a diamond, that it is the hardest substance known.

Fourth, internal-consistency analyses revealed that subjects agreed to a great extent as to what attributes were important, necessary, sufficient, and necessary and sufficient (with internal-consistency reliabilities generally in the mid-.80s; for necessity ratings and sufficiency ratings, reliabilities were generally a bit lower, usually in the mid-.70s).

The second experiment was intended to (a) determine the extent to which people use defining (necessary and sufficient) and characteristic (neither necessary nor sufficient) attributes when deciding whether or not an object is an exemplar of a word; (b) to test four simple models and three mixture models of word meaning; and (c) to determine how generalizable the results were across word domains. Nine of the 10 subjects from the first experiment participated in this experiment. A within-subjects design was used in order to control for possible individual differences in the representation of meaning of specific words. The subjects received booklets with a given word at the top of the page, followed by a list of attributes. The subject's task was to give a confidence rating that the attributes actually described an exemplar of the word at the top of the page. Attribute descriptions were compiled for each subject in order to provide discrimination among alternative models of word representation. The main independent variables were ratings of necessity, sufficiency, necessity and sufficiency, and importance, as taken from Experiment 1. The main dependent variable was the confidence rating that the description described an exemplar of the target word. Subjects rated their confidence that a given word was in fact exemplified by the description appearing below it. For example, one might see the word *tiger* at the top of the page, followed by four attributes: "member of the cat family," "four-legged," "carnivorous," and "an animal." One would rate on a 1–8 scale how likely that list of attributes was to describe a particular tiger.

The alternative representational models tested were those positing (a) use only of defining (necessary and sufficient) attributes; (b) use of an unweighted sum of attributes; (c) use of a weighted sum of attributes; (d) use of a weighted mean of attributes; (e) use of defining attributes as well as a weighted sum of all attributes; and (f) use of defining attributes as well as a weighted mean of all attributes. Models were fit by linear regression with individual data sets concatenated; that is, there was no averaging across either subjects or items, and thus there was just one observation per data point for a total of 863 data points. Proportions of variance accounted for by each of the six respective models in the confidence-rating data were .36 for model a, .01 for b, .02 for c, .11 for d, .45 for e, and .38 for f, concatenated over word types. Data for individual subjects reflected the pattern for the group. It was concluded that in making decisions about whether sets of attributes represent exemplars of specific words, individuals appear to use both defining and characteristic attributes via the weighted-sum model.

The third experiment was parallel to the first, in that it replicated this experiment and provided needed ratings data for the subsequent experiment. Because the results were almost identical to those of the first experiment, they will not be presented separately here.

The fourth experiment was designed to verify the results of the second experiment using converging operations. In particular, response latency and response choice were used as dependent variables, and the subjects' task was to choose which of two attribute lists better described a referent of a given word. For example, subjects might see *sofa,* followed by two lists of attributes: (1) "used for sitting, found in living rooms, slept on, furniture"; and (2) "slept on, rectangular in shape, found in bedrooms." The 32 subjects would have to decide whether list 1 or list 2 was a better exemplar of sofa. Models were fit to group-average data. In this experiment, as in the previous two, natural kinds, defined kinds, and proper names appeared in equal numbers as stimulus terms.

The results again supported the mixture model combining defining attributes with summed characteristic attributes. For response choices, fits of five of the models described earlier were .48 for model a, .57 for c, .46 for d, .65 for e, and .57 for f. Model b, the unweighted variant of model c, was not separately tested.

The data for the four experiments taken as a whole seemed quite strongly to support the mixture model in which defining attributes and characteristic attributes are considered, with the former attributes considered both nonadditively and as a weighted sum combined with the latter attributes. This model was then taken as the representational model on the basis of which to test a process model.

Model of information processing. We have proposed a model that assumes that, in Experiment 4, (a) subjects tested both answer options in order to make sure that they picked the better of the two options and (b) subjects compared answer options on the basis of both defining attributes (when present) and weighted sums of attributes. A flowchart for the model can be found in Figure 8.1.

Quantification of the model. Quantification of the processing model will be explained by referring to the following stimulus item: *"TENT:* (1) Made of canvas, supported by poles, portable, waterproof; (2) A shelter, used for camping, made of canvas." The six parameters of the model and the variables used to estimate them were as follows:

1. *Reading time* was estimated by the total number of words in the two descriptions, excluding the target word. In the example, the total number of words is 16. The value of this variable ranged from 4 to 34 across items (mean = 14.0).

2. *Processing time for negations* was estimated by the number of negated attributes in the descriptions, which is zero for the example. The value of this variable ranged from 0 to 2 across items (mean = .6).

3. *Time for comparison of attributes in the descriptions to attributes of the target word* was estimated by the total number of attributes in the two descriptions. According to the model, each attribute in each description is compared to the attributes of the encoded target word. The weights of matching and mismatching attributes are added to a weighted-sum counter for the description currently being processed (there is a weighted-sum counter for each description). Mismatching attributes are also checked for necessity, and if they are necessary, this information is recorded in a defining-attributes counter for the description currently being processed (there is a defining-attributes counter for each description). When all attributes in a description have been compared to the attributes of the target word, the description is checked for sufficiency. If the description is sufficient, this fact is recorded in the defining-attributes counter for that description. In the example, the comparison variable would take the value 7, the number of attributes in the two descriptions. The comparison variable ranged from 3 to 8 across items (mean = 5.7).

4. *Comparison of options on the basis of defining attributes* was estimated by the absolute difference between the number of subjects for whom the second description was sufficient and the number of subjects for whom the

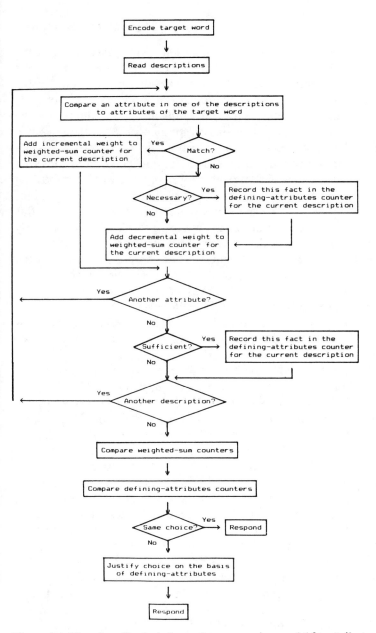

Figure 8.1. Flowchart for the information-processing model for attribute comparison in inferring word meanings. (From "Mental models of word meaning," by Timothy P. McNamara and Robert J. Sternberg, 1983, *Journal of Verbal Learning and Verbal Behavior*, *22*, p. 465. Copyright 1983 by Academic Press, Inc. Reprinted by permission of the publisher.)

first description was sufficient, or by the absolute difference between the number of subjects for whom a negated attribute in the first description was necessary and the number of subjects for whom a negated attribute in the second description was necessary. According to the model, comparison time decreases as the difference between the defining-attributes counter for the first description and the defining-attributes counter for the second description increases; that is, subjects are faster the more dissimilar the options are. We needed to use a continuous variable to estimate a dichotomous construct (the necessity or sufficiency of a set of attributes) because we were modeling group-average data and a given description was not equally good or bad for all subjects. The difference between the two descriptions capitalized on this inherent variability in our stimuli. This comparison variable was linearly scaled so that small values on the variable corresponded to large differences between the two descriptions and hence to fast comparison times. In the example, the first description was sufficient for none of the subjects and the second was sufficient for 11 subjects. Thus, the comparison variable was a linear function of the number 11 (precisely $26 - 11$, or 15).

5. *Comparison of options on the basis of weighted sums of attributes* was estimated by the absolute difference in summed weights between the two descriptions. It was assumed that comparison time decreases as the difference between the weighted-sum counter for the first description and the weighted-sum counter for the second description increases. This variable, like variable 4, was linearly scaled so that small values on the variable corresponded to large differences between the two descriptions. In the example above, the first description had a weighted sum of 11.32 and the second description had a weighted sum of 11.44. Hence, the comparison variable was a linear function of .12 (precisely $17.76 - .12$, or 17.64).

6. *Justification* was relevant when the difference in summed weights and the difference in defining attributes predicted opposite choices. In such cases, the choice of an answer option on the basis of definingness alone had to be justified. The stimulus items were constructed so that for 60 of the 156 pairs of descriptions, there were no differences in definingness between the descriptions. For these items, the justification variable always took the value zero, since there could be no discrepancy between choices. The difference in weighted sums and the difference in definingness predicted opposite choices for 10 of the remaining 96 items. For these items, the justification variable took the value 1. In the example, both the difference in definingness and the difference in weighted sums predict that the second option should be chosen. Thus, the value of the justification variable is zero.

Tests of model of information processing. The model described above was tested in terms of its ability to account for mean response latencies on the 156 items. Responses were included in the mean latencies even if they were errors according to the model. Fits changed trivially when errors were excluded. Fit of the model (R^2) was .79, with a root-mean-square deviation of .66 second. Standardized parameter estimates were .42 for reading time, .37 for processing negations, .33 for comparison to target word, .23 for definingness comparison, .33 for weighted-sum comparison, and .07 for justification. All estimates were statistically significant. The proposed model thus provided a good account of the processing of attribute information, accounting for nearly 80% of the total variance in response latencies (and with only six independent variables on 156 data points). The standardized regression coefficients for the model seemed generally reasonable. They indicated that weighted sums of attributes were somewhat more important than defining attributes in deciding which option was the better exemplar of the target word.

Correlations with ability tests

Correlations were computed between overall mean latencies on the decision task and scores from the Nelson–Denny Reading Test and the Differential Aptitudes Test (DAT). In particular, we used vocabulary, reading comprehension, and reading rate scores from the former test and the verbal reasoning score from the latter test. The only significant correlation involving latency was that between overall mean latency and reading rate (-.37). However, the multiple correlation between mean latency, on the one hand, and both reading rate and comprehension, when taken together, was a significant .47. (The correlation between comprehension and reading rate was .07, and the correlation between comprehension and mean latency was .27; neither correlation was significant.) Both reading rate and comprehension made statistically significant contributions to the multiple correlation, with respective weights of .38 and .30. Thus, reading rate and comprehension, when considered together, were moderately strongly related to latency in our task.

To conclude, the results from the four experiments taken together provide a reasonably coherent picture of both the representation of meaning and the processes used to make reference to a concept. In particular, individuals seem to use an additively based mixture model in their representation of word information and to be able to combine the represented information in a way that enables them to choose synonyms. Obviously, our work on real-time processing is incomplete. It has yet to be extended beyond the level of individual words and is in need of further interface with the theory of learning from context. Nevertheless, the two aspects of the theory of verbal comprehension, taken in combination, seem to provide a relatively comprehensive view of how crystallized intelligence develops and functions.

Metacomponents

Virtually everyone is confronted with much more material to read than they could possibly handle in the time allotted for reading. College freshmen, for example, are often bewildered by a reading load that would seemingly take all of their time if they were to attempt to read with care all of the material they are assigned. Professionals in psychology and other fields often find it impossible to keep up with the latest developments in their field simply because there are so many of them to read about, but not nearly enough time to do the required reading. Clearly, individuals have to allocate their reading time and depth of reading in a way that reflects the realities of their usually overburdened situation.

Earlier (Chapter 4), it was stated that an important metacomponential function in human cognition is that of time allocation. Individuals have to allocate their time across tasks in a way that optimizes (or at least renders adequate) their performance on these tasks. A further metacomponent is strategy selection – selecting a strategy for each of these tasks that enables individuals to accomplish the task in an efficacious way. In Chapter 4, it was shown how metacomponential functioning could be isolated in a relatively structured task, the analogy. But it is important as well to have ways of isolating metacomponential functioning in less structured tasks of equal or greater complexity. We have therefore sought to study metacomponential functioning in real-time verbal comprehension and particularly in reading. Richard Wagner and I have conducted a study of executive processes in reading of narrative texts (Wagner & Sternberg, 1983).

Isolating a time-allocation metacomponent. In a first experiment, subjects were 40 Yale undergraduates. Each subject was presented with 44 untitled passages of about 150 words apiece. One-fourth of the passages were from novels, one-fourth from newspapers, one-fourth from humanities text-books, and one-fourth from science (natural and social) textbooks. Although there were eight different questions per passage, a given subject saw just two of these. These two questions addressed either the gist of the passage (i.e., global theme), the main idea of the passage, specific details in the passage, or analysis and application of points in the passage (i.e., inferences and evaluations from the text). Which subjects received which questions for which passages was counterbalanced across subjects. Subjects also received the Nelson–Denny Reading Test and the Differential Aptitude Test Verbal Reasoning (verbal analogies) subtest.

Subjects received 11 trials of 150 seconds each. Each trial involved 4 reading passages, for a total of 44 passages. Subjects were informed for each passage whether they would be tested for gist, main ideas, details, or analysis and application. Subjects were free to allocate their total time across passages as they wished. Passages were selected by subjects pressing an appropriately designated key on a computer console. Thus, order of presentation of passages within trial and duration of viewing were under subject control. Note, then, that subjects were basically free to allocate their time to the four types of questions as they wished.

Mean latencies for passages read for each of the different purposes (question types) were 38.0 for gist, 37.6 for main ideas, 39.8 for details, and 40.4 for analysis and application. The times differed significantly from each other, with the times for gist and main-idea comprehension significantly shorter than the times for detail comprehension and analysis and application comprehension. Thus, subjects did allocate time systematically so as to spend more time reading passages for which they would receive more demanding questions. Patterns of accuracy in responding to the question types also were systematic: Mean numbers of questions answered correctly (out of 16) for each type of question were 13.3 for gist, 12.6 for main idea, 10.5 for details, and 8.2 for analysis and application. These means, too, differed significantly from one another. The means for gist and main-idea comprehension were significantly higher than those for details, which in turn was significantly higher than for analysis and application.

Overall number of questions correctly answered by each subject for all types of questions was significantly correlated with vocabulary (.57), comprehension (.48), and DAT verbal reasoning (.78). Most of the subscores were also significantly correlated with Nelson – Denny and DAT scores, and all correlations were in the predicted (positive) direction. Thus, our reading questions did seem to measure skills related to those measured by standard tests of reading comprehension.

The most important question, from our point of view, was that of whether time allocation was systematically related to task performance. A time-allocation score was computed for each subject by subtracting the amount of time spent on reading passages for gist and main idea from the amount of time spent on reading passages for details and analysis and application. Presumably, a higher difference score would reflect greater sensitivity in time allocation: the higher the score, the relatively greater the amount of time spent on reading for the more difficult questions and the relatively lesser the amount of time spent on reading for the less difficult questions. Time-allocation score correlated .30 with total number of passage comprehension questions answered correctly. But one might well ask whether this correlation merely reflects some skill already measured by standard reading comprehension tests, which seem to measure primarily performance components rather than metacomponents in reading. We therefore predicted accuracy in answering questions on the reading task from DAT Verbal

Reasoning score, Nelson – Denny total score (reading comprehension + vocabulary), Nelson – Denny reading rate, and time allocation. The question addressed was whether time allocation would make a significant contribution to the regression after the other, standard test variables were added to the equation. In fact, it did. The semipartial regression weight for the time-allocation parameter was .30, which was statistically significant. The overall multiple correlation was .85. Thus, our metacomponential measure of reading time allocation makes a significant contribution in predicting task performance over and above that made by standardized test scores (including vocabulary, comprehension, verbal reasoning, and reading rate). Again, metacomponential processing seems to be important in real-time verbal comprehension.

Strategies in using adjunct information. In a second experiment, 90 Yale undergraduates were divided into three groups. In a control group, subjects received 8 passages and 44 questions taken from the reading comprehension sections of two editions of the Graduate Record Examination of the Educational Testing Service. The passages were of two lengths. Four of the passages were approximately 175 words in length. There were three questions on each of these passages. The other four passages were approximately 500 words in length. There were eight questions on each of these passages.

In a difficulty-information group, subjects received the identical passages and questions to those used in the control group, but with two kinds of difficulty information added. General difficulty information informed subjects of the average difficulty of the set of questions associated with each passage. This information was conveyed through a table containing the average difficulty of the questions associated with each passage and the number of questions per passage (either three or eight questions per passage). Specific difficulty information informed subjects of the difficulty level of each question. This information was conveyed by labeling each question on a scale of relative difficulty. Both general and specific difficulty information was presented through use of the phrases "very difficult," "moderately difficult," "moderately easy," and "very easy." Difficulty level was determined by the proportions of the examinees who passed the question when it was administered nationwide as part of the Graduate Record Examination.

In an importance-information group, subjects received the identical passages and questions to those received in the other two groups (but without any difficulty information). However, the most important sentences in the passages (as determined by the judgment of the experimenters) were highlighted with a yellow marker pen. Approximately 45% of the text was highlighted.

Subjects in the difficulty-information condition were instructed to use the difficulty information so as to maximize their performance. They were not told how to do so, however. Examples of questions labeled as to their difficulty were provided. Subjects in the importance-information condition were instructed to use the importance information so as to maximize their performance. Again, they were not told how to do so. An example of a highlighted text was provided.

In all conditions, subjects reported the time (from an easily visible clock) that they started work on each reading passage. At the conclusion of the task, subjects in all groups provided written descriptions of their task strategies. Subjects in the two experimental conditions additionally described whether they made use of the adjunct difficulty or importance information, and if so, how.

Reference ability measures of reading and reasoning abilities were the same as those employed in the previously described experiment.

Task performance in terms of total number of questions answered correctly was 25.7, 23.6, and 21.6 for the control, difficulty-information, and importance-information conditions. These means did not differ significantly. Written reports of task strategies provided by subjects were scored for presence of explicit mention of revising strategy during task performance. Twenty-eight percent of subjects reported strategy revision during task performance. This percentage remained essentially constant across conditions: 30%, 30%, and 23% for the control, difficulty-information, and importance-information conditions, respectively. Two reasons were given for strategy revision: A strategy chosen before beginning the task was not working out, or a strategy was changed when time began to run out so that the subject would have a chance of answering the remaining questions. Subjects who reported strategy revision performed significantly better on the task than subjects who did not, achieving a mean total score of 26.1, compared to 22.7 for subjects who did not report strategy revision. Subjects who reported strategy revision also attained significantly higher scores on the DAT Verbal Reasoning Test than did subjects who did not (45.7 versus 44.1); scores on the Nelson–Denny Reading Test did not differ significantly between groups, however.

Recall that subjects marked down the time when they began work on each passage, producing a record of the order in which passages were read. This record was used to score the presence or absence of the strategy of reading passages in their order of difficulty. No attempt was made to distinguish between subjects who followed this strategy exclusively and subjects who followed this strategy for only part of the reading task. Fifty-three percent of subjects in the difficulty-information condition used this strategy. Subjects using this strategy obtained higher average task scores than subjects who did not (26.3 versus 20.6). Subjects using this strategy also obtained marginally significantly higher scores on the Nelson–Denny Reading Test (136.3 versus

123.9) and had a higher reading rate as measured by the Nelson–Denny (348.8 versus 286.8). Performance on the DAT Verbal Reasoning Test did not differ between the two types of subjects (43.9 versus 44.1). More able subjects, then, used general difficulty information in planning their order of passage reading to correspond with the order of passage difficulty. It was possible to determine the validity of subjects' written reports of task strategies by comparing actual strategy as determined from the record of passage order with written reports of strategy. All subjects who used the strategy of reading passages in order of their difficulty reported doing so; conversely, no subjects who did not use this strategy reported doing so.

Subjects' written reports of task strategy were scored for (a) the presence of a strategy of using the specific difficulty information and (b) indications that the specific information was distracting. Twenty-seven percent of subjects reported using the specific difficulty information. Subjects who reported using the specific difficulty information described a strategy of matching how much effort they spent searching for and evaluating possible answers to the difficulty level of the questions. Subjects who reported using the specific difficulty information actually performed more *poorly* on the task than did subjects who did not report use of specific difficulty information (18.8 versus 25.4). These subjects also obtained lower Nelson–Denny Reading Test scores (111.0 versus 136.5), but performance on the DAT Verbal Reasoning Test did not differ significantly across groups (41.6 versus 44.8). Twenty percent of subjects reported that the specific difficulty information was distracting. One commonly given reason for the general unhelpfulness of the specific difficulty information was that the difficulty rating of a particular question did not coincide with a subject's personally perceived difficulty. Subjects also reported that they disliked being told how difficult a question was; in some cases, knowing that a question was very difficult made them anxious. Subjects who reported the specific difficulty information as distracting performed better on the task than did subjects who did not (31.2 versus 21.8). No reliable differences were found on the reference ability tests, however, for this comparison. Overall, then, more able subjects were (a) more likely to use *general* difficulty information for planning order of passage selection, (b) less likely to use *specific* difficulty information, and (c) more likely to find the *specific* difficulty information distracting.

Three strategies for using importance information were identified. Twenty-seven percent of subjects reported using a strategy of reading highlighted sections exclusively. Task performance for subjects using this strategy was comparable to that of subjects who did not use the strategy (21.8 versus 21.6), as was performance on the Nelson–Denny Reading Test (125.0 versus 130.1). Subjects who used this strategy did perform better on the DAT Verbal Reasoning Test, however (46.9 versus 44.3). A second strategy, related to the previous one, was reading the highlighted sections more carefully than the nonhighlighted sections, but not exclusively. Forty-three percent of subjects reported using this strategy, but performance on the task and reference ability measures was comparable for subjects who reported using this strategy and those who did not. A final identifiable strategy was one of searching for unknown answers in the highlighted portions. This was an understandable strategy because a majority of the answers were to be found in the highlighted sections and subjects were informed of this fact. Thirty-three percent of subjects reported using this strategy. Task performance was comparable for subjects who reported using this strategy and those who did not (23.8 versus 20.6). Subjects who reported using this strategy performed better on the Nelson–Denny Reading Test, however (139.8 versus 123.7). Their performance on the DAT Verbal Reasoning Test was comparable to that of subjects who did not use this strategy (46.1 versus 44.4).

To conclude, the proposed theory of real-time verbal comprehension appears to give a good account of processing both at the word level and for time allocation at the passage level. The theory is by no means a complete theory of real-time processing, but it may at least provide a step in that direction.

9 Social and practical intelligence

When both experts and laypersons were queried regarding their views of intelligence, a clear factor of social competence emerged, in addition to the factors of problem-solving and verbal abilities. In Chapters 5 and 6, the nature of problem-solving abilities was reviewed under the rubric of "fluid intelligence." In Chapters 7 and 8, the nature of verbal abilities was reviewed under the rubric of "crystallized intelligence." The present chapter goes beyond the conventional kinds of cognitive abilities that have formed the bases for most theories and investigations of intelligence and considers possible directions for the study of social competence. In my theory and research, I have divided social competence into two kinds of intelligences: social and practical intelligence. Although social intelligence can be viewed as a subset of practical intelligence, both historically and theoretically it seems to deal with a somewhat different set of abilities from those that best fit under the notion of practical intelligence. Hence, the two sets of abilities are considered separately.

Social intelligence

The search for a construct of social intelligence has had a long and, some might say, checkered history. As noted by Walker and Foley (1973) in a thorough review of the literature to that date, social intelligence is a cyclical concept, seeming to come in and go out of favor in repeated cycles over time. Part of the reason for the periodic changes in the fashionability of the construct may be due to uncertainties regarding both what the construct is and how it might best be studied. Consider four major approaches to understanding the construct of social intelligence.

Brief review of the literature

The first of the four major approaches to understanding social intelligence is what might be called a *definitional approach*. The investigator simply defines what he or she believes social intelligence to be. This approach dates back at least to Thorndike (1920), who defined social intelligence as comprising the abilities to understand others and to act or behave wisely in relation to others. Related definitions were proposed by Moss and Hunt (1927), who defined social intelligence as the ability to get along with others, and by Hunt (1928), who defined the construct in terms of one's ability to deal with people. Strang (1930) expanded upon Hunt's definition by emphasizing the role of prior knowledge (about people) in the exercise of social intelligence. Vernon (1933) combined aspects of past definitions with some new ideas when he defined social intelligence as including the ability to get along with people in general, knowledge of social matters, ease with other people, susceptibility to stimuli from other members of a group, and insights into the states and traits of others. Wedeck (1947) expanded upon the last aspect of Vernon's definition by defining social intelligence as one's ability to judge correctly the feelings, moods, and motivations of others. Perhaps all of these various definitions are best and most succinctly summarized by Wechsler's (1958) definition of social intelligence as one's facility in dealing with human beings. (See Walker & Foley, 1973, for a further explication of these and other definitional views.) The definitional approach gives us some basis for understanding the construct of social intelligence. It does not readily lend itself to empirical tests, however. The approaches considered below, in contrast, are empirically testable, and have in fact served as the bases for a number of empirical studies.

A second approach to understanding social intelligence might be characterized as an *implicit theoretical approach*. In this approach, one seeks to discover what various groups of people mean by social intelligence by investigating their implicit and usually tacit theories of the construct. For example, studies by Bruner, Shapiro, and Tagiuri (1958) and by Cantor (1978) of people's conceptions of intelligence – where people were simply asked to list or rate characteristics of intelligent people – revealed many characteristics that were highly social in nature. This kind of approach was formalized by Sternberg, Conway, Ketron, and Bernstein (1981) in a study described in Chapter 2. Briefly, these investigators factor-analyzed both experts' and laypersons' ratings of how distinctively characteristic various behaviors are of intelligent, academically intelligent, and everyday intelligent people. In all of the factor analyses – for both experts on intelligence and laypersons – a factor emerged that was labeled "social competence." Behaviors exhibiting high loadings on this factor were ones such as "accepts others for what they are," "admits mistakes," "displays interest in the world at large," "is on time for appointments," and "has social conscience." Ford and Miura (1983) used a related approach to studying social intelligence. They had university students list behaviors characteristic of ideally socially competent individuals and then had other students sort behaviors into groups. Four main dimensions of what we are calling social intelligence emerged from their study: *prosocial skills*, including characteristics such as "responds to needs of others," "is emotionally supportive," and "is genuinely interested in others"; *leadership skills*, including characteristics such as "has leadership ability," "knows how to get things done," and "likes to set goals"; *social ease*, including characteristics such as "is easy to be around," "opens up to people," and "enjoys social activities and involvement"; and *self-efficacy*, including characteristics such as "has good self-concept," "has own identity and values," and "has a good outlook on life."

The third and fourth approaches to understanding social intelligence are both *explicit theoretical approaches*, in that they involve standard kinds of psychological theorizing. One approach involves psychometric theorizing; the other involves social-experimental theorizing.

In the third, *psychometric approach* to understanding social intelligence, social intelligence is understood in terms of scores on various kinds of psychometric tests. Perhaps the best known of these tests is the George Washington Social Intelligence Test of Moss, Hunt, Omwake, and Woodward (1949). This test includes subtests involving judgment in social situations, recognition of the mental state of the speaker, memory for names and faces, observation of human behavior, and sense of humor. Another such test, the Social Insight Test (Chapin, 1967), requires individuals to read about problem situations, most of which involve fictitious people trying to avoid embarrassment or to achieve some satisfaction to offset a frustration, and then to select the best of four alternative interpretations of the situation. Guilford (1967; Guilford & Hoepfner, 1971) has also devised a series of tests of social intelligence that fit into the framework of his structure-of-intellect (SI) model of intelligence. Included in his tests are instruments such as Faces, which requires individuals to match two from among several faces for the similarity of the mental state the faces portray; Inflections, which requires an individual to choose one from among four sketched facial expressions that represents the same feeling as a tape-recorded vocal expression; and Missing Cartoons, which requires individuals to fill in a blank in a missing cartoon with the best of four alternative completions.

In the fourth, *social-experimental approach* to understanding social intelligence, tests of social-intelligence skills are used, but these tests are based upon experimental social–psychological rather than psychometric theorizing. The social-experimental approach can be subdivided into two subapproaches that use rather different theoretical bases and instruments for assessing social-intelligence skills.

The first subapproach is based upon the literature in *social–developmental psychology* on *social competence* (see, e.g., Flavell, Botkin, Fry, Wright, & Jarvis, 1968; Gough, 1966; Gresham, 1981; Kurtines &

Greif, 1974). This subapproach uses measures such as self-ratings, teacher ratings, and interviewer ratings of social competence, peer nominations, and measures of goal directedness, empathy, social maturity, moral–developmental level, and the like (e.g., Ford, 1982; Ford & Tisak, 1983; Keating, 1978) to assess social-intelligence skills. The results of the subapproach are mixed: Keating (1978) failed to find substantial intercorrelations between social-competence measures and was unable to obtain any nontrivial social-competence factors in a factor analysis of his intercorrelation matrix for social-intelligence measures; Ford (1982; Ford & Tisak, 1983), however, using what was probably a more refined selection of social-intelligence measures, did find substantial evidence of an underlying social-intelligence ability.

The second subapproach is based upon the literature in *social psychology* on *nonverbal communication* (see, e.g., Argyle, 1969; Cook, 1971; Ekman, 1964; Ellsworth & Carlsmith, 1968; Mehrabian, 1972). This subapproach uses measures of nonverbal decoding (and occasionally, encoding) skills as bases for assessing social intelligence (e.g., Rosenthal, 1979; Rosenthal, Hall, DiMatteo, Rogers, & Archer, 1979). Much of this research has used the Profile of Nonverbal Sensitivity (PONS) Test of Rosenthal et al. (1979). The PONS presents a single woman in a variety of poses. The subject's task is to decode the implicit signals being emitted and to figure out which of two alternative descriptions better describes what the test taker has just seen and/or heard. The test isolates 11 nonverbal channels, including ones that are visual only, auditory only, and visual plus auditory. Rosenthal et al. (1979) found the test to have satisfactory reliability and weak to moderate correlations with other measures of social and cognitive competence. Halberstadt and Hall (1980) found moderate correlations between children's PONS scores and measures of academic ability.

A second instrument along the lines of the PONS is the Social Interpretations Test (SIT), formulated by Archer (see Archer, 1980; Archer & Akert, 1977a, 1977b, 1980). In this test, subjects are presented with visual and in some cases auditory information regarding a social situation. For example, subjects might see a picture of a woman talking on the phone and hear a fragment of the woman's conversation. The subjects' task is to judge whether the woman is talking to a man or to a woman. In another situation, subjects are asked to venture a judgment as to whether a man and a woman shown in a picture are strangers who have never talked before, acquaintances who have had several conversations, or friends who have known each other for at least six months. Archer and Akert have found substantial individual differences in people's abilities to perform these tasks.

The approach we have taken (Sternberg & Smith, in press) attempts to apply some of the techniques of componential analysis to the understanding of social intelligence. The particular direction we have taken continues in the tradition of the Archer and Akert work on social intelligence. In our particular instantiation of it, we sought to assess people's abilities to decode nonverbal messages in two very different kinds of interpersonal situations involving two people. In one set of pictures, a man and a woman were shown posed together in an interactive way. The subject's task was to determine whether the two individuals were an actual couple involved in a close relationship or strangers who had just met each other but who had been asked to pose as though they were a genuine couple in a close relationship. In the other set of pictures, two same-sex or mixed-sex individuals were also shown interacting. The subject's task was to indicate which of the two individuals was the other's work supervisor. We were interested in determining whether we could model people's judgments about the relation between two people (stimulus variance) and whether individual differences in judgments on the two tasks were systematic within and across tasks (subject variance).

Judgmental cues

On the basis of previous research and our own intuitions, we hypothesized that as many as 15 cues regarding the individuals and their interactions might be relevant to ascertaining the relationship between each of the pairs of individuals:

1. How pleasant is each person's facial expression?
2. To what extent is each person looking at the other?
3. To what extent is each person leaning toward the other person?
4. Overall, how relaxed is each person?
5. How physically attractive is each person?
6. How formally dressed is each person?
7. How old is each person?
8. How naturally (comfortably) is each person holding his/her arms and/or legs (depending upon visibility of extremities)?
9. How tense are each person's hands?
10. How tall is each person?
11. What sort of build does each person have?
12. What is the socioeconomic class of each person?
13. How far apart are the bodies of the two people in the photograph?
14. How much physical contact are the two people making?
15. How similar in appearance are the two people?

Method

Fifty-two townspeople (nonstudents) ranging in age from 18 to 70 years (mean = 33 years) were asked to view 136 pictures of pairs of individuals. Pictures were equally divided into two books, one of which contained pic-

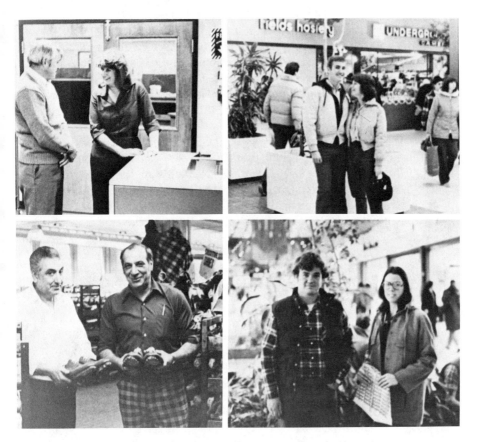

Figure 9.1. Examples of stimuli used in experiment studying decoding of nonverbal cues. The two left pictures are of supervisor–supervisee pairs; the two right pictures are of couples. In the top left picture, the supervisor is on the left; the p value (proportion of subjects correctly identifying the supervisor) for this item was .63. In the bottom left picture, the supervisor is on the right; the p value for this item was .60. In the top right picture, the couple is genuine; the p value for this item was .77. In the bottom right picture, the couple is artificial; the p value for this item was .70.

tures of the heterosexual couples (half of which were genuine and half of which were fake couples posing as real couples) and the other of which contained pictures of the supervisors and supervisees. Some typical pictures are shown in Figure 9.1. All pictures were $3\frac{1}{2} \times 5$-inch black-and-white glossy photographs. Subjects were asked to answer two questions about each of the two kinds of pictures.

For the heterosexual couples, the first question required the subject to indicate for each couple "whether the couple in the photo is a real couple or a fake couple." A real couple was defined as "one with an ongoing relationship," whereas a fake couple was defined as one "which was artificially posed for this study; the two persons had never met before." Subjects circled "yes" for a real couple and "no" for a fake couple. The second question asked for a confidence rating on a scale of 1 (not at all sure) to 7 (extremely sure) regarding the yes – no judgment that had just been made. Thus, higher ratings corresponded to greater confidence that the yes – no judgment had been correct.

For the supervisors and supervisees, the first question required the subject to indicate "whether the person on the (left, right) is the supervisor or not." (Half the subjects were asked to make judgments about the person on the left, and half to make judgments about the person on the right.) Subjects circled "yes" if the person on the left (or right) was the supervisor, and "no" if the person on that side was not the supervisor. The second question asked for a confidence rating (on the same 1 – 7 scale as above) regarding the yes – no judgment that had just been made. Again, higher ratings corresponded to greater confidence that the yes – no judgment had been correct.

Subjects also received several standard psychometric-type tests of social and cognitive intelligence. These tests were the photo version of the PONS, which required decoding of visual nonverbal cues; the Social Insight Test, which required "appropriate, intelligent, or logical comments" about situations "in which individuals are trying to avoid embarrassment or to achieve some satisfaction as an offset to frustration"; the George Washington Social Intelligence Test (second edition), with subtests requiring judgment in social situations, recognition of the mental state of the speaker, memory for names and faces, observation of human behavior, and sense of humor; the Group Embedded Figures Test, which required individuals to detect a given figure embedded in a more complex figure; and the Cattell Culture-Fair Test of g, with subtests requiring solution of figural series problems, figural classification problems, figural matrices, and figural topology problems.

Order of the two judgment tasks was counterbalanced, but these tasks always preceded the psychometric ability tests, which were administered in a fixed order.

Other subjects were asked to rate each of the pictures in terms of the 15 cues described earlier. The purpose of these ratings was to serve as independent variables in predicting the subjects' yes – no and confidence ratings in the main part of the study described above.

Results

The mean proportions of items answered correctly were .60 for the couples task and .74 for the supervisors task. Both proportions differed significantly from the chance proportion of .50. Reliabilities across all possible split halves of subjects were .90 for the couples task and .96 for the supervisors task, indicating that there was considerable consistency in subjects' strategies for performing each of the tasks. Reliabilities across all possible split halves of items, however (the standard kind of psychometric internal-consistency reliability), were lower: .62 for the couples task and .59 for the supervisors task. Thus, it appears that internal consistency across the various items within a given set was not particularly high. Such a result suggests that subjects tended to use or emphasize different cues on different pictures.

Independent variables (ratings) corresponding to each of the 15 cues were correlated with subjects' evaluations of whether each pair was or was not a true couple and whether or not a given individual was the supervisor in a given pair. For the couples task, statistically significant correlations were obtained for the extent to which each person was leaning toward the other, the amount of relaxation each person showed, the naturalness of each person's position of arms and legs, the tenseness of the hands of the more tense person, the socioeconomic class of the person with lower perceived socioeconomic class, the distance between the bodies of the individuals, the amount of physical contact between individuals, and the similarity in appearance of the individuals. All correlations were in the predicted directions (e.g., greater amounts of relaxation were associated with real couples), and the significant correlations ranged in magnitude from .27 to .57, with a median of .45. For the supervisors task, statistically significant correlations were obtained for the differences between the extent to which each person was looking at the other, the physical attractiveness of the individuals, the formality of the dress of the individuals, the ages of the individuals, the tenseness of the hands of the individuals, and the socioeconomic classes of the individuals. Again, all correlations were in the predicted directions (e.g., the supervisor was seen to be of higher socioeconomic class), and the significant correlations ranged in magnitude from .30 to .86, with a median of .42.

We also used forward stepwise multiple regression to predict the subjects' judgments in the two tasks. In order to reduce capitalization upon chance, we allowed only variables with significant simple correlations to enter into the equations and then allowed a maximum of only three variables into each equation. For the couples task, the multiple correlation was .73. The three variables in the equation, all with significant regression weights, were naturalness of individuals' arms and legs (beta = .43), amount of physical contact (beta = .27), and similarity in appearance (beta = .41). For the supervisors task, the multiple correlation was .92. The three variables in the equation, all of them with significant weights, were all differences: in formality of dress of the individuals (beta = .46), ages of the individuals (beta = .25), and socioeconomic class of the individuals (beta = .35). Thus, we were able to predict responses in both tasks, but especially the supervisors task, with a high level of accuracy.

Although the results of the internal validation were promising, the results of the external validation were not. Performance on the two tasks was not significantly correlated ($r = .09$), and correlations with the reference tests were significant only for the Embedded Figures Test ($r = .40$). Thus, we had no evidence that our judgment task was measuring a consistent individual-differences dimension.

Implications

Does the measurement of decoding skills in nonverbal communication provide a promising avenue for the measurement of social intelligence? This question should be answered from two perspectives. Recent theoretical work on cognitive intelligence has suggested that adequate measures of intelligence should be both internally valid – that is, capable of decomposition of stimulus variance – and externally valid – that is, demonstrating subject variance related to other purported measures of the same construct (Carroll, 1976; Hunt, 1980; Sternberg, 1977b, 1980f). The nonverbal decoding measures used in the research described above passed the first test but failed the second one. The present work was consistent with previous work, such as that of Archer (1980), Ekman (1964), Mehrabian (1972), Rosenthal et al. (1979), and others, in suggesting that it is possible to decompose decoding judgments for nonverbal communications into individual decision elements. The present work indicated, perhaps even more so than this past work, just how successful this decomposition can be. In essence, it sought to discover the components of information evaluation in a particular social–cognitive task, nonverbal decoding, and seems pretty well to have succeeded.

But only one variable proved related to the nonverbal decoding task in the external validation. This variable, performance on the Embedded Figures Test, must be viewed as essentially "cognitive" rather than "social" in nature. As in previous studies, correlations with external measures were generally positive (see, e.g., Halberstadt & Hall, 1980; Rosenthal et al., 1979). But also as in these previous studies, the magnitude of the relationship between nonverbal decoding measures and other measures of social and cognitive intelligence was far from impressive.

If there exist measures of some generalized skill or set of skills that might properly be labeled "social intelligence," then certainly these skills must yield measurements that pass the test of external validation as well as that of internal validation. Indeed, conventional psychometric notions of "intelligence," dating back to Spearman (1927), emphasize cross-subject correlations (such as those assessed in external validation) almost wholly at the expense of cross-item correlations (such as those assessed in internal valida-tion). I thus find myself unwilling, at least at the present, to accept the notion advanced by Archer (1980) and others that nonverbal decoding skills pro-vide a valid measure of some construct of "social intelligence," which is not to say that they are not of considerable interest in their own right and, perhaps, as measures of other constructs.

I would emphasize the tentative nature of my doubts regarding the rele-vance of nonverbal decoding skills for understanding social intelligence, because at present as in the past, it is not clear exactly what reference tests should be used for external validation. It may be that some other set of measures, not used in this study, would show more promising results. The present data, of course, are far from definitive with respect to the question of whether decoding of nonverbal messages is a general skill and possibly a part of a generalized construct of social intelligence. Pictures were only black and white, they were not accompanied by an auditory channel, and there was no temporal dimension to stimulus presentation, as can be achieved with, for example, videotape. Moreover, the two kinds of situations we used represent an extremely limited sampling of the kinds of situations one might use in this kind of research. And it is possible, of course, that encoding skills (i.e., skills used in communicating nonverbally to others) would result in a different outcome. My pessimism regarding the existence of a stable decoding ability results from my reading of the entire literature and not just this one study. At the same time, I am prepared to accept the notion that there exists a set of skills that is stable across subjects and situations and that goes beyond the concept of academic intelligence. In the next section of the chapter, I de-scribe what I believe this set of skills to be.

Practical intelligence

Attempts to measure practical intelligence in the real world have been nota-bly scarce when compared to the large number of tests of more academic kinds of intelligence. One reason for this scarcity may be a sense that it is not clear that there is any generalized construct of practical intelligence that extends beyond particular classes of tasks or situations.

Brief review of the literature

A first approach is essentially *psychometric* in nature. A good example of the psychometric approach is the ETS Basic Skills Test (1977). The test is a 65-item measure originally designed to assess real-life competencies that should have been attained by high school seniors. The items are of eight basic kinds: understanding labels on bottles of household goods, reading street maps, understanding charts and schedules, paragraph comprehension, filling out forms, reading newspaper and telephone directory advertisements, understanding technical documents, and comprehension of news text. Willis, Schaie, and Lueers (1982) studied performance on the Basic Skills Test in relation to performance on other, more conventional psychometric tests. Correlations between performance on this test and other more conventional tests were quite high. Correlations tended to be higher with fluid-ability tests (such as figural relations and induction) than with crystallized-ability tests (such as verbal meaning and social knowledge). These results suggest that the ETS test is not just a measure of acquired knowledge of the real world or ability to deal with real-world events, but is also a measure of fluid abilities of the kind measured by more academic kinds of intelligence tests.

A second, and perhaps the best-known, approach to measuring practical intelligence, involves the *simulation of real-world performance*. In this approach, subjects (often job applicants) are presented with tasks that are similar to those required in the real world. The best-known instantiation of this approach may be the "in-basket" technique devised by Norman Frederiksen (1962; Frederiksen, Saunders, & Ward, 1957). Typically, the applicant for an executive job is presented with letters, memoranda, notes on telephone calls, and other documents that have supposedly accumulated in the in-basket of an executive. The applicant is also given background information concerning the organization and his or her role in it. The applicant's task is to respond as well as possible to the contents of the in-basket. The applicant's responses are then graded for their quality. Frederiksen has scored individuals on 70 different categories of in-basket behavior. Forty of these categories have produced the most reliable scores. A factor analysis of these categories has revealed three major dimensions of task performance (Frederiksen, 1962; see also Blum & Naylor, 1956): preparing for action, amount of work accomplished, and seeking guidance. People who are high on the first factor tend to defer decisions and actions on problems and instead spend greater amounts of time preparing to make important decisions. People high on the second factor tend to have greater work output than people low on the factor. People high on the third factor tend to be eager to please superiors and frequently seek advice from others. Frederiksen has done fairly extensive validation on the in-basket, and the results are mixed. The instrument seems to be weakly predictive of executive performance, but even these low levels of prediction tend to be erratic.

A third approach makes use of *trait and behavioral checklists* (e.g., Ghiselli, 1966). Ghiselli's self-report checklist is intended to measure 13 characteristics: supervisory ability, intelligence, initiative, self-assurance, decisiveness, masculinity – femininity, maturity, working-class affinity, need for occupational status, need for self-actualization, need for power, need for high financial reward, and need for job security. Ghiselli studied these attributes in a series of investigations over a 15-year period and found some to be more important for success than were others. For example, supervisory ability, need for occupational status, and intelligence were found to be most important, and need for power over others, maturity, and masculinity–femininity were found to be least important.

Ghiselli's approach to measuring personality needs was through checklists. Another approach, made famous by McClelland (1953, 1961), involves the assessment of needs, and particularly of need for achievement, via *projective testing* through the Thematic Aperception Test. In this test, one is shown a picture of an emotionally charged situation and asked to construct a story about it, including a beginning, a middle, and an end. McClelland's approach to assessing practical abilities thus focuses more on motivation than on intelligence per se. A long series of studies conducted over the years suggests that need for achievement is at least somewhat predictive of managerial and other kinds of success. Indeed, McClelland (1973) has suggested that conventional intelligence testing badly needs supplementation by testing of competence, including projective tests that can be used to measure needs such as need for achievement.

The list of approaches given above is incomplete but conveys some sense of the variety of approaches that have been used to assess practical intelligence among individuals. Our own approach (Wagner & Sternberg, in press) combines some aspects of the simulation approach with other aspects of the psychometric approach but emanates from a theoretical focus somewhat different from that which has motivated previous investigations.

Theoretical framework

The basic idea underlying our approach to practical intelligence is that underlying successful performance in many real-world tasks is *tacit knowledge* of a kind that is never explicitly taught and in many instances never even verbalized. Interviews with successful business executives and academic psychologists revealed a striking level of agreement that a major factor underlying success in each occupation is a knowledge and understanding of the ins and outs of the occupation. These ins and outs are generally bits of information one learns on the job rather than in any preparatory academic or other work. In academia, for example, abilities to write grant proposals, to ascertain what is considered important by one's department for promotion, to delegate authority in research, and so on, can be critical to success but do not constitute part of the training in most graduate programs. To measure potential for job success, therefore, one might wish to go beyond conventional ability and achievement tests, measuring as well an individual's knowledge and understanding of the hidden agenda in his or her field of endeavor.

In particular, we have found three kinds of tacit knowledge to be particularly important for success. Our categorization is not intended to be either mutually exclusive or exhaustive but rather to capture major aspects of what it is that leads to real-world occupational success in many fields:

1. *Managing people:* knowing how to direct the work of others and what constitute effective interpersonal and supervisory skills.
2. *Managing tasks:* knowing how to manage the day-to-day tasks that confront one in one's work.
3. *Managing self:* knowing how to maximize one's performance on the job.
4. *Managing career:* knowing what activities lead to the enhancement of one's reputation and success in one's field of endeavor.

Consider, in the domains of business and academic psychology, some examples of items that measure these kinds of tacit knowledge. In each case, one's task is to rate the importance of each of several behaviors for a given goal:

First, consider the management of people in the business domain:

In business as in other fields, there are often several people who are acknowledged to do extraordinary work. Rate the following characteristics by how important you believe them to be for the success of these individuals:
a. Very good at selling their ideas to others.
b. Socially adept.
c. Always the leader in group situations.

Second, consider the management of tasks in the academic psychology domain:

Rate the following strategies of working according to how important you believe them to be to doing well at the day-to-day work of an academic psychologist:
a. Think in terms of tasks accomplished rather than hours spent working.
b. Delegate tasks to competent others whenever possible.
c. Carefully consider the optimal strategy before beginning a task.

Third, consider the management of one's self in the academic psychology domain:

Rate the following motivations in terms of their importance as incentives for pursuing a career in academic psychology:
a. I enjoy the subject matter of the areas I am pursuing.
b. I want recognition from my peers in the field for my accomplishments.
c. I like having a job with no "boss."

Fourth and finally, consider the management of one's career in the business domain:

You are looking for several new projects to tackle. You have a list of possible projects and desire to pick the best two or three among them. Rate the importance of each of the following considerations when selecting projects:
a. The scope of the project goes beyond my present responsibilities.
b. The project will bring favorable attention to my superiors.
c. The project will require working directly with several senior executives.

In each case, one is presented with a brief orienting paragraph and then must rate how important each of several considerations would be in order to achieve some goal. Our approach to measuring practical intelligence has used items such as these as a basis for assessing tacit knowledge.

To date, we have conducted three experiments. The first involved development and construct validation of a questionnaire relevant to success in academic psychology. The second involved development and construct validation of a questionnaire relevant to success in business. The third involved cross-validation of the business questionnaire to new subjects and a new setting. Below, I describe the methodology we used in these experimental pursuits. (See Wagner & Sternberg, in press, for further details.)

Experiment 1

The purpose of our first experiment was to test our theory and methodology on an initial occupational group. We chose as our first group academic psychologists.

Method. In the first experiment, our subjects were 187 individuals having some connection with academic psychology. Fifty-four of these individuals were faculty members in psychology departments. Of the 54, some 27 were from 10 of the "top 15" departments according to available ratings, and 21 were from 10 other departments pseudorandomly selected from schools other than those in the top 15. An additional 6 faculty members failed to identify their school and so were unclassifiable. Of the remaining 133 subjects, 104 were graduate students in psychology and 29 were Yale undergraduates in a variety of fields. Of the graduate students, 53 were from 11 of the "top 15" departments, 49 were from 10 other departments, and 2 failed to identify their school and hence were unclassifiable.

Each subject received the psychology tacit knowledge questionnaire as well as questions about performance in school and career (except for undergraduates). Fifty-eight questionnaire items were retained for final analyses.

The criterion for retention in the final data analysis was that responses to the item showed a statistically significant correlation with level of expertise in the field of psychology, where levels of expertise were coded on a three-point scale (undergraduate student, graduate student, faculty member). Sample items from the questionnaire are presented in Table 9.1.

Retained items were classified in terms of whether they measured tacit knowledge regarding management of (a) others, (b) tasks, (c) self, (d) career, or (e) miscellaneous. These categories provided the basis for subscores as well as a full-scale score on the questionnaire. These various scores were used to predict a variety of external criteria of success.

All questionnaires were sent out by mail except for those administered to the Yale students. The return rates were 28% for faculty members and 47% for graduate students.

Results. Mean questionnaire scores were 290.4 ($SD = 20.8$) for faculty members, 268.7 ($SD = 25.8$) for graduate students, and 227.1 ($SD = 23.1$) for undergraduate students. The basic statistics for the faculty members are probably those of most interest. The mean number of citations of published work was 52.9 ($SD = 92.0$), but the distribution of citations was extremely right-skewed, with a range in number of citations from zero to 396 during a one-year period. The mean number of publications per year was 3.2 ($SD = 2.2$). The mean number of conventions attended per year was 2.3 ($SD = 1.5$), and the mean number of convention papers presented per year was 1.9 ($SD = 2.0$). Faculty members were asked to estimate how they allocated their time among various pursuits, and the mean percentages were 30.8 for teaching, 34.9 for research, 11.2 for advising students, 5.3 for editorial work, 12.8 for administrative work, and 5.1 for other kinds of activities. The average year of Ph.D. was 1964.

For faculty members, composite questionnaire scores were significantly correlated with self-reported number of publications in the present year (.32), number of conferences attended (.34), and level of school – top 15 versus all the rest (.40). Moreover, scores were negatively correlated with percentages of time spent on teaching (-.29) and administrative duties (-.41) but positively correlated with time spent on research (.39). Questionnaire scores were not significantly correlated with number of years in the profession, suggesting that it is what one learns from experience, rather than experience per se, that affects questionnaire scores. An analysis of subscores revealed 5 significant correlations with external criteria of success for managing people, 3 for managing tasks, 2 for managing self, and 5 for managing career (all out of 13 computed). These results suggest, then, that the questionnaire did predict with some success several of the major criteria for faculty member performance.

Table 9.1. *Sample items from tacit knowledge questionnaires*

Psychology

1. It is your second year as an assistant professor in a prestigious psychology department. This past year you published two unrelated empirical articles in established journals. You don't, however, believe there is yet a research area that can be identified as your own. You believe yourself to be about as productive as others. The feedback about your first year of teaching has been generally good. You have yet to serve on a university committee. There is one graduate student who has chosen to work with you. You have no external source of funding, nor have you applied for funding.

Your goals are to become one of the top people in your field and to get tenure in your department. The following is a list of things you are considering doing in the next two months. You obviously cannot do them all. Rate the importance of each by its priority as a means of reaching your goals.
   a. Improve the quality of your teaching
   b. Write a grant proposal
   c. Begin long-term research that may lead to a major theoretical article
   d. Serve on a committee studying university–community relations
   e. Begin several related short-term research projects, each of which may lead to an empirical article
   f. Write a paper for presentation to an upcoming American Psychological Association convention
   g. Ask for comments from senior members of the department on future papers

2. Rate the importance of the following in deciding to which journal to submit an article for possible publication:
   a. Reputation of the journal in your field of expertise
   b. Number of years the journal has been in existence
   c. Publication lag of the journal
   d. Rejection rate of the journal
   e. Overall circulation of the journal
   f. Appropriateness of the journal for content of your paper

3. An undergraduate student has asked for your advice in deciding to which graduate programs in psychology to apply. Consider the following dimensions for rating the overall quality of a graduate program in psychology and rate their importance:
   a. Breadth of the program
   b. Prestige of the faculty
   c. Quality of the undergraduate student population
   d. Job placements of recent graduates of the program
   e. Number of required courses
   f. Current grants and research projects underway

Business

1. It is your second year as a midlevel manager in a company in the communications industry. You head a department of about 30 people. The evaluation of your first

Table 9.1 *(cont.)*

year on the job has been generally favorable. Performance ratings for your department are at least as good as they were before you took over, and perhaps even a little
better. You have two assistants. One is quite capable. The other just seems to go
through the motions but to be of little real help.

You believe that although you are well liked, there is little that would distinguish
you in the eyes of your superiors from the nine other managers at a comparable level
in the company.

Your goal is rapid promotion to the top of the company. The following is a list of
things you are considering doing in the next two months. You obviously cannot do
them all. Rate the importance of each by its priority as a means of reaching your goal.

    a. Find a way to get rid of the "dead wood," e.g., the less helpful assistant and three
       or four others
    b. Become more involved in local public service organizations
    c. Find ways to make sure your superiors are aware of your important accom-
       plishments
    d. As a means of being noticed, propose a solution to a problem outside the scope
       of your immediate department that you would be willing to take charge of
    e. When making decisions, give a great deal of weight to the way your superior
       likes things to be done
    f. Accept a friend's invitation to join the exclusive country club that many higher-
       level executives belong to
    g. Ask for comments from superiors about important decisions you need to make
    h. Adjust your work habits to increase your productivity

2. Rate the following strategies of working according to how important you believe
them to be for doing well at the day-to-day work of a business manager:
    a. Always have a variety of projects in progress – many "irons in the fire"
    b. Do not force yourself to do tasks you don't feel like doing
    c. Use a daily list of goals arranged according to your priorities
    d. Don't try to do everything well – many tasks are trivial
    e. Delegate tasks to competent others whenever possible
    f. Carefully consider the optimal strategy before beginning a task

3. You have just been promoted to head an important department in the company.
The previous head had been transferred to an equivalent position in a less important
department. Your understanding of the reason for the move is that the performance
of the department as a whole was mediocre. There were not any glaring deficiencies,
just a perception of the department as so-so rather than as very good. Your charge
was to shape up the department. Results are expected quickly. Rate the following
pieces of advice colleagues have given you by their importance to succeeding in your
new position:
    a. Always delegate to the most junior person who can be trusted with the task
    b. Make people feel completely responsible for their work
    c. Be intolerant of your own mistakes and of the mistakes of others

Table 9.1 *(cont.)*

---

d. Be careful to avoid the company's "sacred cows"
e. Do not try to do too much too soon
f. Promote open communication

Note: Ratings were made on a scale of 1 to 7, where 1 signified "not important" and 7 signified "extremely important." Items of a given question varied in number from 9 to 20.

For graduate students, composite questionnaire scores were significantly correlated with years of graduate study completed (.39), level of school (.52), number of publications (.31), and number of research projects participated in (.31). Of five possible correlations computed, one was statistically significant for managing people, two for managing tasks, one for managing self, and five for managing career. Not only were there more significant correlations for the managing career subscore, but the correlations tended to be higher: Whereas significant correlations for other subscores were generally in the .20s, those for managing career were generally in the .30s and .40s. For an undergraduate sample different from that in the main experiment (but from the same population – Yale students – as we used in the main experiment), correlations between scores on an IQ test and on our tacit knowledge measure differed only trivially from zero.

The combined results for the faculty members and graduate students (we had no viable measures of criterion performance for undergraduate students, who generally have not yet done anything to prove themselves in the field of psychology) suggest that the composite questionnaire score provides a useful predictor of some of the criteria usually associated with professional success and, moreover, that questions pertaining to career management were those most relevant for prediction. Naturally, we would not want to claim that tacit knowledge is all that is involved in professional success: Certainly, academic intelligence, creativity, motivation, and a host of other factors are responsible as well. But it does appear that tacit knowledge is one of the factors that should be considered when attempting to account for individual differences in success of professional performance in the domain of academic psychology.

Experiment 2

The purpose of this experiment was to extend the theory and methodology of Experiment 1 to a different occupational group. The occupational group we chose was that of business executives.

Method. A total of 127 individuals were involved in Experiment 2. Of these, 54 were business executives. Included in this group were 19 executives from among the "top 20" of Fortune 500 companies, 28 executives from companies outside the Fortune 500, and 7 executives who did not indicate their company and hence could not be identified with respect to group. Another 51 participants in the study were students in graduate schools of business administration. Of these students, 28 were from top-rated business schools, 15 were from a middle-rated business school, and 7 were from modestly-rated business schools. One student failed to identify his or her school. An additional 22 subjects were Yale undergraduates (in a variety of fields).

All subjects received the business questionnaire. Thirty-nine items were retained for the final business data analyses. Sample items from the questionnaire are shown in Table 9.1. Items were retained only if they discriminated significantly (as with the psychology questionnaire, a significant correlation between questionnaire score and level of expertise) among the three levels of business experience (business executives, graduate students in business administration, and undergraduates). This criterion for selecting items was probably a bit less successfully applied in the present experiment than in the first due to the fact that most business students have at least some experience in business firms (whereas virtually no psychology graduate students have had experience as professors).

Items were classified, as in Experiment 1, according to whether they required tacit knowledge regarding management of others, tasks, self, career, or miscellaneous. As before, all questionnaires were sent by mail except those administered to the Yale undergraduates.

Results. Mean questionnaire scores were 171.9 ($SD = 18.0$) for business executives, 150.0 ($SD = 12.6$) for graduate students of business administration, and 138.6 ($SD = 12.2$) for undergraduates. Mean salary for the business executives was in the range of $50,000 to $59,000 ($SD =$ approximately $30,000). The distribution of salaries was highly skewed and ranged from a category of $10,000–$19,000 to a category of $100,000+.

Composite scores on the business questionnaire proved to be predictive of several of the criteria we measured for business success. Significant correlations were obtained for three of six correlations computed, those with level of company (.34), years of formal schooling (.41), and salary (.46). For sub-scores, no significant correlations were obtained between the managing people and self dimensions and our criteria. Three significant correlations were obtained for each of managing tasks and managing career. Unfortunately, no significant correlations were obtained for questionnaire scores and criteria used to assess performance among the business administration students. In this experiment, we administered to undergraduates the Verbal Reasoning subtest of the Differential Aptitudes Test in order to determine whether our questionnaire was simply a fancy measure of verbal reasoning ability: The correlation was a nonsignificant .16, suggesting that whatever our questionnaire measures, it is something beyond mere *"g."*

To conclude, our questionnaire shows some predictive validity in measuring success among business executives. It did not work, however, for business graduate students. Whatever success the questionnaire may have had, it is not due to overlap with verbal reasoning ability: The abilities measured by our business questionnaire, as by our psychology questionnaire, are statistically orthogonal to those measured by a well-known standardized test of verbal reasoning ability.

Experiment 3

The purpose of the third experiment was to cross-validate the results for the business questionnaire to a new sample of subjects for whom we would have better measures of performance than were available from the executives to whom we had mailed our business questionnaire.

Method. Subjects in our third experiment were 29 managers at a New Haven bank. All subjects received the business questionnaire administered by the head of personnel for the bank. In this experiment, we were able to obtain somewhat more interesting criteria of success than we had been able to obtain in the previous experiment: We had for each executive a measure of percentage salary increase over the past two years (which was determined on a merit basis); a global performance rating; specific performance ratings for "managing personnel," "generating business," and "following bank policy" (our categorization); and level of title in the bank.

Results. Significant correlations were obtained between questionnaire scores (using the same items as in Experiment 2) and percentage salary increase (.48), global performance rating (.37, significant at the .06 level), and the generating business derived rating (.56). For the particular questionnaire subscores, no significant correlations were obtained between criterion measures and the managing people and managing tasks subscores. Of six correlations computed, one significant correlation was obtained for the managing self score, and four significant correlations were obtained for the managing career subscore. Thus, in this experiment, as in the others, the managing career subscore seems to be the most diagnostic one in predicting external performance criteria.

Conclusions

The results of our three initial studies of practical intelligence lead us to believe that tacit knowledge is, in fact, a useful measure of practical intelligence. Although it is certainly not all that matters to occupational success, it appears to be one important factor in real-world performance. Moreover, we expect that its importance would generalize to domains other than the ones we have studied, an expectation we plan to test in subsequent research. The two questionnaires we used are only preliminary, of course, but they appear to have some construct validity for the purposes for which they were intended. Tacit knowledge relevant to managing one's career appears to be more important to career success than does tacit knowledge relevant to managing people, tasks, or self.

In sum, we believe that one important aspect of practical intelligence – tacit knowledge – is measurable and that the extent of such knowledge is predictive of real-world occupational success. This conclusion regarding practical intelligence obviously differs markedly from that regarding social intelligence as measured by nonverbal decoding skills: For the present, I believe that the tacit knowledge approach to practical intelligence is likely to be more productive than the nonverbal decoding approach to social intelligence.

Part IV

The triarchic theory: some implications

Part IV contains two chapters presenting some implications of the triarchic theory of human intelligence for issues of contemporary importance in research and practice.

Chapter 10, "Exceptional intelligence," discusses the implications of the triarchic theory for understanding intellectual giftedness and retardation. Although all aspects of the triarchic theory have some relevance to understanding both giftedness and retardation, their relevance may not be equal. It is suggested that a particularly important aspect of intellectual giftedness is exceptional insight skills, which are understood in terms of the facet of the experiential subtheory of intelligence concerning adjustment to novelty; a particularly important aspect of intellectual retardation appears to be inadequate metacomponential functioning, as dealt with in the componential subtheory.

Chapter 11, "Implications of the triarchic theory for intelligence testing," discusses how the triarchic theory accounts for the successes (and failures) of current intelligence tests and describes the kinds of intelligence tests that would follow from the each of the subtheories of the triarchic theory. These new tests are not suggested as a replacement for current tests but would seem to provide useful supplements for them. Most importantly, they would broaden considerably the domain of abilities sampled in the measurement of intelligence.

10 Exceptional intelligence

Viewing intelligence on a unidimensional scale, such as IQ, typically leads to the view that exceptional intelligence, as represented by intellectual giftedness and retardation, are opposite ends of a single scale. In some quantitative sense, this may be true. But I doubt that the attributes that best distinguish the intellectually gifted are truly the same as those that best distinguish the retarded. Rather, the gifted are probably above average, but not necessarily exceptional, in those attributes that distinguish the retarded from the normal. At exceptional levels of intellectual talent, qualitatively different attributes start to matter from those that distinguish normal from retarded performance. In particular, it is proposed that giftedness derives especially from unusual ability to deal with novel kinds of tasks and situations (as covered by the experiential subtheory), whereas retardation derives largely from inadequate functioning of componential subsystems (as covered by the componential subtheory), inadequate automatization of componential subsystems (as covered by the experiential subtheory), or both. This is not to say that intellectual giftedness is limited to ability to deal with novelty, or retardation to inability to perform executive functions. Rather, these aspects are proposed to be those that are most distinctive. I will discuss in turn each of these two kinds of exceptional intelligence.

Intellectual giftedness: insight and the ability to deal with novelty

Janet Davidson and I have proposed that a key psychological basis of intellectual giftedness resides in what might be referred to as "insight skills" (Sternberg & Davidson, 1982, 1983). We refer to our account as a "subtheory" of intellectual giftedness in order to emphasize our view that, although insight skills represent an important part of the story of intellectual giftedness, they do not represent the whole story. Certainly other psychological functions constitute other parts of the story as well (see, e.g., Renzulli,

1976; Sternberg, 1981b). We do believe, however, that insight skills form a particularly important part of intellectual giftedness.

Before proceeding to a presentation of our views, it would be helpful to put them in historical context by considering two major views of the nature of intellectual giftedness. These two (which of course are not the only ones) are the psychometric and the information-processing views. (For a further discussion of alternative psychological views of intellectual giftedness, see Feldman, 1982.)

On the psychometric view, intellectual giftedness consists of the possession of greater amounts of (and thus higher scores on measures of) latent mental abilities. These latent mental abilities are usually identified through the statistical method of factor analysis. For example, gifted children might be seen as superior to average children in their level of general intelligence (*"g"*), or in their levels of major mental abilities such as verbal comprehension, reasoning, or spatial visualization. Psychometric theorists and practitioners have given the lion's share of attention to the underlying factors of intelligence but have also paid some attention to factors of creativity. Intelligence and creativity tests have been widely used as bases for assessing intellectual giftedness.

The information-processing approach to intelligence arose in large part in reaction to a perceived failure of advocates of the psychometric approach to specify the *processes* that constitute intelligent performance; however, advocates of the information-processing approach have had little to say about the nature of giftedness per se, at least so far. Presumably, gifted individuals would be those who are superior to others in the exercise of information-processing skills. In my earlier theoretical work (e.g., Sternberg, 1981b), intellectual giftedness was viewed as attributable primarily to superior componential skills. Some theorists, such as Hunt (1978), would probably emphasize the role of speed of mechanistic process execution in giftedness. For example, one would expect gifted individuals to be more rapid than ordinary individuals in retrieving the name codes of objects from long-term memory. The view presented below is an example of an information-processing view, one that emphasizes processes in insightful thinking.

Motivation for the subtheory

Why use the study of insight skills as a preferred entree for studying intellectual giftedness? We believe at least two bases exist for this preference.

First, significant and exceptional intellectual accomplishment - for example, major scientific discoveries, new and important inventions, and new and significant understandings of major literary, philosophical, and similar works - almost always involve major intellectual insights. The thinkers' gifts seem directly to lie in their insight abilities and abilities to do nonentrenched thinking rather than in their IQ-like abilities or their mere abilities to process information rapidly (Sternberg, 1981h, 1982d, 1982f, 1984d).

Second, it is possible, in studying insight, to study problems in a wide variety of content domains. Insight is not a skill limited to any one particular domain. One need not, say, discriminate against those with primarily verbal talents by concentrating only on mathematical problems or discriminate against the mathematically oriented by studying only verbal problems. Indeed, it seems important to show that a theory of giftedness that claims to be general does extend beyond any one content domain. If one's goal is to avoid pitfalls of past theory and measurement, insight seems at least like a good starting point for studying giftedness.

Proposed view of insight

We believe that a main reason psychologists (and others) have had so much difficulty in isolating insight is that it involves not one but three separate yet related psychological processes (Sternberg & Davidson, 1982, 1983). These processes are extensions of the knowledge-acquisition components to novel tasks and situations. As the processes are described in some detail in Chapter 3, I will review them only briefly here.

1. *Selective encoding.* An insight of selective encoding involves sifting out relevant information from irrelevant information. Significant problems generally present one with large amounts of information, only some of which is relevant to problem solution. In my journal editing, for example, I have found that a major distinguisher of better from lesser scientists is the ability of the better scientists to recognize what is important in their data. They seem to know what findings to emphasize and what findings to deemphasize or ignore. The lesser scientists seem almost to weight their findings with a uniform distribution of weights. They are unable to distinguish what matters more in their data from what matters less.

2. *Selective combination.* An insight of selective combination involves combining what might originally seem to be isolated pieces of information into a unified whole that may or may not resemble its parts. Whereas selective encoding involves knowing which pieces of information are relevant, selective combination involves knowing how to put together the pieces of relevant information. In my journal editing, for example, I have found that the more competent scientists seem better able to fit their findings together into a coherent package, or story. They are able to see how the various findings fit together. Lesser scientists often seem not to see how their various findings are interrelated. They present them as isolated facts rather than as part of a finely woven story about the phenomenon under investigation.

3. *Selective comparison.* An insight of selective comparison involves relating newly acquired information to information acquired in the past. Problem solving by analogy, for example, is an instance of selective comparison: One realizes that new information is similar to old information in certain ways (and dissimilar from it in other ways) and uses this information better to understand the new information. In my journal editing, for example, I have found that better scientists seem better able to relate their new work to past work that has been done in the field. They have a sense of where their work fits into the current scientific picture and of just what its contribution is to ongoing scientific research. Less able scientists often seem to have little conception of how their research fits into the current scientific picture and may do their work without a clear understanding of why it is, or is not, really worth doing.

In sum, we have proposed a three-process view of insight that constitutes what we believe to be a well-specified theory of insightful information processing. This theory forms the basis for our subtheory of what it is that makes for intellectual giftedness. The theory does not deal with all of what makes an individual gifted. At present, we are not in a position to evaluate the differential importance, if any, of the three kinds of insights in gifted performance, nor can we say whether the three kinds of insights constitute three distinct sources of individual differences or rather fewer sources by virtue of their derivation from some "higher-order" insight ability, of which selective encoding, selective combination, and selective comparison are special cases. These questions remain open for empirical determination of their answers.

Tests of the subtheory

We have sought to test our subtheory of intellectual giftedness on fourth-, fifth-, and sixth-grade normal and gifted subjects (Davidson & Sternberg, 1984). The subjects, students in an upper-middle-class suburban school district, had been identified as either gifted (minimum IQ 140) or nongifted on the bases of IQ test scores, Torrance creativity test scores, teacher recommendations, and parental comments. Three experiments were performed – examining, respectively, the nature of selective encoding, selective combination, and selective comparison – using both mathematical and verbal insight problems. Because there is some doubt as to whether our verbal problems (sentence completions) actually succeeded in measuring insight, and because we experienced ceiling effects on the part of the gifted with respect to these problems, I shall confine my discussion of results to the data for the mathematical problems. In addition to the insight problems, subjects were also given a test battery including mystery problems (requiring subjects to figure out how a detective knew the identity of the perpetrators of various crimes), inductive reasoning problems, and deductive reasoning problems. We also had available IQ test scores for all of the subjects on a group-administered IQ test. The mathematical insight problems were similar to those described earlier in Chapter 3 – for example, "If you have black socks and brown socks in your drawer, mixed in the ratio of 4 to 5, how many socks will you have to take out to make sure of having a pair of socks the same color?"

I think it important to note that the kinds of problems we have used to date in our studies of insight clearly depart from the kinds of large-scale scientific, mathematical, literary, and other problems that give rise to major intellectual insights. Thus, the data I report here can be regarded as only of the most preliminary kind. They very much need to be followed up by data based upon problems requiring much more significant kinds of insights. Our present work is, we hope, headed in this direction.

Our first concern was whether performance on the insight problems showed the predicted pattern of convergent–discriminant validation. In particular, we expected performance on the insight problems (a) to be better for gifted children than for nongifted children and (b) to correlate most highly with performance on the mystery stories, which require insights; next most highly with inductive problems, which require the subject to go beyond the information given; and least highly with deductive problems, which provide all information needed for solution. In fact, the respective mean numbers of problems correct (out of 15 possible) were 8.45 for the gifted children and 5.36 for the nongifted children, a difference that was statistically significant for the 86 children involved in this comparison. Correlations with the respective reference tests were .56 with mysteries, .53 with letter sets, and .43 with nonsense syllogisms. The correlation with a group IQ test administered by the school was .55. Although the differences between correlations were not significant, they seemed to fall at least into the pattern we had expected.

In a first experiment, which investigated selective encoding, subjects were either precued as to what information in each of a set of insight problems was relevant for problem solution or not so precued. For example, the following problem would either be given in normal form or with solution-relevant parts underlined, as follows: "A farmer buys 100 animals for $100. Cows are $10 each, sheep are $3 each, and pigs are 50 cents each. How much did he pay for 5 cows?" Eighty subjects participated in this experiment: All of them received half of the problems with cueing and half without. Which problems were or were not cued was counterbalanced. In addition, some of the problems were designated as "encoding" problems, in that they contained both relevant and irrelevant information; other problems contained only relevant information, and were thus designated as "nonencoding" problems (because selective encoding was not needed). When these problems were presented in cued form, the entire problem was underlined.

There were five major predictions regarding the results. First, it was predicted that gifted children would perform better than nongifted ones. This prediction was confirmed, with respective mean insight-problem scores (out of 12 possible) of 4.08 and 2.45. Second, it was predicted that performance on the cued problems would be better than performance on the uncued problems. This prediction was also confirmed. Mean scores were 3.63 for cued problems and 2.89 for uncued problems (out of 12 possible). Third, it was predicted that encoding problems, for which the underlining manipulation would be expected to provide facilitation, would be easier than nonencoding problems, for which the underlining manipulation would be expected to provide no facilitation. Again, the prediction was confirmed: Respective means were 3.42 for encoding problems and 3.10 for nonencoding problems (out of 12 possible). Fourth, it was predicted that there would be a significant Cueing × Encoding interaction. This interaction would follow from cueing having more of a facilitatory effect for encoding problems (where only some information was underlined) than for nonencoding problems (where all information was underlined). If the cueing information did genuinely facilitate selective encoding, then, this interaction should be significant. This prediction was also confirmed. Means were 2.99 for uncued nonencoding problems, 3.22 for cued nonencoding problems, 2.80 for uncued encoding problems, and 4.04 for cued encoding problems (all out of 6 possible). Finally, it was predicted that there would be a significant Group × Cueing × Encoding triple interaction. Such an interaction would follow if there was a greater facilitation by cueing for encoding than for nonencoding problems and if this facilitation was greater for nongifted than for gifted subjects. We expected such a difference across groups in facilitation in that, according to our view of giftedness, the primary difficulty of the nongifted subjects in solving insight problems is in having the proper insight. Thus, providing them with the insight should be quite helpful; as the gifted subjects are more likely to have the insight without cueing, providing the cueing should be less helpful to them. This prediction, too, was confirmed. Examination of the eight relevant means confirmed that the interaction resulted from the predicted pattern of results. In this experiment and in the ones that follow, differential performance of gifted and nongifted was not due to ceiling effects, which did not occur in any of the experiments.

To conclude, the results of the selective encoding experiment were wholly consistent with our five major predictions. The results thus supported the proposed role of selective encoding as critical to solution of insight problems and as an important factor in distinguishing the performance of the gifted from the nongifted.

Our second experiment had as its target the role of selective combination in insightful problem solving. The 74 subjects in the experiment received mathematical insight problems presented either in the standard format or with cueing intended to facilitate selective combination processes. Consider an example of a problem and how it was cued.

There are five people sitting in a row at a table at a dinner party:

Scott is seated at one end of the row.
Ziggy is seated next to Matt.
Joshua is not sitting next to Scott or Ziggy.
Only one person is sitting next to Walter.
Who is sitting next to Walter?

In its uncued form, the problem was presented just as above. In its cued form, the subject was shown a horizontal grid of five contiguous rectangles. The name "Scott" was written in the leftmost rectangle. The subject was thereby both shown how to form a grid that would represent the table arrangement and was given a clue as to the location of one individual at the table. Again, all subjects received both cued and uncued problems in a counterbalanced order.

Three major predictions were made regarding the results. First, it was predicted that the gifted subjects would perform better than the nongifted. This prediction was confirmed. Respective means (out of 16 possible) were 6.50 and 4.16 for the gifted and nongifted subjects. Second, it was predicted that performance on the cued problems would be superior to performance on the uncued problems. This prediction, too, was confirmed. Mean scores were 5.82 on the cued problems and 4.84 on the uncued problems (out of 8 possible). Finally, it was predicted that there would be a significant Group × Cueing interaction, with the nongifted group profiting more from the cueing than the gifted group. This prediction, too, was confirmed. Relevant means were 6.56 for the gifted on uncued problems, 6.44 for the gifted on cued problems, 3.11 for the nongifted on the uncued problems, and 5.20 for the nongifted on the cued problems (all out of 8 possible). Thus, once again, the nongifted profited more from receiving the insight than did the gifted.

In sum, the selective combination experiment also supported our theory. In particular, selective combination appears to play an important role in solving insight problems (not all of which involved seats at a table, as did the sample). Moreover, it appears to be a primary source of difficulty for nongifted but not for gifted subjects: Gifted subjects did not benefit from cueing, whereas nongifted ones did.

Our third experiment was designed to assess the role of selective comparison in insightful problem solving. In this experiment, most subjects received two different example problems prior to receiving the insight problems. For example, the subject might see as an example: "You are flipping a fair coin. So far, it has come up heads 10 times and tails 1 time. What are the chances that it will come up tails the next time that you flip the coin?" After subjects read the example problems, the nature of the problems was explained to them, and they were given a fairly detailed explanation of how to solve each problem. Later, subjects received a set of insight problems. Some of these problems, in fact, drew upon the principle taught in one example; other problems drew upon the principle taught in the second example; still other problems drew upon neither principle. Problem solving would clearly be facilitated if the subject recognized (via selective comparison) that one of the examples was relevant to solution of certain ones of the test problems. For instance, a test problem corresponding to the above example would be: "There are an equal number of red, white, and blue gum balls in a penny gum machine. Sandy spent 6 pennies last week and got 5 red gum balls and 1 white one. What are the chances that if she puts in one penny today she will get a red gum ball?"

The experiment actually involved four conditions of item presentation. In one condition, "No Examples," subjects received no examples prior to the actual test problems. In a second condition, "Examples – No Relevance Information," subjects received two example problems that they could later draw upon in their solution to test problems. They were not told, however, that the examples would later be directly helpful to them. In a third condition, "Examples – Limited Relevance Information," subjects received two relevant examples and were further told that the examples were relevant to the solution of some of the test problems. They were not told, however, to which test problems each of the examples was relevant. In the fourth condition, "Examples – Full Relevance Information," subjects were given two examples, told that they would be relevant to their solution of some of the test problems, and were explicitly told to which problems each example was relevant.

There were three main predictions in this experiment. First, it was predicted that gifted children would perform better than nongifted ones. This prediction was confirmed. Mean scores (out of 6 possible) were 4.08 for the gifted children and 3.17 for the nongifted children. Second, it was predicted that problems would become easier as more selective comparison information was provided to the subjects. This prediction, too, was confirmed. Relevant means (all out of 6 possible) were 1.63 for the "No Examples" condition, 3.76 for the "Examples – No Relevance Information" condition, 4.32 for the "Examples – Limited Relevance Information" condition, and 4.79 for the "Examples – Full Relevance Information" condition. Finally, it was predicted that there would be a significant Group × Condition interaction, with the nongifted benefiting more than the gifted from successive amounts of relevance information. This prediction, too, was confirmed. Respective condition means (for the four conditions of successively more information) were 1.82, 4.60, 5.00, and 4.91 for the gifted subjects, and 1.44, 2.92, 3.64, and 4.67 for the nongifted subjects (all out of 6 possible). Note that the gifted benefited only from the receipt of examples. Relevance information seemed to have little or no further effect upon their performance. The nongifted, in contrast, benefited incrementally as each further amount of information was given them.

In sum, the third experiment supports our contention of the importance of selective comparison in insightful problem solving as well as its role in differentiating the performance of gifted from nongifted subjects. In particular, gifted subjects seem to perform spontaneously the selective comparison that nongifted subjects perform only when prompted.

To conclude, then, the results of our experiments are wholly consistent both with our information-processing theory of insight and with our contentions regarding the roles of selective encoding, selective combination, and selective comparison in distinguishing the performance of gifted from nongifted elementary school students. Of course, the theory needs to be tested on more consequential kinds of insight problems before any strong conclusions can be drawn.

Benefits of the proposed approach

We believe that the proposed approach to understanding and assessing intellectual giftedness has several potential benefits over alternative psychometric and information-processing approaches.

First, our approach is theoretically based and draws upon a theory that seems to apply particularly well to the understanding of giftedness. It is not merely an extension of a theory that might, say, as well be applied to understanding intellectual retardation as to understanding intellectual giftedness. Rather, it seems to deal with what it is that makes the gifted special.

Second, the measurement of insight skills can take place in the absence of items that make heavy demands upon prior knowledge. For individuals with standard middle-class backgrounds, assessing intellectual skills by items that draw heavily upon knowledge may be quite reasonable. But for individuals with nonstandard backgrounds, heavy demands upon the knowledge base may result in "misses" in identification that could otherwise be prevented.

Because there already exist many measures of various kinds of intellectual skills that are appropriate for those from standard middle-class backgrounds, we think it particularly important to develop instruments that can spot exceptional talent in those from nonstandard backgrounds.

Third, we have avoided the extreme emphasis on speed of processing that characterizes many psychometric and information-processing assessments of intellectual skills. We believe that despite the many fine features of reaction time or speeded responses, in general, as dependent variables, they need supplementation when one's goal is to understand or assess intellectual giftedness. We believe that what primarily distinguishes the intellectually gifted in their performance is not that they are faster, but that they are better in their insightful problem-solving skills.

Fourth, we do not use the kinds of low-level information-processing tasks that characterize much experimental-psychological research on intelligence. Tasks such as speed at naming letters of the alphabet may give us certain insights into the nature of intelligence in general, but it remains to be shown that they give us much insight into the nature of intellectual giftedness in particular. Skills such as rapidity of lexical access to items in memory may be one basis for differentiating levels of intelligence, but they seem not to be the basis for distinguishing, say, highly original thinkers from more ordinary ones.

Finally, our approach differs from many psychometric and information-processing approaches in starting with a theory and proceeding to task selection rather than the other way around. Factor theories of intelligence have traditionally been derived as a function of the tasks selected. One starts with a standard battery of conventional psychometric tests and then proceeds to factor-analyze them in one way or another and to rotate the obtained factors. Information-processing theories of intelligence have often started either with the standard psychometric tasks (e.g., Sternberg, 1981j, 1984f), or the standard information-processing tasks (Hunt, 1978) and then developed theoretical accounts on the basis of performance on these tasks. The advantage of such an approach is that one starts with tasks that are "time-honored" and whose properties are well known. The disadvantage is that the possibility for discovering new insights about giftedness may be restricted. In effect, one wishes to understand "nonentrenched" performance in "entrenched" ways, and it is not clear that such an approach is optimally likely to work.

Other aspects of intellectual giftedness

As noted earlier, it would be foolish to maintain that insight skills are *all* of the skills involved in intellectual giftedness. The triarchic theory posits other sources of difference between the intellectually gifted and other individuals.

First, the gifted will, in most cases, show superior performance to others on standard kinds of intelligence tests. According to the present view, such superiority is attributable to better metacomponential, performance-componential, and knowledge-acquisition-componential skills (Sternberg, 1981b). Indeed, the three components of insight are special cases of the application of knowledge-acquisition components where the application of these components is particularly nonobvious and of some consequence. Second, the gifted can be expected to be superior in dealing with novel kinds of tasks and situations in general (Sternberg, 1982f). Indeed, insight skills are a subset of those skills used to deal with nonentrenchment in one's environment (see Chapter 3). Third, the gifted are likely to have automatized highly practiced performances to a greater extent than the nongifted, as well as being more adept at automatization than are others. Fourth and finally, the gifted are individuals who are particularly adept at applying their intellectual skills to the task or situational environment in which they display their gifts. Although they may or may not be above average in everyday kinds of real-world skills, they are exceptional in the everyday skills of the pursuits in which they have shown their gifts. Thus, they have unusual ability to adapt to, select, or shape at least that environment in which they distinguish themselves. Such skills will not necessarily generalize to other environments and kinds of environments.

These other aspects of giftedness can be seen in the performance of individuals identified as gifted through various means. Moreover, they are by no means perfectly correlated. For example, many of us are familiar with people who have exceptionally high IQs and are outstanding in componential kinds of performances, but who seem to lack insightful or creative ideas. They seem to be "analyzers" rather than "synthesizers." Although they may obtain very high grades in school and be considered to be extremely bright, they lack the spark of originality that distinguishes exceptional people in the arts and sciences. Similarly, many of us are familiar with people whose contextual skills are outstanding but who seem to fall down in other areas. In every profession, for example, there seem to be people who get ahead – who are highly visible and regarded – but who seem to lack the intellectual skills of others who have attained their positions. Sometimes, such people are referred to as "operators." According to the present view, it is perhaps unfair to fail to give them the credit they are due. They may be people with unusual skills in adapting to their environments or in selecting or shaping environments so as to make themselves valued, but whose other intellectual skills do not match their contextually oriented ones. They are unusually intelligent, although not in the sense that everyone feels comfortable rewarding: Their "visibility" in a field of endeavor may well overpower their "reputation." Thus, intellectual giftedness can be of many kinds. In highlighting insight, we by no means wish to ignore other kinds of skills in which individuals can be gifted.

In short, the triarchic theory specifies several loci of intellectual giftedness. We believe, however, that the locus of insight is the one of primary importance for understanding what, in particular, distinguishes the intellectually gifted from others.

Intellectual retardation

A triarchic view of retardation

Intellectual retardation is not well understood in terms of the relative absence of striking insights. People of normal intelligence rarely or never have such insights either. Rather, according to the present view, retardation is understood in terms of inadequate functioning of componential subsystems, inadequate automatization of componential subsystems, or both. The degree of impairment will depend upon the range of task domains to which the impairment extends. This range will in turn depend on things such as an individual's motivation (or lack thereof) in different task domains; kind and extent of organic damage, if any; compatibility of teaching methods with a given individual's set of abilities; and quantity, quality, and timing of exposure to materials in various task domains.

Consider the loci of intellectual retardation suggested by the triarchic theory, and particularly the componential subtheory, and how these could be applied to understanding deficient performance on a typical IQ test (see also Sternberg, 1981a, in press-d).

1. *Impaired activation by metacomponents of each other and of other kinds of components.* A person has all the necessary procedural and declarative knowledge necessary to solve a problem but is unable to bring this knowledge to bear upon the problem. There is a gap in communication between the metacomponents that "know" what to do and the performance components that actually do it. This kind of impairment seems closely analogous to what Flavell and Wohlwill (1969) have referred to as a "performance deficit," in contrast to a "mediation deficit." If, for example, a child knows how to solve a certain kind of reasoning problem but is unable to bring that knowledge to bear upon problems of that kind, impaired activation of performance components by metacomponents might be a source of difficulty.

2. *Impaired feedback to metacomponents from other metacomponents and other kinds of components.* A person is unable to use information acquired during the course of information processing to alter his or her performance. For example, if, during the course of reading an algebra word problem, one encodes the information that a certain item costs a certain amount but one is

unable to feed this information into one's decision-making processes about how the problem should be solved or further analyzed, an impairment in feedback might be indicated. This situation is, in a sense, the reverse of the one described immediately above. In the above case, communication from metacomponents to other kinds of components (activation) was impaired; in this case, communication to metacomponents from other kinds of components (feedback) is impaired.

3. *Impaired functioning of components of one or more kinds, either through (a) unavailability of components, (b) inaccessibility of components, (c) slowness of component execution, or (d) inaccuracy in the results of component execution.* A person either lacks certain components needed for task performance, cannot access these components (although they are available), or uses those components in an inefficacious way. For example, a young child is unable to map second-order relations because the component is unavailable to him or her; or a child is able to encode information but tends to do it either incompletely or sloppily.

4. *Impaired automatization of componential subsystems.* A person is unable to make, or makes only excessively slowly, the transition from controlled to automatic processing in a task. For example, slow or otherwise disabled readers often show reading processes characterized by excessive amounts of controlled processing and by failures in automatization of bottom-up processes that peers would have automatized long ago (Sternberg & Wagner, 1982).

5. *Impaired coordination between controlled and automated componential subsystems, such that control of processing does not pass readily between the two kinds of subsystems.* A person is unable to effect a smooth transition between controlled and automated information processing of different parts of a task. For example, in reading, it is often necessary to move back and forth quickly between relatively well automatized bottom-up processing (such as phoneme recognition) and relatively controlled top-down processing (such as recognizing the main idea of a paragraph). A person who is unable smoothly to transit between controlled and automated processing will be at a disadvantage in reading any material of nontrivial complexity.

6. *Inadequate knowledge base.* The various components are constantly drawing upon old information in their processing of new information. If, either for reasons of inadequate environmental opportunities or for reasons of componential inadequacies (and especially inadequacies in the functioning of knowledge-acquisition components), the knowledge base is poorly stocked with information or poorly organized with respect to the information it has, then the outcomes of componential processing will be impaired, possibly independently of actual inadequacies in the components.

7. *Inadequate or inappropriate motivation for componential functioning.* If

the individual lacks the motivation to utilize his or her componential system to the best of his or her ability, or if the motivations the individual has are nonoptimal for maximal task performance, then the level of functioning of the componential system will be reduced accordingly.

8. *Structural limitations upon componential functioning.* Although we know surprisingly little about individual differences in structural capacities, it is at least plausible to postulate that some individuals may be faced with structural deficits relative to peers – for example, reduced working memory capacity. Such deficits would be likely to interfere with optimal componential functioning.

Clearly, these are not the only possible sources of intellectual retardation. (See Sternberg & Spear, in press, for a much more detailed discussion of these and other sources of deficit and of how the present theory relates to other theories.) According to the triarchic theory, a retarded individual would also show difficulty in adjusting to novel kinds of tasks and situations and would demonstrate at least some difficulty in adapting to the environments in which he or she lives. To the extent that adaptive functioning is unimpaired, the retardation would be of importance, presumably, only in academic kinds of situations.

Implications of the triarchic theory for current controversies

The theoretical and empirical claims of the triarchic theory have direct implications for several of the major current controversies among researchers in the field of mental retardation. Consider just a few of these controversies.

The developmental versus difference controversy. Zigler (1982; Zigler & Balla, 1982) has claimed that accounts of mental retardation, or at least that kind of mental retardation that is cultural – familial in nature (as opposed to acutely organic), can be divided into two kinds: developmental and difference. The distinction between these two positions is not easily stated in a compact way, because of its complexity. In essence, though, the developmental position, which is the one Zigler has championed, holds that

the cognitive performance of individuals of differing IQs who are at the same cognitive level and, therefore, at different chronological ages, should [be] exactly the same on cognitive tasks. Cognitive performance is thus viewed as totally a function of the cognitive level of the individual, irrespective of the amount of time it took that individual to reach that cognitive level. (Zigler, 1982, p. 167)

The idea, then, is that mentally retarded individuals of a given mental age will perform, on the average, identically to normal individuals of the same mental age but lower chronological age. In contrast, difference positions hold that retarded individuals differ from normal ones in more than just a slower rate of development and a lower asymptote of performance. Rather, there is alleged to be some difference in the "hardware" or "software" of such individuals that transcends mere differences of rate or asymptote of development. According to Zigler, a developmental theorist, "the etiology of the postulated defect or difference must inhere in the low IQ itself" (Zigler, 1982, p. 178). If two individuals of equal mental age but different chronological age are compared, where one is retarded and the other not, the two individuals will still show differences in performance, with the retarded individual showing the poorer performance.

There are a number of "difference" positions (e.g., Brown, 1974; Ellis, 1963, 1970; Kounin, 1941a, 1941b; Zeaman & House, 1979). The question that must be raised here is whether, from the standpoint of the triarchic theory, the distinction between "developmental" positions, on the one hand, and "difference" positions, on the other, is a viable one. I believe that it is not: The viability of the distinction depends upon certain measurement assumptions that I am not ready to accept.

The developmental–difference distinction hinges upon the notion of "cognitive level," which Zigler holds can be roughly measured by mental age. Although the triarchic theory does not itself postulate "cognitive levels," such levels are not inconsistent with the theory. Levels would refer to qualitative differences in observable performance that arise from qualitative changes in mental functioning. For example, the performance component of mapping seems first to become available (or at least accessible) to children about the age of 10 or 11, or, in Piagetian terms, roughly at the onset of formal operations (Sternberg & Rifkin, 1979). The mapping component, used to discover second-order relations between relations, is of critical importance to a number of thinking tasks, but particularly those that distinguish Piagetian "formal-operational" thinking. Hence, one might view the acquisition of mapping as marking the entrance into a "stage." But from a componential point of view, such a stage notion is more a heuristic than an explanatory construct. A retarded individual is one who, for a given chronological age, lags behind age peers in sufficient numbers of loci (as described earlier) or sufficiently seriously in a small number of loci to result in performance that is well below the norm for that age level.

From this point of view, a "mental age" is nothing more than a composite of performance on some set of cognitive components that typifies the performance of individuals at a certain chronological age. Individuals who are matched in mental age will invariably differ in their profiles of component skills (as well as in their abilities to handle nonentrenched tasks and to automatize information processing); but on the average, their performances will be the same by definition. One might well find some tasks on which retarded individuals, compared to typical college students, perform worse than the college students; but one can also find tasks in which the reverse would be true (Spitz, Borys, & Webster, 1982; Weisz, Yeates, & Zigler, 1982). The reason, of course, is that mental age is no more than a convenient summary value representing an average over tasks within a given universe of tasks; hence, the obtained differences reflect the expected sampling variability around the mean.

I do not believe that my position on the cognitive bases of mental retardation differs in any fundamental psychological respect from Zigler's. At least, I have been unable to find any difference. It is for this reason that I believe that the developmental–difference distinction is predicated upon acceptance of the measurement procedures associated with the ratio IQ. When one views mental phenomena in information-processing terms, these constructs become conveniences rather than fundamental psychological measurements, and they can no longer support the developmental–difference distinction Zigler proposes. Hence, I accept the basic psychology of Zigler's position without accepting his distinction as a psychological one. Indeed, my own position is both developmental and differential in character: At a given chronological age, retarded individuals differ from normals quantitatively and possibly qualitatively; at a given mental age, they differ in the universe of tasks defining the mental age only as a function of differences in task sampling. Once one goes outside that task universe, of course, other differences may emerge as well.

Differences among "difference" positions. There are, of course, many theories of differences between normals and the retarded. To name just a few, there is Kounin's (1941a, 1941b) theory of rigidity, Luria's (1961) theory of verbal mediation, Butterfield and Belmont's (1977) theory of executive functioning, Brown and DeLoache's (1978) related theory of executive functioning, Zeaman and House's (1963) theory of attentional processing, and Ellis's (1963) stimulus trace theory.

The triarchic theory implies that it is futile to look for just a single locus of mental retardation. What studies supporting these theories typically show is that retardates differ from normals in the locus specified by the theory. The convergent validation of each of these theories is usually at least somewhat convincing. What is less convincing, and usually nonexistent, is discriminant validation with respect to the alternative positions. The problem is not one that is confined to the literature on mental retardation. There are any number of theories of intelligence that have been constructed on the basis of the usually moderate correlation between performance on a single task or class of tasks and IQ. And similarly, studies of the effects of aging upon intelligence have tended to confine themselves to limited aspects of intelligence, so that one gains only an incomplete picture of what happens to intelligence with increasing age. Often, for example, either contextual or cognitive factors are ignored. The problem arises when single correlates are taken to tell the "whole story." The outcome is a set of seemingly competing theories that compete only because they look at only a limited aspect of the whole phenomenon. Mental retardation, and intelligence in general, are multifaceted phenomena that cannot be understood by taking a task, showing a difference between groups and then formulating an ad hoc theory on the basis of differences for that one task. Such theories are not wrong so much as they are incomplete; because their formulators may be enchanted with the task or tasks that give rise to the observed differences, they may fail to take into account all of the other tasks that also show group differences.

The role of motivation. Zigler has sometimes been interpreted as offering a "motivational" theory of mental retardation. As he has pointed out on several occasions (e.g., Zigler, 1982), this interpretation of his position is incorrect. His theory is a cognitive one that nevertheless postulates differences in performance due to differential patterns of motivation between retarded and nonretarded individuals. I think it highly probable that differences in motivational patterns exist between retarded and normal individuals, just as they are likely to exist between members of different cultures and subcultures, and even individuals within a given culture. The contextual subtheory suggests that differences in motivational patterns might well lead to differences in performance on real-world (and probably laboratory) tasks. For example, to shape one's environment, one needs first to be motivated to do so, just as to select a new environment, one first has to decide that it is worth the effort to do so. Moreover, I believe that at least part of the observed differences in people's abilities to handle nonentrenched tasks may derive from differences in their preferences for and interests in nonentrenched kinds of tasks (and situations). In sum, motivation no doubt plays a large role in observed individual differences in intelligence, including those that distinguish retarded from normal individuals.

General retardation versus specific learning disabilities. Difficulties in distinguishing retarded from learning disabled subjects have led some to question whether there is any legitimate distinction at all to be made between these two groups (see, e.g., Wolford & Fowler, 1982). I believe that there is a valid distinction to be made: The mentally retarded show generalized deficits, especially in metacomponential functioning. Indeed, to the extent that retarded individuals differ from normal ones in general intelligence, or g, I see this primarily as a metacomponential deficit. In contrast, I believe that learning disabilities arise primarily, although not exclusively, from automatization failures in certain specific domains, such as reading (Sternberg & Wagner, 1982). Thus, specific disabilities will tend, on the average, to be more "bottom-up" than "top-down" deficits; retardation, on the other hand, will tend more to be a top-down deficit or set of deficits.

To summarize, then, intellectual retardation is understood primarily in terms of inadequate functioning and automatization of componential skills, whereas giftedness is understood primarily in terms of exceptional functioning in adapting to novelty, particularly via insight. Although the two levels of exceptional intelligence can be understood as representing two different ends of a quantitative continuum, such an understanding does not do full justice to their complexity and, I believe, to their inherently asymmetrical nature.

11 Implications of the triarchic theory for intelligence testing

IQ tests work only for some people some of the time. There has been an upper limit on the validity coefficients of IQ tests – generally around .5 – that has not changed for many years (Ghiselli, 1966), and this upper limit results in large part from the very limited portion of intelligence that IQ tests measure and from the inappropriateness of the tests for many people in the prediction of intelligent behavior in a variety of situations.

The triarchic theory accounts for why IQ tests work as well as they do and suggests ways in which they might be improved. In this chapter, I consider implications of the triarchic theory for evaluating current tests and for improving or supplementing the tests we now have. I will consider in turn the implications of each of the componential, experiential, and contextual subtheories for intelligence testing.

Implications of the componential subtheory for intelligence testing

The componential subtheory posits three kinds of information-processing components that are critical to individual differences in intelligence: metacomponents, performance components, and knowledge-acquisition components. Do existing tests measure these components, and if so, how might their measurement be improved? Consider each kind of component in turn.

Metacomponents

I would argue that to the extent that existing IQ tests do in fact measure intelligence and predict consequential real-world performance, it is in large part because they implicitly measure metacomponential functioning (Sternberg, 1980a). Consider a typical IQ test and how it measures such functioning:

1. *Deciding upon the nature of the problem.* Most IQ tests contain a variety of types of problems, and part of the examinee's task is to figure out just what

is required of him or her by each type of problem. Once such a decision has been made at a global level (the problem requires analogical reasoning, finding opposites, unscrambling words, etc.), many local decisions must be made as well. For example, in arithmetic and algebra word problems, the examinee must figure out exactly what question is being posed. Answering the wrong question is a major source of errors in such problems, and distractors are often constructed so as to fool people who misread the question and answer correctly a question other than the one asked. Very low scores on IQ tests and especially subtests often result from an examinee not quite understanding what is required by the tasks at hand.

2. *Deciding upon performance components relevant for task solution.* Once the examinee has figured out what a problem is asking, the examinee must decide how to solve the problem. Typical fluid ability tasks, such as analogies, matrix problems, and series problems, require selection of a rather large set of performance components. Selecting the wrong components or only a partial set of components will result in a considerable number of problems incorrectly solved.

3. *Deciding upon a strategy into which to combine performance components.* Fluid ability tasks require not only selection of the right components but also proper sequencing of these components. The models of analogical reasoning described earlier (Chapter 5; see also Sternberg, 1977a, 1977b), for example, are complicated, and they no doubt represent simplifications of what examinees actually do. Examinees who are unable to sequence components in an efficacious way will be likely to find themselves unable to solve correctly items having complicated structures.

4. *Selecting a mental representation for information.* In some types of problems, the way in which information is represented can have a crucial effect upon the solution reached. Many apparently spatial problems, for example, can be solved either verbally or spatially, and the examinee's choice of representation, given his or her own pattern of abilities, may critically affect whether or not the examinee is able to solve given problems correctly. In arithmetic reasoning items, the right representation, whether done as a diagram, set of equations, or both, can result either in a right or wrong answer. In figural reasoning items, examinees sometimes find that none of the answer options appears to be correct; such an outcome often results from representing the geometric structure of the item in a way different from that intended by the item writer.

5. *Allocating resources for problem solution.* The large majority of tests are timed either in whole or in part. Deciding how to allocate time can be critical to maximizing the number of items reached and solved correctly. Spending too much time on excessively difficult problems, or too little time on problems that appear easy on the surface but that have nonobvious complexities associated with them, can result in suboptimal test performance.

6. *Monitoring solution processes.* Very often, the strategy that examinees have chosen for test performance, whether the global strategy they use for allocating their time among all of the items, or the local strategy they use for solving a single item, is unsuccessful. The ability to monitor one's solution processes and recognize that the strategy is failing is an important ingredient in successful test performance.

7. *Being sensitive to external feedback.* Group IQ tests often involve no external feedback at all. Individual tests do, however, involve some feedback. The extreme case is Feuerstein's (1979) Learning Potential Assessment Device (LPAD), where the ability to use feedback is central to the examinee's performance. The ability to understand and act upon feedback can be important in success on tests where such feedback is given.

Because of the importance of successful metacomponential functioning for high test performance, I believe existing tests could, for the most part, be improved by better taking into account what we know about metacomponential functioning. For purposes of illustration, I will concentrate upon what I see as one critical shortcoming of most existing tests, namely, their reliance upon the common but, I believe, incorrect view that speed of mental functioning is in and of itself a critical aspect of intelligence.

The assumption that "smart is fast" permeates our entire society. When we refer to someone as "quick," we are endowing him or her with one of the primary attributes that we perceive an intelligent person to have. Indeed, in a recent study of people's conceptions of intelligence, when we asked people to list behaviors characteristic of intelligent persons, behaviors such as "learns rapidly," "acts quickly," "talks quickly," and "makes judgments quickly" were commonly listed (Sternberg, Conway, Ketron, & Bernstein, 1981; see Chapter 2). It is not only the man in the street who believes that speed is associated with intellect: Several prominent contemporary theorists of intelligence base their theories in large part upon individual differences in the speed with which people process information (Brand & Deary, 1982; Eysenck, 1982; Hunt, 1980; Jensen, 1979).

The assumption that more intelligent people are rapid information processors also underlies the overwhelming majority of tests used in identification of the gifted, including creativity as well as intelligence tests. It is rare to find a group-administered test that is not timed or a timed test that virtually all examinees are able to finish by working at a comfortable rate of problem solving. I would argue that this assumption is a gross overgeneralization: It is true for some people and for some mental operations, but not for all people or all mental operations. What is critical is not speed per se but rather speed selection – knowing when and being able to function rapidly or slowly according to task or situational demands. Thus, it is resource allocation, in addition to the resource itself, that is central to general intelligence.

Almost everyone knows people who, although often slow in performing tasks, perform the tasks at a superior level of accomplishment. Moreover, we all know that snap judgments are often poor ones. Indeed, in our study of people's conceptions of intelligence, "does not make snap judgments" was listed as an important attribute of intelligent performance. Moreover, there are theoretical reasons for believing that to be quick is not always to be smart. In his classic but little-known book on the nature of intelligence, Thurstone (1924) proposed that a critical element of intelligent performance is the ability to withhold rapid, instinctive responses and to substitute for them more rational, well-thought-out responses. According to this view, the impulsive responses one makes to problems are often not the optimal ones for problem solution, and the ability to inhibit these responses and to consider more rational forms of response is a critical one for high levels of task performance. More recently, Stenhouse (1973) has arrived at the same conclusion via a comparative analysis of intelligence across different species of animals. Interestingly, his conclusion appears to be wholly independent of Thurstone's, in that there is no evidence that Stenhouse was aware of Thurstone's book.

A number of findings from psychological research undermine the validity of the assumption that smart is always fast. I will cite just a few of the findings that indicate the fallacy of this view.

First, it is well known that, in general, a reflective rather than impulsive cognitive style in problem solving tends to be associated with more intelligent problem-solving performance (see Baron, 1981, 1982, for reviews of this literature). Jumping into problems without adequate reflection is likely to lead to false starts and erroneous conclusions. Yet timed tests often force the examinee to solve problems impulsively. It is often claimed that the strict timing of such tests merely mirrors the requirements of our highly pressured and productive society. But for most of us, there seem to be few significant problems encountered in work or personal life that permit no more than the 5 to 50 seconds allowed for a typical test problem on a standardized test. Of course, there are some people, such as air traffic controllers, who must make consequential split-second decisions as an integral part of their everyday lives. But such people seem to be the exception rather than the rule.

Second, in our study of planning behavior in problem solving (Sternberg, 1981d), we found that more intelligent persons tend to spend relatively more time than do less intelligent persons on global (higher-order) planning and relatively less time on local (lower-order) planning. In contrast, less intelligent persons seem to emphasize local rather than global planning (relative to the more intelligent persons). The point is that what matters is not total time spent, but rather distribution of this time across the various kinds of planning one can do. Although for the problems we used (complex forms of analogies), quicker problem solving was associated, on the average, with higher intelligence, looking simply at total time masked the compensating relations for the two kinds of planning.

Third, in studies of reasoning behavior in children and adults, it has been found that although greater intelligence is associated with more rapid execution of most components of information processing, problem encoding is a notable exception to this trend. The more intelligent individual tends to spend relatively more time encoding the terms of the problem, presumably in order to facilitate subsequent operations on these encodings (see Mulholland, Pellegrino, & Glaser, 1980; Sternberg, 1977b; Sternberg & Rifkin, 1979). Similar outcomes have been observed in comparisons of expert versus novice problem solvers confronted with difficult physics problems (Chi, Glaser, & Rees, 1982; Larkin, McDermott, Simon, & Simon, 1980). Siegler (1981, 1984; see Sternberg, 1984c) has also found that intellectually more advanced children are distinguished especially by their superior ability fully to encode the nature of the problem being presented to them. The point, again, is that what matters is not total time spent but rather distribution of this time across the various kinds of planning one can do.

Fourth, in a study of people's performance in solving insight problems (arithmetical and logical problems whose difficulty resided in the need for a nonobvious insight for problem solution rather than in the need for arithmetical or logical knowledge), a correlation of .75 was found between the amount of time people spent on the problems and measured IQ. The correlation between time spent and score on the insight problems was .62 (Sternberg & Davidson, 1982). Note that in these problems, individuals were free to spend as long as they liked solving the problems. Persistence and involvement in the problems was highly correlated with success in solution: The more intelligent individuals did not give up, nor did they fall for the obvious, but often incorrect, solutions.

Fifth and finally, in a study on executive processes in reading (Wagner & Sternberg, 1983), we found that although faster readers, on the average, tended to have higher comprehension and to score higher on a variety of external ability measures, simply looking at overall reading time masked important differences between more and less skilled readers. In the study, which employed standard texts of the kinds found in newspapers and textbooks, we found that relative to less skilled readers, more skilled readers tended to allocate relatively more time to reading passages for which they would be tested in greater detail and relatively less time to reading passages for which they would be tested in lesser detail.

Obviously, it would be foolish to argue that speed is never important. In dangerous situations one confronts when driving a car, slow reflexes or thinking can result in an accident that otherwise could have been averted. In many other situations, too, speed is essential. But the large majority of consequential tasks one faces in one's life do not require problem solving or decision making in the small numbers of seconds typically allotted for the solution of IQ test problems. Instead, they require an intelligent allocation of one's time to the various subproblems or problems at hand. Ideally, IQ tests would stress allocation of time rather than total time or speed in solving various kinds of problems.

To the extent that simple tasks such as those used by Jensen (1982), Hunt (1978), and others correlate with IQ, it may be in part because of the shared but ecologically unrealistic time stress imposed on performance in both kinds of tasks. I doubt, however, that the speed demand is the only source of the correlation. What correlation is left after sheer shared speed requirements are removed may be accounted for in part by metacomponential processing. A finding in Jensen's (1982) research, for example, is that the correlation between choice reaction time and IQ increases as the number of choices in the reaction-time task increases. This result suggests that the more that metacomponential decision making is required in selecting from among alternative choices, the higher the correlation is with tested intelligence. A finding in the Hunt (1978) research paradigm, which is based upon the Posner and Mitchell (1967) letter-comparison task, is that as the complexity of the comparison that needs to be made increases, so does the correlation between performance on the comparison task and measured intelligence (Goldberg, Schwartz, & Stewart, 1977). Again, the result suggests that it is higher-level decision making, rather than sheer speed of simple functioning, that is responsible for obtained correlations between performance on cognitive tasks and performance on psychometric tests. Moreover, cognitive tasks such as these may well become automatized over the large number of trials they require for subject performance and thus will measure efficacy of automatization as well, another key ingredient of intelligent performance (see Chapter 3).

To conclude, what needs to be measured by intelligence tests is not overall time or speed of functioning, but time or speed of functioning for individual components of intelligence. Some components should be performed relatively more rapidly, others relatively more slowly. Imposing an overall time limit on a test hides the most important information about time – how it is allocated.

Performance components

Although I believe metacomponents to be centrally responsible for correlations between cognitive tasks and psychometric tests and for the limited success of psychometric tests in predicting real-world performances of various kinds, metacomponents do not account for all of the obtained correlations. Performance components, especially those that are general across substantial ranges of tasks, can also have an influence.

In Chapter 5, I claimed that the performance components of inductive reasoning – encoding, inference, mapping, application, comparison, justification, and response – are quite general across test formats and are also important in real-world task performance. The data presented in that chapter (from Sternberg & Gardner, 1983) showed that high correlations (with magnitudes as high as .7 and .8) can be obtained between component scores and performance on psychometric tests of inductive reasoning, and high correlations are also obtained between corresponding component scores across various inductive tasks. To the extent that IQ tests measure these performance components and others of equal centrality and generality in intellectual functioning, they are indeed likely to be good measures of intelligent behavior. Most of the existing tests of fluid abilities do in fact stress measurement of these performance components.

Again, however, I believe there is room for improvement in the measurement we are now getting. Existing tests do not separate out scores for the various performance components of intelligence. Such separation is important because there is evidence that different components behave in various ways.

One kind of difference, discussed above, is in terms of speed allocation. For most performance components, greater speed of processing is associated with superior overall task performance. But for at least one component, encoding, the opposite pattern appears.

A second kind of difference is in the kinds of mental representations upon which the various components act. Consider syllogistic reasoning tasks, for example. As discussed in Chapter 6, some of the components of syllogistic reasoning operate upon a linguistic representation, others upon a spatial representation. Overall scores on syllogistic reasoning tests, whether expressed in terms of latencies or errors, are therefore confounded with respect to the linguistic and spatial abilities involved. An individual could achieve a given score through different combinations of information-processing components and strategies. To the extent one wishes to understand the cognitive bases of task performance, componential decomposition of task performance is desirable and even necessary.

A third kind of difference is in the centrality of the components of the task to what it is the examiner actually wishes to measure. Most tasks contain components that are of greater and lesser interest for measuring a particular construct. By separating out component scores, it is possible to obtain purer measures of the construct of interest. In the case of inductive reasoning, for example, one would probably wish to separate out the reasoning components (inference, mapping, application, justification) from the other components.

Such separation becomes especially important for purposes of diagnosis and remediation. Consider, for example, the possibility of a very bright person who does poorly on tests of abstract reasoning ability. It may be that the person is a very good reasoner but has a perceptual difficulty that leads to poor encoding of the terms of the problem. Because encoding is necessary for reasoning upon the problem terms as encoded, the overall score is reduced not by faulty reasoning but by faulty encoding of the terms of the problem. Decomposition of scores into performance components enables one to separate out, say, reasoning difficulties from perceptual difficulties. For purposes of remediation, such separation is essential. Different remediation programs would be indicated for people who perform poorly on reasoning items because of deficiencies in reasoning, on the one hand, or deficiencies in perceptual processing, on the other.

Finally, componential decomposition can be important if the individual's problem is not in the components at all but rather in the strategy for combining them. A person might be able to execute the performance components quite well but still do poorly on a task because of nonoptimal strategies for combining the components. By modeling the examinee's task performance, it is possible to determine whether the person's difficulty is in the performance components per se or in the way the person combines those performance components.

Knowledge-acquisition components

If one examines the contents of the major intelligence tests currently in use, one will find that most of them measure intelligence as last year's (or the year before's, or the year before that's) achievement. What is an intelligence test for children of a given age would be an achievement test for children a few years younger. In some test items, like vocabulary, the achievement loading is obvious. In others, like verbal analogies and arithmetic problems, it is disguised. But virtually all tests commonly used for the assessment of intelligence place heavy achievement demands upon the individuals tested.

The emphasis upon knowledge is consistent with some current views of differences in expert versus novice performance that stress the role of knowledge in performance differences (e.g., Chase & Simon, 1973; Chi, Glaser, & Rees, 1982; Keil, 1984; Larkin et al., 1980). Indeed, there can be no doubt that differences in knowledge are critical to differential performance between more and less skilled individuals in a variety of domains. But it seems to me, at least, that the critical question for a theorist of intelligence to ask is that of how those differences in knowledge came to be. Certainly, just sheer differences in amount of experience are not perfectly correlated with levels of expertise. Many individuals play the piano for many years but do not become concert-level pianists; chess buffs do not all become grandmasters, no matter what the frequency may be of their play. And simply reading a lot does not guarantee a high vocabulary. What seems to be critical is not sheer amount of experience but rather what one has been able to learn from and do with that experience. According to this view, then, individual differences in knowledge acquisition have priority over individual differences in actual knowledge. To understand expertise, one must understand first how current individual differences in knowledge evolved from individual differences in knowledge acquisition.

Consider, for example, vocabulary. It is well known that vocabulary is one of the best predictors, if not the best single predictor, of overall IQ score (Jensen, 1980; Matarazzo, 1972). Yet few tests have higher achievement load than does vocabulary. Can one measure the latent ability tapped by vocabulary tests without presenting children with what is essentially an achievement test? In other words, can one go beyond current individual differences in knowledge to the source of those individual differences, that of differences in knowledge acquisition?

As noted in Chapter 7, there is reason to believe that vocabulary is such a good measure of intelligence because it measures, albeit indirectly, children's ability to acquire information in context (Jensen, 1980; Sternberg & Powell, 1983; Werner & Kaplan, 1952). Most vocabulary is learned in everyday contexts rather than through direct instruction. Thus, new words are usually encountered for the first time (and subsequently) in textbooks, novels, newspapers, lectures, and the like. More intelligent people are better able to use surrounding context to figure out the words' meanings. With time, the better decontextualizers acquire the larger vocabularies. Because so much of one's learning (not just vocabulary) is contextually determined, the ability to use context to add to one's knowledge base is an important skill in intelligent behavior. We have attempted to measure these skills directly by presenting children with paragraphs written at a level well below their grade level. Embedded within the paragraphs are one or more unknown words. The children's task is to use the surrounding context to figure out the meanings of the unknown words (see Chapter 7). Note that in this testing paradigm, differential effects of past achievements are reduced by using reading passages that are easy for everyone but that contain target vocabulary words that are unknown to everyone. We have found that the quality of children's definitions of the unknown words is highly correlated with overall verbal intelligence, reading comprehension, and vocabulary test scores (about .6 in each case). Thus, one can measure an important aspect of intelligence –

knowledge acquisition – directly without heavy reliance upon past achievement.

Consider, second, another common type of intelligence test item – arithmetic word problems (and at higher levels, algebra and geometry word problems as well). Again, performance is heavily dependent upon one's mathematical achievements and, indeed, opportunities. Can one measure the main skills tapped by such tests without creating what is essentially an achievement test? We believe we have done so through the insight problems mentioned in Chapters 3 and 10. Consider again two typical examples of such problems:

1. If you have black socks and brown socks in your drawer, mixed in the ratio of 4 to 5, how many socks will you have to take out to make sure of having a pair the same color?
2. Water lilies double in area every 24 hours. At the beginning of the summer there is 1 water lily on a lake. It takes 60 days for the lake to become covered with water lilies. On what day is the lake half-covered?

Solution of problems such as these requires a fair amount of insight but very little prior mathematical knowledge. In most of these problems, common elements of performance are what were earlier called the three "knowledge-acquisition components": selective encoding, selective combination, and selective comparison. Performance on such problems is correlated about .6 to .7 with IQ. Thus, it is possible to use word problems that are good measures of intelligence but that directly measure knowledge acquisition rather than merely accumulated knowledge.

The achievement-testing orientation exhibited in intelligence tests may be acceptable and even appropriate when the tests are administered to children who have had fully adequate educational opportunities in reasonably adequate social and emotional environments. But for children whose environments have been characterized by deprivation of one kind or another, this orientation may lead to invalid test results. There is no fully adequate solution to the problem of assessment of intelligence among such youngsters, especially if the youngsters will have to function in a normal sociocultural milieu. But the knowledge-acquisition approach seems to be a step in the right direction in terms of creating tests that are fairer and more appropriate for the people to whom tests are likely to be given.

Implications of the experiential subtheory for intelligence testing

The experiential subtheory suggests that tasks requiring metacomponents, performance components, and knowledge-acquisition components will measure intelligence to the extent that they involve coping with novelty or automatization of task performance. Most intelligence tests require at least some of each of these skills. Tests with greater amounts of novelty (such as Raven matrix problems) or that better measure skill automatization (such as reading comprehension tests) are likely to be especially useful for the measurement of intelligence. The tasks mentioned in Chapter 3 – conceptual projection, used for the assessment of novelty in task acquisition, and insight problems, used for the assessment of novelty in task performance – would seem to be particularly appropriate as measures of intellectual abilities. As mentioned earlier, most cognitive tasks administered in the laboratory probably show correlations with IQ in part because they measure the degree to which performance is automatized over large numbers of trials.

The experiential view suggests one reason why it is exceedingly difficult to compare levels of intelligence fairly across members of different sociocultural groups. Even if a given test requires the same components of performance for members of the various groups, it is extremely unlikely to be equivalent for the groups in terms of its novelty and the degree to which performance has been automatized prior to the examinees' taking the test. Consider, for example, the by now well-known finding that nonverbal reasoning tests, such as the Raven Progressive Matrices or the Cattell Culture Fair Test of *g*, actually show greater differences between members of different sociocultural groups than do the verbal tests they were designed to replace (Jensen, 1982). The nonverbal tests, contrary to the claims that have often been made for them, are *not* culture-fair (and they are certainly not culture-free). Individuals who have been brought up in a test-taking culture are likely to have had much more experience with these kinds of items than are individuals not brought up in such a culture. Thus, the items will be less novel and performance on them more automatized for members of the standard U.S. culture than for its nonmembers. Even if the processes of solution are the same, the degrees of novelty and automatization will be different, and hence the tests will not be measuring the same skills across populations. As useful as the tests may be for within-group comparisons, between-group comparisons may be deceptive and unfair. A fair comparison between groups would require comparable degrees of novelty and automatization in test items as well as comparable processes and strategies.

Implications of the contextual subtheory for intelligence testing

Intelligence tests should measure or at least predict behaviors that are relevant to the sociocultural context in which an individual lives. Even creators of the seemingly artificial kinds of problems found on intelligence tests have often defined intelligence in terms of adaptation to one's real-world environment (e.g., Binet & Simon, 1905; Pintner, 1921; Wechsler, 1958). I would add the notions of purposive selection and shaping of environments to this definition (see Chapter 2). What this means is that there may be no one set of behaviors that is "intelligent" for everyone, in that people can adjust to their environments in different ways.

What does seem to be common among people mastering their environments is the ability to capitalize upon strengths and to compensate for weaknesses (see Cronbach & Snow, 1977). Successful people are able not only to adapt well to their environments, but actually to modify the environments they are in so as to maximize the goodness of fit between the environment and their adaptive skills.

Consider, for example, the "stars" in any given field of endeavor. What is it that distinguishes such persons from all the rest? Of course, this question, as phrased, is broad enough to be the topic of a book. But for present purposes, the distinguishing characteristics to which I would like to call attention are (a) at least one extraordinarily well-developed skill and (b) an extraordinary ability to capitalize upon this skill or set of skills in their work. For example, generate a short list of "stars" in your own field. Chances are that the stars do not seem to share any one ability, as traditionally defined, but rather share a tendency toward having some set of extraordinary talents that they make the most of in their work. In my own list, for example, are included a person with extraordinary spatial visualization skills (if anyone can visualize in four dimensions, he can!), a person with a talent for coming up with almost incredibly counterintuitive findings that are of great theoretical importance, and a person who has an extraordinary sense of where the field is going and repeatedly tends to be just one step ahead of it so as perfectly to time the publication of his work for maximum impact. These three particular persons (and others on my list) share little in terms of what sets them apart, aside from at least one extraordinary talent upon which they capitalize fully in their work. Although they are also highly intelligent in the traditional sense, so are many others who never reach their heights of accomplishment.

Because what is adaptive differs at least somewhat, both across people and across situations, the present view suggests that intelligence is not quite the same thing for different people and for different situations. The higher-order skills of capitalization and compensation may be the same, but what is capitalized on and what is compensated for will vary. The differences across people and situations extend beyond different life paths within a given culture.

Consider an example of where it becomes clear that intelligence tests are not wholly adequate as measures of environmental mastery. Seymour Sarason has described to me the rather bizarre situation that confronted him when he went to work at his first job as a psychologist in a school for the mentally retarded. He arrived just as the students executed a successful escape from the school's restricted grounds. When the escapees were caught,

Sarason was left to do his job, namely, to give the students the Porteus Maze Test. Curiously, the very persons who had plotted and executed the some-what successful escape were unable successfully to complete even the first problem on the test. This enigmatic situation left Sarason, as it leaves us all, with the puzzle of trying to figure out which was the better measure of intelligence, the problem of escape or the Porteus Maze Test. Clearly, the IQ test was missing something! Tests such as Frederiksen's (1962) "in-basket" test and the measures of practical intelligence described in Chapter 9 attempt to measure at least part of this something. In my opinion, the most critical need in ability testing today is to develop measures that are more sensitive to real-world kinds of intelligence. These tests would supplement the academic kinds of intelligence measured by traditional tests.

Current IQ tests not only lack some of the elements relevant to real-world performance but also introduce other elements of doubtful relevance. Consider, for example, the level of stress involved in testing, especially on tests such as the Scholastic Aptitude Test (SAT), Law School Admission Test (LSAT), or Medical College Admission Test (MCAT), each of which can be, in some cases, the most important criterion for admission to the program of one's choice. Few situations in life are as stressful as the situation confronting the examinee receiving a standardized test. Most examinees know that the results of the test are crucial for their future and that one to three hours of testing may have more impact on the future than many years of school performance. The anxiety generated by the test-taking situation may have little or no effect on some examinees and even a beneficial effect on other examinees. But there is a substantial proportion of examinees – the test-anx-ious – whose anxiety will cripple their test performance, possibly severely. Moreover, because the anxiety will be common to standardized testing situa-tions (although often not to other testing situations), the error in measure-ment resulting from a single testing situation will be compounded by error in measurement in other testing situations. With repeated low scores, a bright but test-anxious individual may truly appear to be stupid. What is needed is some kind of standardized assessment device that is fair to the test-anxious, as well as to others, and that does not impose a differential penalty on individuals as a function of a form of state anxiety that may have no coun-terpart in situations other than that of standardized testing. I believe that we have some promising leads in this direction.

One lead is testing based on the notion of intelligence as, in part, a function of a person's ability to profit from incomplete instruction (Resnick & Glaser, 1976). A measure of this ability is now provided by Feuerstein's (1979) Learning Potential Assessment Device (LPAD), which, although originally proposed as an assessment device for retarded performers, can be used for performers at varying levels of performance, including advanced ones. The device involves administration of problems with graded instruction. The amount of instruction given depends upon the examinee's needs. Moreover, the test is administered in a supportive, cooperative atmosphere, where the examiner is actually helping the examinee solve problems rather than impassively observing the examinee's success or failure. The examiner does everything he or she can to allay anxiety (rather than to create it!). Feuerstein has found that children who are intimidated by and unable to perform well on regular standardized tests can demonstrate high levels of performance on his test. Moreover, their performance outside the testing situation appears to be better predicted by the LPAD than by conventional intelligence tests (see Feuerstein, 1979).

A second lead is based on the notion that intelligence can be measured with some accuracy by the degree of resemblance between a person's behavior and the behavior of the "ideally" intelligent individual (see Neisser, 1979). In Chapter 2, I reported on a behavioral checklist measure that showed correlations at the .5 level with standard intelligence tests. Such a checklist seems like a desirable supplement to conventional tests, especially for individuals who are test-anxious. Although it would not be adequate as a "stand-alone" measure, it may be a useful addition to a testing battery. Someone who scored high on such a measure but low on a conventional measure would at least be worth follow-up evaluation in order to see whether the conventional test might have undervalued his or her potential performance.

Conclusions

To conclude, I believe that intelligence tests would be better than they are now if they took into account the implications for testing of the three subtheories of the triarchic theory. No existing test satisfies all of the criteria that have been discussed, nor is it clear that any one test could satisfy them all. Indeed, to the extent that intelligence comprises somewhat different skills for different people there is no one, wholly appropriate test of it. Rather, the ideal instrument for assessing intelligence would probably be one that combines measurements of different kinds that together take into account the considerations above. No one or combination of the measurements would yield a definitive IQ, because any one instrument can work only for some of the people some of the time. Which instruments work for which people will be variable across people within and between sociocultural groups. The best one can hope for is a battery of assessments that, when interpreted intelligently, can tell us more about intelligence than any one kind of assessment and than any of the measures presently available.

Given the fallibility of present tests, is the only viable solution to the problem of test interpretation to stop using tests altogether? I do not believe so. Used judiciously, test scores have almost always been found to provide some incremental validity over assessments made in their absence. But what is important is that the tests be used prudently. If they are not used in this way, I believe their use is worse than their nonuse. There is an allure to exact-sounding numbers. An IQ score of 119, an SAT score of 580, a mental ability score in the 74th percentile – all sound very precise. Indeed, social psychologists have found that people tend to weigh accurate-sounding information highly, almost without regard to its validity (see Nisbett & Ross, 1980). But the appearance of precision is no substitute for the fact of validity. Indeed, a test may in fact be precise in its measurements – but not of whatever it is that distinguishes the more from the less intelligent. IQ tests usually account for between 5% and 25% of the variance in scholastic performance, rarely more. When more consequential kinds of criteria are used (success in various real-world pursuits), the degree of relationship is even less. Yet school administrators and teachers blithely go on as though the tests were highly accurate predictors of interesting criterion performances.

Few people are willing to admit that they are entranced by test scores. When they hear the results of experiments showing that people overvalue precise-sounding information of low validity, they tend to think of these results as applying to others. Because of this tendency to discount the experimental evidence, I would like to offer some anecdotal evidence to back up my claim.

When I worked one summer at the Psychological Corporation, distributors of the Miller Analogies Test (a widely used test for graduate admissions and financial aid decisions), we heard what I considered then, and still consider, to be an amazing story: A teachers' college in Mississippi required a score of 25 on the Miller Analogies Test for admission. The use of this cutoff was questionable, to say the least, in that 25 represents a chance score on this test. (There are 100 items with 4 answer options per item, and no penalty for guessing is subtracted for wrong answers.) A promising student was admitted to the college despite a sub-25 Miller score and went through the program with distinction. When it came time for the student to receive a diploma, she was informed that the diploma would be withheld until she could take the test and receive a score of at least 25. I am pleased to say that she did in fact retake the test and receive a score slightly above the requisite chance score. But I am less pleased with the logic behind the readministration: The predictor had somehow come to surpass the criterion in importance! The test had become an end rather than a means. I told this pathetic story to a large meeting of teachers of the gifted, showing them how bad things could be at an isolated teachers' college in Mississippi. Afterward, a teacher came up to me and told me an essentially identical story (except for a higher cutoff score) as it pertained to her own quite reputable university in southern Connecticut (not my own, I am happy to say).

That variants of this kind of logic are not limited to isolated cases is shown by the fact that I have encountered personally, and heard about innumerable times, similar experiences at major universities. Consider, for example, the cases of applicants to graduate (and often, undergraduate) programs with stellar credentials except for reduced test scores. In my experience, these applicants have a way of getting a "full and open discussion" of their full set of credentials and then of getting rejected. Often, people know in their hearts, right from the beginning of the discussion, that the decision will be negative. The discussion seems more to alleviate people's feelings of guilt at going with test scores than to do anything else. These negative decisions are particularly frustrating when the applicants have shown excellent competence at the criterion task (in my profession, psychological research) and yet are rejected on the basis of test scores that are at best highly imperfect predictors of performance on the criterion task. Again, the means becomes the end, and people forget which is the criterion and which the predictor. The test becomes more important than the performance it is supposed to predict. When criterion information is unavailable or scanty, test scores can serve a very useful function; people who might otherwise be denied admission to programs on the basis of inadequate evidence may be admitted because their test scores show them capable of high-level performance. But when criterion information is available, the tests may be superfluous or even counterproductive. The criterion information in these cases should receive the lion's share of attention in making decisions about future performance.

To conclude, tests work for some people some of the time; but they do not work for other people much of the time. Moreover, the people for whom they do not work are often the same ones, again and again. Applied conservatively and with full respect for all of the available information, tests can be of some use. Misapplied or overused, they are worse than nothing. I believe we do have some promising leads for the tests of the future, however, that eventually may enable us to test intelligence in ways superior to those of conventional IQ tests. In the meantime, we must remember that the fact that a test score is (or appears to be) precise does not mean that it is valid.

Part V

Concluding remarks

Part V contains a single chapter, Chapter 12, which presents the integration and implications that follow from the material in the previous chapters. This chapter briefly discusses implications of the triarchic theory of intelligence for some general issues regarding (a) theories, (b) measures, (c) training, and (d) the field of intelligence as they exist today and may exist in the future.

12 Integration and implications

In concluding this presentation of the triarchic theory of human intelligence, there are a number of issues in need of resolution. At least some of these issues are discussed in this final chapter. First, I will deal with issues relating directly to the triarchic theory; then I will deal with issues pertaining to the study of intelligence in general.

The triarchic theory

Goal of the triarchic theory

The triarchic theory of human intelligence seeks to specify the loci of human intelligence and to specify how these loci operate in generating intelligent behavior. It provides a somewhat broader conceptualization of intelligence than do most conventional theories. This broader conceptualization may help us understand not only the 10–25% of variance in real-world performance accounted for by traditional intelligence tests but also a sizable chunk of the remaining variance. No matter how.well traditional psychometric or cognitive theories account for performance on intelligence tests, they seem not to go much beyond the tests in terms of their ability to account for intelligence in the everyday world.

The triarchic theory of intelligence is a theory of individuals and their relations to their internal worlds, their external worlds, and their experiences as mediators of the individuals' internal and external worlds. Whereas laboratory psychologists, in their desire for simplicity, elegance, and detail, have in some cases removed their theories from any consequential involvement in real-world intelligence, contextual theorists, in their desire for ecological validity, have in some cases provided theories that lack any detail regarding what the internal mechanisms are that lead to intelligent behavior. With a few exceptions, theorists have been reluctant to acknowledge the need for both contextual and cognitive constraints when theorizing about what constitutes intelligent behavior.

The triarchic theory will not totally satisfy those theorists of intelligence who seek the locus of intelligence only in the individual, or only in behavior, or only in the contexts of behavior. The reason for this is that the triarchic theory postulates the locus of intelligence to be in all three. I believe that it has been and continues to be important to study how these loci contribute to and interact in defining intelligence; but I believe it counterproductive to seek a unique locus of the nature of origins of intelligence when no single locus exists.

The literature in psychology is replete with instances of fruitless "either-or" debates: propositional versus imagery theories of mental representation; process versus knowledge accounts of expertise in problem solving; spatial versus linguistic accounts of transitive inference; featural versus nonfeatural accounts of psychological meaning; factorial versus process theories of intelligence; and so on. In each of these instances, and in many other instances as well, the debates became far more productive when the issue became not one of which account was uniquely correct, but one of those particular circumstances under which one kind of account was correct or preferred and those other particular circumstances under which the other kind (or kinds) of account was correct or preferred. In each of these debates, the original arguments were fruitless because it was so easy for either side to amass evidence in its favor. And the reason it was so easy to amass evidence in favor of either side was that each side was correct, but only part of the time and under a particular set of circumstances. Useful progress resulted only when views that had formerly seemed in opposition to each other were recognized to be complementary and even mutually supportive rather than exclusive. The same is true for the nature of intelligence: Die-hard contextualists will continue to argue that intelligence inheres only in the environment; die-hard mentalists will seek to understand intelligence only with respect to the mental structures and processes of the individual. The debate will never be resolved in this form, because the debate is only in the minds of the theorists and in the contexts they create. Contextual and mentalistic views of intelligence are complementary, not contradictory. Intelligence inheres in both the individual and the environments that the individual inhabits.

Structure of the triarchic theory

The subtheories. The triarchic theory of human intelligence seeks to understand intelligence in terms of three subtheories: a contextual subtheory that relates intelligence to the external environment of the individual, a componential subtheory that relates intelligence to the internal environment of the individual, and an experiential subtheory that applies to both the internal and external environments. Of course, this distinction is one of convenience: The components specified by the componential subtheory provide the mental bases for dealing with the external world; thus, the contextual theory can be seen as specifying particular domains in which individuals may have greater or lesser expertise in applying componential functions. Behavior is intelligent to the extent that it is (a) used in adaptation to, selection of, or shaping of one's environment; (b) responsive to a novel kind of task or situation or in the process of becoming automatized; and (c) the result of metacomponential, performance-componential, or knowledge-acquisitional functioning of the kind specified by the componential subtheory. The overall structure of the theory and subtheories is shown in Figure 12.1.

It is important to note the hierarchical structure of the triarchic theory. The theory as a whole is divided into three subtheories, and these three subtheories are in turn divided into successively narrower sets of subtheories. In this scheme, it is the theoretical structure, rather than the mind itself (cf. Vernon, 1971), that is viewed hierarchically.

The hierarchical structure of the triarchic theory of intelligence is what prevents it from being a throwback to the "grand style" theorizing of the early 1900s, whether in the field of intelligence, personality, learning, or whatever. The grand style theories, including most of the psychometric (factorial) theories of intelligence considered in Chapter 1, were essentially top-down in character. Their advantage was the breadth and scope of the questions they addressed. Their disadvantage was their extreme dependence upon the correctness of the superstructure. If the superstructure crumbled, the whole theory went along with it. Too much of the informational and heuristic value lay at the top of the theoretical superstructure. When those theories toppled, they toppled mightily, starting at the top. More recent psychological theorizing has been more "bottom-up." In the 1980s, we have little in the way of contemporary theories that deal with the wholes of intelligence, personality, or learning. Rather, the theories tend to deal with limited aspects of these constructs. Such theories are more closely tied to empirical data and generalizations than were their predecessors, and thus are less susceptible to toppling down. But what these more bottom-up theories gain in stability they lose in scope and breadth: They are addressed to narrower problems. Most contemporary cognitive theories of intelligence, for example, are quite a bit narrower in scope than were the psychometric theories. The triarchic theory of human intelligence is both top-down and bottom-up in its formulation. The theories at lower levels of the theoretical hierarchy are narrower in scope and closely tied to data. These theories are merged at successively higher levels of the hierarchy to form theories that are

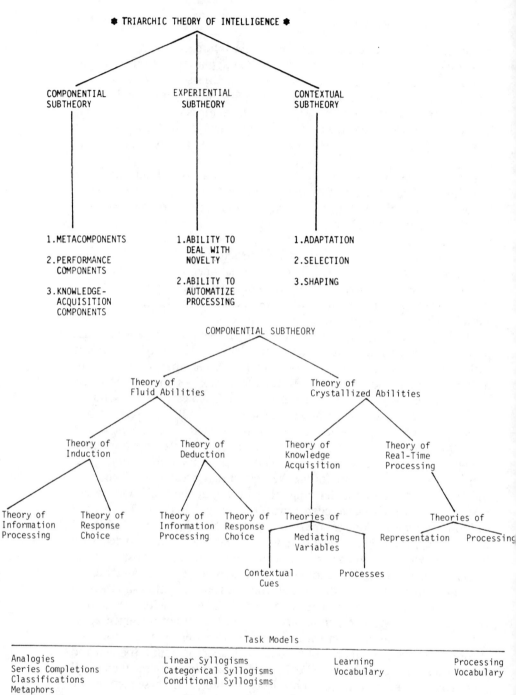

● TRIARCHIC THEORY OF INTELLIGENCE ●

COMPONENTIAL SUBTHEORY	EXPERIENTIAL SUBTHEORY	CONTEXTUAL SUBTHEORY
1.METACOMPONENTS	1.ABILITY TO DEAL WITH NOVELTY	1.ADAPTATION
2.PERFORMANCE COMPONENTS	2.ABILITY TO AUTOMATIZE PROCESSING	2.SELECTION
3.KNOWLEDGE-ACQUISITION COMPONENTS		3.SHAPING

COMPONENTIAL SUBTHEORY

Theory of Fluid Abilities

Theory of Crystallized Abilities

Theory of Induction

Theory of Deduction

Theory of Knowledge Acquisition

Theory of Real-Time Processing

Theory of Information Processing

Theory of Response Choice

Theory of Information Processing

Theory of Response Choice

Theories of

Mediating Variables

Theories of

Representation   Processing

Contextual Cues

Processes

Task Models

Analogies
Series Completions
Classifications
Metaphors
Causal Inferences

Linear Syllogisms
Categorical Syllogisms
Conditional Syllogisms

Learning
Vocabulary

Processing
Vocabulary

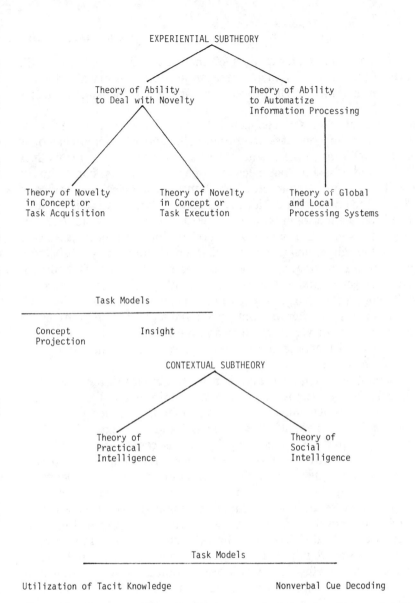

EXPERIENTIAL SUBTHEORY

Theory of Ability
to Deal with Novelty

Theory of Ability
to Automatize
Information Processing

Theory of Novelty
in Concept or
Task Acquisition

Theory of Novelty
in Concept or
Task Execution

Theory of Global
and Local
Processing Systems

Task Models

Concept
Projection

Insight

CONTEXTUAL SUBTHEORY

Theory of
Practical
Intelligence

Theory of
Social
Intelligence

Task Models

Utilization of Tacit Knowledge

Nonverbal Cue Decoding

Figure 12.1. Structure of the triarchic theory and subtheories of human intelligence.

broader in scope, but less closely tied to data. The simultaneous construction
of the theoretical structure from the top, down, and from the bottom, up,
enables the triarchic theory to be broad in its scope, but nevertheless firm in
its links to data. If the superstructure goes, as well it eventually might, then
the lower-order, narrower theories can still stand on their own merits, and

vice versa. For example, the "triarchic" character of the theory could still hold even if the theory of induction were wrong, or the theory of induction could hold even if the triarchy proved to be wrong. The theory as a whole is thus robust.

All three requirements of intelligent behavior (a, b, and c, above) may not be met fully in any one task requiring intelligent behavior: Behavior is viewed as intelligent to the extent that it partakes of these elements. It is possible to find behaviors that meet only one or two of these constraints in any significant degree, as a result of which they are not clearly identified as "intelligent" behaviors. Eating, for example, meets criterion a (it is certainly adaptive!), but neither of criteria b or c. Hence, it is not a useful basis for assessing intelligence. Learning how to perform simple motor tasks, such as turning on the light switch when one enters a dark home, may satisfy criterion b and even a, but does not involve any nontrivial exercise of the components of intelligence. Some of the simple laboratory tasks used by investigators of intelligence, such as choice reaction time, may well satisfy criterion b and even c but satisfy criterion a only in a trivial sense. The environment to which one is adapting is one set up by an experimenter for measuring performance on a task that probably has very little to do with the demands of the world in which one lives.

It is essential again to note that no claim is being made that the structure of the triarchic theory in some way represents or mirrors the structure of the mind. For example, it would be erroneous to infer that the theory claims the existence of "componential," "experiential," and "contextual" faculties. Rather, the structure of the theory highlights three central aspects of intelligence. The basic unit of intelligence is the cognitive component (componential subtheory). The use of components is most relevant to understanding and assessing intelligence when the components are applied to contextually appropriate tasks and situations (contextual subtheory) that are either relatively novel or in the process of becoming responded to in an automatic way. Figure 12.2 shows a three-dimensional map of the circumstances under which cognitive components are most relevant to understanding and assessing intelligence. A task or situation is viewed as measuring intelligence to the extent that it meets the full set of constraints specified by the triarchic theory. Obviously, few if any tasks or situations will meet all of the constraints, so that tasks and situations will, in practice, measure intelligence in greater or lesser degrees.

Is the triarchy specified by the triarchic theory the only way to slice the "intelligence pie"? Certainly not. There is nothing psychologically absolute about this particular division. I would claim, however, heuristic usefulness for this particular slicing. Consider how this slicing relates to previous theoretical accounts of intelligence.

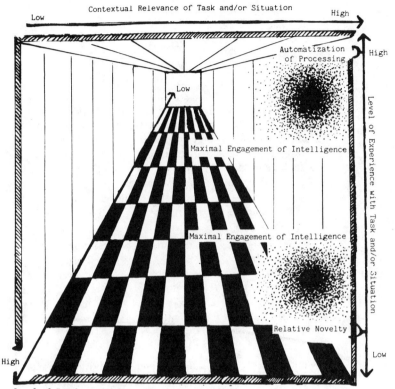

Figure 12.2. Circumstances under which cognitive components most aptly measure intelligent performance.

Table 12.1 describes some previous attempts to understand the nature of intelligence, and characterizes them in terms of (a) the domain about which theorizing takes place and (b) the source of information about this domain. With respect to domains, a surprisingly large number of previous attempts (only a small sample of which are listed here) can be characterized as dealing with either the internal world of the individual (as dealt with by the componential subtheory), the external world of the individual (as dealt with by the contextual subtheory), or the experience of the individual (as dealt with by the experiential subtheory). With respect to sources of information, theories can generally be characterized as deriving from definitions, empirical analyses of subject variance (e.g., psychometric accounts of intelligence), or empirical analyses of stimulus variance (e.g., cognitive accounts of intelligence). Certainly, these are not the only dimensions along which previous theories of

Table 12.1. *Scheme for classification of theories of intelligence*

Source of information	Domain		
	Internal world	External world	Experience
Definitional	Ability to carry on abstract thinking (Terman) Power of good responses from point of view of truth or fact (Thorndike)	Ability to learn to adjust oneself to environment (Colvin) Ability to adapt to relatively new situations in life (Pintner)	Capacity to learn or profit by experience (Dearborn) Capacity to acquire capacity (Woodrow)
Subject variance	Mental energy (Spearman) Primary mental abilities (Thurstone)	Cognitive styles adaptation (Berry) Level of involvement in subsistence activities (Munroe & Munroe)	Individual differences in Piagetian (e.g., conservation) tasks (Tuddenham, J. Hunt)
Stimulus variance	Mental speed (Jensen) Speed of lexical access (E. Hunt)	Culturally targeted cognitive tasks (Cole, Wagner)	Equilibration: assimilation and accommodation (Piaget) Ability to deal with novelty (Cattell, Raaheim)

intelligence might be characterized, nor are the assignments of investigators to cells necessarily unique. Some cognitive investigators, for example, have tried to integrate psychometric thinking into their accounts. But I believe the table may be useful in pinpointing what I see as a potential contribution of the triarchic theory – namely, its integration of domains and sources of information. The triarchic theory explicitly attempts to deal with all three domains and to utilize data from experiments analyzing both subject and stimulus variance.

The table also carries some implications regarding the evolution of the triarchic theory. Early psychometric theorizing concentrated upon subject variance. The major contribution of the cognitive research of the 1970s (e.g., Carroll, 1976; Hunt, 1978; Sternberg, 1977b), seen from the present point of view, was methodological rather than substantive: This research focused upon stimulus variance instead of or in addition to subject variance. But the domain of inquiry – the functioning of the internal mechanisms of intelligence – was essentially the same as that of psychometric theorizing. It is thus perhaps not surprising that the cognitive and psychometric theorizing basically converged in their findings. These two approaches provided different ways of studying essentially the same phenomena. The triarchic theory seeks to provide a substantive as well as a methodological integration, expanding the domain of inquiry to the contextual and experiential domains that have not received adequate attention in traditional psychometric or cognitive work (although they have received attention in other streams of research).

Among previous theories, perhaps the most comprehensive has been that of Piaget (1972), whose full theory dealt with both the internal world of the individual (via stages and structures of intellectual development) and the experience of the individual (via assimilation and accommodation). The theory has less to say about contextual effects upon the individual and upon the nature of intelligence itself.

With few exceptions, the history of theories of intelligence has been one of theories constrained by, and even dictated by, available measures of intelligence. I believe the fundamental mistake that has been made by many theorists has been to start with measures and then to develop theories on the basis of these existing or preferred measures. Sometimes this starting point has been obvious; other times it has been subtle or even concealed. But a careful consideration of existing theories will show, I believe, that the measures usually dictate the theories rather than the other way around. The time has come to turn the tables around: The theory should come first, and the measures follow from the theory. If there are unmeasurables at a given time, then instrumentation should be a priority for future research and development. But we should not let available instruments canalize our thinking.

In sum, then, the triarchic theory is an attempt to account for, in a single theory, what in the past has been accounted for by multiple theories often perceived to be in conflict with each other. According to the present view, past theories were often subsets of what a comprehensive theory of intelligence should have comprised. The triarchic theory seems to be at least a step toward such a more comprehensive theory.

Interrelations among the subtheories. The three subtheories that constitute the triarchic theory of intelligence each make independent contributions to the total theory. Nevertheless, the subtheories are highly interconnected.

The interface between the contextual and experiential subtheories is in the role of novelty and automatization in intelligence expressed in context. One's life is filled with automatized behaviors of which one is hardly aware – bottom-up processes in reading, certain aspects of driving an automobile, scripted behavior in social interaction that can be performed almost "without thinking," and so on. Similarly, everyone encounters in his or her life numerous situations that are novel. Our first encounter with an experience is bound to carry with it some adjustment to novelty. Visiting new environs, learning new kinds of academic material, dealing with new kinds of situations and stresses in interpersonal relationships, and the like all involve coping with novelty. Thus, the two levels of experience of novelty and automatization form an important part of what is required in environmental adaptation, selection, and shaping. From the standpoint of the triarchic theory, the regions of environmental experience involving coping with novelty and automatization of processing are those most critical to intelligence.

The interface between the contextual and componential subtheories is in the fact that environmental adaptation, selection, and shaping are "macrocomponents" that are constituted of the "microcomponents" specified by the componential subtheory. In other words, "adaptation" is no more a basic process than is "dealing with novelty." Rather, adaptation is constituted of more elementary processes, such as recognizing the nature of a problem and knowing what steps to use to solve it (metacomponents), properly encoding the terms of a problem and inferring relations among elements of a problem (performance components), and knowing how to put together the information in one's environment in a proper way (a knowledge-acquisition component). As with the experiential subtheory, there is a need to identify those components of human intelligence that are involved in adaptation to, selection of, and shaping of environments.

The interface between the experiential and componential subtheories is in the fact that some, but not all, components of information processing (a) can be involved in dealing with novelty (at least for a given individual) and (b) are susceptible to automatization of functioning (again for a given individual). For example, the performance component of processing a negation in linear syllogistic (and other forms of) reasoning is not applied to novel material (except in very young children, who are first learning the meaning of *not*) and is probably also not susceptible to complete automatization. Thus, one goal of empirical research is to determine exactly which metacomponents, performance components, and knowledge-acquisition components can be used in dealing with novel tasks and situations and which of these components can become automatized in their functioning. At one level, then, one understands the ability to deal with novelty in terms of the components that constitute this ability; similarly, one understands automatization at one level in terms of those components that can or cannot become automatized via the mechanisms described in the earlier chapters.

Combination rule for abilities specified by the three subtheories. An important issue concerns the combination rule for the abilities specified by the three subtheories. How does the intelligence of a person who is average in the abilities specified by all three subtheories compare to the intelligence of a person who is, say, high in some abilities but low in others? Or what can one say of the intelligence of a person whose environmental opportunities are so restricted that he or she is unable to adapt to, select, or shape any environment? I am very reluctant to specify any combination rule at all, in that I do not believe that a single index of intelligence is likely to be very useful. Consider, for example, the comparison between (a) a person who is very adept at componential functioning, and thus likely to score well on standard IQ tests, but who is lacking in insight or, more generally, in the ability to cope well with nonentrenched kinds of tasks or situations versus (b) a person who is very insightful but not particularly adept at componential operations. The first individual might come across to people as "smart" but not very "creative"; the second individual might come across as creative but not terribly smart. Although it might well be possible to obtain some average score on componential abilities and abilities to deal with nonentrenched tasks and situations, such a composite would obscure the critical qualitative differences between the functioning of the two individuals. Or consider (c) a person who is both componentially adept and insightful but who makes little effort to fit into the environment in which he or she lives. Certainly one would not want to take some overall average that hides the person's academic intelligence (or even brilliance) in a combined index that is reduced because of reduced adaptive skills. The point to be made, then, is that intelligence is not a single thing: It comprises a very wide array of cognitive and other skills. Our aim in theory, research, and measurement ought to be to define what these skills are and to learn how best to assess and train them, not to figure out a way to combine them into a single, possibly meaningless number.

Many people will be uncomfortable with the notion that comparisons between the intelligence of groups or even individuals will always be at least slightly amiss because intelligence is not quite the same thing for different groups and individuals. Yet we are all aware, at least implicitly, that intelligence is not quite the same thing for different individuals. Both in their everyday lives and even in taking tests, people draw upon different skills in order to solve problems. Two business executives, scientists, lawyers, accountants, or whatever may be equally successful but for quite different reasons. Similarly, two students may receive identical scores on intelligence tests but for different reasons. This is not to say that comparisons never can or should be made. If, for example, there is a slot for a senior scientist at a university, a rank-ordering may become necessary, even though one often has the feeling when doing such a rank-ordering that one is comparing "apples and oranges." Similarly, in writing letters of recommendation for graduate students seeking jobs, one often becomes aware that two of the students may be quite able, but in different ways. Moreover, the differences in their abilities are scarcely captured by the traditional kinds of patterns of abilities measured by multiple-aptitude tests. In sum, although we often need to make comparative judgments of people's intelligence or other skills, we ought to keep in mind that we are placing on a unidimensional scale attributes that are intrinsically multidimensional, with the possibility that the relevant dimensions for performance differ from one individual or group to another. The resulting comparisons may be pragmatically useful, but they are not wholly valid.

Present status of the triarchic theory

Each of the three subtheories of the triarchic theory has received at least some empirical validation and elaboration, although more empirical research and theory development are clearly needed. The utility of a theory is seriously impaired if the theory is not falsifiable. To the extent that falsifiability is a problem for the triarchic theory, it is a problem for all other theories of intelligence as well: Theories of intelligence (like theories of many other psychological constructs, such as extraversion, motivation, or paranoia) define the construct that is their object. And definitions, or at least stipulative definitions, are not falsifiable. Thus, there is a sense in which no theory of intelligence is falsifiable.

Fortunately, the picture is not as bleak as it might first appear to be. Although theories of intelligence may not be falsifiable as theories of intelligence, specific models generated by these theories can and should be falsifiable. The question therefore becomes one of whether the theory generates models of human performance, which in turn generate empirically falsifiable predictions. From this point of view, the triarchic theory certainly does generate falsifiable predictions. Indeed, the bulk of this volume is devoted to an exposition of the models generated by the theory and the results of empirical tests of these models.

The contextual subtheory is the least elaborated of the three subtheories, and it is also the one most in need of further research. This subtheory seeks to account for contextual fit to the environment in terms of adaptation to, selection of, and shaping of relevant or potentially relevant environments.

By *context*, I refer to the full set of environments in which an individual lives. By *relevance*, I refer to those aspects of the environmental context that impinge upon an individual's life. Such aspects may be potentially relevant to an individual's life, in that at a given time they do not impinge upon that individual's life but might in the future. By *adaptation*, I refer to the mental events involved in individuals' attempts to adjust to their given environmental contexts. By *selection*, I refer to the mental events involved in individuals' placing themselves in new environments, which then change the contexts in which the individuals reside. And by *shaping*, I refer to the mental events involved in individuals' attempts to adjust their environmental contexts to their own desires or preferences for the way those contexts should be.

Note that the contextual subtheory, like the componential and experiential subtheories, is a theory of mental events. This restriction is necessary in order to keep the conception of intelligence within mental (and manageable!) bounds. One might achieve contextual success by virtue of good looks, wealthy parents, athletic prowess, or any of a number of forms of sheer good luck. Similarly, contextual failure might eventuate from any of a number of forms of bad luck, such as time, place, or other circumstances of birth. The contextual subtheory does not attempt to deal with these factors in contextual success or failure. If it did, it would cease to be a subtheory of intelligence. Rather, it deals with the mental events that mediate, in part, contextual success or failure. Thus, good or bad physical appearance is not within the scope of the contextual subtheory, but the ways in which one exploits good physical appearance or compensates for bad physical appearance (or even turns poor physical appearance into an asset) are within the scope of this subtheory. Level of wealth is not within the scope of the subtheory, but the ways in which one exploits whatever monetary funds one has are within this scope, and so on.

Research emanating out of the contextual subtheory has proceeded along two general lines, based upon explicit and implicit theories of intelligent behavior. The research based on explicit theorizing was presented in Chapter 9. This research seeks to understand social and practical aspects of human intelligence. The research on social intelligence has focused upon decoding of nonverbal cues. Although this research yielded potentially fruitful models of decoding task performance, the external measures used for convergent–discriminant validation did not yield an easily interpretable pattern, and the two decoding tasks used did not even correlate with each other. The research on practical intelligence has focused upon the role of tacit knowledge in professional expertise. In particular, we examined people's tacit knowledge regarding management of self, others, and career. We found that although all three kinds of tacit knowledge are of at least some importance, tacit knowledge regarding one's career seems to be most important in visible measures of career success. In general, tacit knowledge of the kind one tends to pick up on the job (e.g., to what journals to send articles, how to budget one's time) is moderately correlated with criteria for professional success, but not with general intelligence as measured by a psychometric test of verbal reasoning. We are currently following up this work in two ways: by trying to develop a measure of tacit knowledge that more explicitly measures adaptive, selective, and shaping abilities and by trying to formulate process models for how learning of tacit knowledge occurs.

A researcher must acknowledge that the criteria used in studies of contextual intelligence, whatever greater ecological relevance they may have over conventional criteria such as test scores and school grades, are nevertheless flawed. A worker may achieve high performance ratings, substantial merit raises, or placement in a prestigious firm through means having nothing to do with intelligence, just as a student may achieve high grades by nonintellectual means. Moreover, any set of criteria chosen, whatever its ecological relevance, will reflect a value system that a given, evaluated individual may not share. It is thus essential to remember that *all* criteria are flawed. They serve as external validators of theories of intelligence, but they, like the theories, are imperfect. The locus of contextual intelligence is in the mental processes and structures used to attain contextual success, not in the highly imperfect criteria used to assess the success actually obtained.

The research based on implicit theorizing was presented in Chapter 2. In this research, we sought to characterize the implicit theories of intelligence characterizing adults in the mainstream U.S. culture. Three factors - problem-solving ability, verbal ability, and social–practical competence – seemed to characterize the implicit theories of laypersons as well as experts in the field of intelligence. These factors are used in evaluating one's own intelligence as well as the intelligence of others. The first two factors correspond quite closely to factors that have emerged from research on the measurement of intelligence (as generated by explicit, psychometric theories). The third factor has generally not appeared in psychometric theories of intelligence, although there are exceptions, such as Guilford's theory (Guilford, 1967). We are currently following up this work in two ways. In one study, we have examined conceptions of intelligence, wisdom, and creativity both in laypersons and in artists, business professors, physicists, and philosophers. In a second study, we are looking at people's conceptions of intelligence over the life span, using subjects of varying adult ages (from early adulthood to old age).

The experiential subtheory seeks to understand the relations between a person's level of experience with tasks and situations and his or her intelligent behavior. According to this subtheory, intelligence is best measured (a) when a task or situation is relatively (but not completely) novel or (b) when performance on a task or in a situation is in the process of becoming auto-matized. Only the first facet of the subtheory has been directly addressed by our research.

We have examined two kinds of novelty in task performance. This work is discussed in Chapters 3 and 10 of the book.

The first kind pertains to novelty in understanding the structure of a task. A concept projection task was used to assess how well people could learn and apply new conceptual systems for understanding aspects of the world. In one study, for example, subjects had to make projections of future events in a world in which people either are born young and die old, are born old and die young, are born young and die young, or are born old and die old. We were able to model reasoning performance on this kind of task quite successfully and, moreover, found that those parameters of task performance that re-quired thinking in nonentrenched ways were the parameters most closely related to psychometrically measured inductive reasoning abilities. We are currently doing two follow-up studies on the concept projection work. In one study, we are seeking to understand to what extent people's difficulties in handling nonentrenched concepts are due to the strangeness of the concepts themselves and to what extent their difficulties are due to nonentrenchment of the language in terms of which the concepts are expressed. This study therefore relates closely to the time-honored issue in cognitive psychology of the relation between language and thought. In the second study, we are seeking to introduce nonentrenched elements into standard kinds of psy-chometric test items, such as analogies, so as to make them better measures of the ability to deal with novelty.

The second kind of novelty is involved in performing, rather than under-standing, a task. In research investigating this kind of novelty, the problems are straightforward in their appearance but require individuals to think about the problems in novel ways. We have used primarily quantitative insight problems in this kind of work and have obtained preliminary valida-tion of a theory according to which insight can be characterized as involving three separate but related processes – selective encoding, selective combina-tion, and selective comparison. Scores on the insight tasks we have used have shown predicted patterns of convergent and discriminant validation with respect to external psychometric measures of abilities: For example, insight scores tend to be more highly correlated with inductive than with deductive reasoning tasks. Presently, we are following up our reseach on insight using tasks that require more consequential kinds of insights than those required by the quantitative problems we have used to date.

The componential subtheory seeks to understand the mechanisms under-lying intelligent behavior (i.e., behavior that is used in environmental adap-tation, selection, and shaping, particularly at points where the task or situation confronted is novel or being automatized) in terms of three kinds of information-processing components. These kinds of components are (a) metacomponents, which are used to plan, monitor, and evaluate performance; (b) performance components, which are used to execute the plans formulated by the metacomponents; and (c) knowledge-acquisition components, which are used to learn new information. The componential subtheory is by far the most elaborated of the three subtheories of the triarchic theory.

The role of metacomponents in the subtheory is discussed primarily in Chapters 4 and 8. In one study – involving complex forms of analogies – it has been found that more intelligent people (as defined by analogy task scores and psychometric tests) tend to spend relatively more time on global planning and relatively less time on local planning than do less intelligent people (as defined by the same criteria). In the second study, it was found that better readers tend to allocate their time more effectively across different reading passages as a function of the level of comprehension required by the passage. Although metacomponents have been explicitly investigated in these two particular experiments, their effects on task performance have been evident in a large number of studies reviewed in the book, and especially in Chapter 5 on inductive reasoning.

The role of performance components in the subtheory is discussed primarily in Chapters 5–8, which deal with performance components in the context of tasks assessing both fluid and crystallized abilities.

Performance components play a key role in inductive reasoning, as discussed in Chapter 5. In particular, the components of encoding, inference, mapping, application, comparison, justification, and response seem to be generalizable across a variety of induction tasks. Explicit information-processing models of performance have been formulated for analogies (both of the second order and of the third order), series completions, classifications, and metaphorical reasoning tasks. These models have accounted for substantial proportions of the variance in reaction-time as well as response-choice data. The performance components of inductive reasoning seem to be the most central ones in the various psychometric tests, such as the Raven Progressive Matrices and the Cattell Culture Fair Test of g, that have been used to measure g or general intelligence. The research we have done shows that individual differences in latencies of these components can account for large proportions of variance on psychometric tests of g (convergent validation) but have little to do with individual differences on tests of such abilities as perceptual speed (discriminant validation).

The performance components of deductive reasoning, discussed in Chapter 6, appear to be somewhat less consistent across tasks than do the components of inductive reasoning. This finding is consistent with psychometric findings suggesting that deductive reasoning, unlike inductive reasoning, does not comprise a unitary factor of mental ability. Two theories are proposed in Chapter 6 to account for reasoning in three types of syllogisms.

The first theory, a mixture theory of linear-syllogistic reasoning, accounts for linear-syllogistic reasoning in terms of a set of performance components (such as premise encoding, processing of marked adjectives, processing of negations, and seriation of premises) that operates upon both linguistic and spatial representations for information but at different points during the course of problem solution. The theory is applicable across a wide range of item contents and formats, experimental manipulations, and ages of subjects. It does not apply to everyone, however. There is clear evidence of individual differences in subjects' strategies for solving linear-syllogism problems.

The second theory, a transitive-chain theory of categorical- and conditional-syllogistic reasoning, accounts for information processing and response choices in terms of four kinds of operations – those involved in (a) encoding of premises, (b) combination of information expressed in the premises, (c) comparison of mental representations for the premises to mental representations for possible solutions, and (d) response. The theory places a heavy emphasis upon the role of working memory limitations and response biases in the solution of both categorical and conditional syllogisms. Deep-structural spatial representations appear to play a much more important part in these kinds of syllogistic reasoning than do linguistic representations of information, despite the surface-structural form of the problems, which is usually linguistic.

The mixture and transitive-chain theories have stood up under fairly extensive testing of both internal validity (ability of the theory to account for variance in stimulus difficulty) and external validity (ability of the theory to account for individual-difference variance). In combination, the theories seem to give a fairly thorough account of how individuals make deductive inferences.

Some of the performance components involved in verbal comprehension are discussed in Chapter 8. Our treatment of this aspect of information processing is quite limited, in that we have dealt only with performance components in word identification and comparison. Our theory of representation and processing of word meanings suggests that people represent words in terms of both defining and characteristic attributes and that the characteristic attributes are treated as a weighted sum of the importances assigned to each attribute. People's latencies in choosing between alternative attribute sets as better representations of word meanings are significantly correlated with their verbal comprehension abilities as measured by a psychometric test of reading skills. We are currently following up on this work by trying to identify and understand the performance components involved in synonym and antonym judgments of the kinds required on standardized tests of vocabulary.

The role of knowledge-acquisition components in the componential subtheory is discussed primarily in Chapter 7 in the context of theory and research on verbal comprehension. We have sought, in particular, to understand how people acquire meanings of new words. Our theory takes into account (a) the textual cues people use in decontextualization of meanings, (b) the mediating variables that affect how well textual cues can be exploited, and (c) processes of knowledge acquisition that can be applied to the textual cues. Our theory of verbal comprehension provides a fairly good account of what it is that makes some words harder to learn in context than others. Moreover, scores on the task to which the theory has been applied – learning vocabulary from context – are highly correlated with psychometric measures of verbal intelligence. Currently, we are conducting more refined tests of the theory that will identify the weights of various kinds of textual cues in a variety of situations involving vocabulary acquisition.

In order for the triarchic theory to be viewed as reasonably comprehensive, it should be able to account for extremes of intelligence as well as for more typical levels of it. Chapter 10 considers implications of the triarchic theory for understanding exceptional levels of intelligence. Although all aspects of the theory can be applied to understanding both giftedness and retardation, it is claimed that the ability to deal with novelty (as specified by the two-facet subtheory) is particularly crucial to intellectual giftedness and that inability to make metacomponential decisions is particularly crucial to intellectual retardation. Research from both my own studies and the studies of others seems to support these contentions. These claims are being subjected to further empirical testing in work currently being conducted in my research group.

Although the triarchic theory was formulated for scientific purposes, it does seem to have practical implications for the technology of intelligence testing. These implications are discussed in Chapter 11. The triarchic theory can account, in terms of psychological theory, for at least some of the reasons that intelligence tests are reasonably successful for a variety of selection and placement decisions. More importantly, perhaps, it also suggests domains of human intelligence that have not been sufficiently tapped by existing tests and that perhaps should be tapped by the tests of the future. We are attempting to contribute to the formulation of such tests. The domains in which we believe supplementation of existing tests is most critical are the measurement of (a) metacomponential abilities, (b) the ability to deal with novelty, and (c) the abilities involved in attaining contextual fit.

Our research, like that of others, is hindered by the lack of wholly satisfactory external criteria against which to validate our theories and measures.

The standard kinds of criteria – psychometric test scores, school grades, and even on-the-job performance – all have apparent weaknesses. The test scores, for example, assume the validity and completeness of psychometric conceptions of intelligence, whereas school grades and job performance ratings are likely to be affected by many other psychological attributes besides intelligence. Clearly, there is a pressing need for better criteria as well as better measures. Unfortunately, it is easier to recognize the need for better criteria than it is to suggest what such criteria might be. At present, the interests of intelligence research seem best to be served by the use of multiple criteria, none of which is wholly adequate by itself but which in combination seem to tell us something about the domains to which theories of intelligence should apply and generalize.

The study of intelligence

Theories of intelligence

A theory of intelligence should specify the nature of intelligence in terms of the external world, the internal world, and the interrelation between them. Contextual theories have been limited to the former, most other theories to the latter. For example, factorial theories and cognitive theories have generally concentrated on internal mechanisms without regard to the environmental consequentiality of the behaviors studied. Oddly enough, the early theorists in a given area have tended to be most cognizant of the requirements for a broad theory of intelligence; their disciples have chosen, however, only to dwell on limited aspects of their theories. Thus, for example, Binet, Spearman, and Wechsler all dealt in some detail with both the internal mechanisms of intelligence and the role of intelligence in the world. Cattell's (1971) triadic theory also touches on aspects of both the internal and external worlds of the individual. One would often not recognize the breadth of some of these seminal theorists, however, from the work that has followed from the original contributions of these and other individuals.

One implication of the present view, discussed especially in Chapters 1–4, is that many existing theories of intelligence are incomplete rather than incorrect. Indeed, as noted earlier, many of them say essentially the same thing in different languages. Especially within a given paradigm for theorizing, competitive theorists seem to have devoted too much attention to highlighting the differences among their theories, which are not great, and not enough attention to highlighting the ways in which their theories are similar or identical. Factor theories and certain cognitive theories, for example, say pretty much the same things, but in terms of different units of analysis (see Sternberg, 1980c).

There is an unfortunate tendency on the part of many psychologists to view intelligence in an overly restrictive way, although progress is now being made toward broader conceptualizations of intelligence (e.g., Gardner, 1983). Intelligence is not ontologically comparable to cognitive processes such as perception, learning, and problem solving, but neither is it totally different from them. A wholly cognitive theory that tries to equate intelligence to some aspect or aspects of cognition fails to recognize the "stipulative" nature of the concept: *Intelligence* is a concept we invented in order to provide a useful way of evaluating and, occasionally, ordering people in terms of their performance on tasks and in situations that are valued by the culture; however, this performance *is* based upon cognitive (as well as motivational and affective) functioning, a point that seems not explicitly to be dealt with by many existing contextual accounts, although it is a point that has certainly not been totally ignored in contextual theorizing (e.g., Rogoff, 1982).

I believe that the most important task for future theorizing about intelligence is to specify better the interrelations between environmental context, on the one hand, and mental functioning, on the other. It is not enough merely to pick a set of tasks, task-analyze them, and then claim that the result is a theory of intelligence. Such a theory fails to account for the fact that the very same behavior that might be intelligent in one situation might be unintelligent in another. As noted in the preceding chapter, for example, speed may be adaptive or maladaptive, depending upon the task and the reward system under which it is performed.

Measures of intelligence

Even the most highly regarded of the currently available measures of intelligence, such as the Wechsler and Stanford–Binet intelligence tests, fail to do justice to their creators' conceptions of the nature of intelligence. They certainly fail to do justice to the conception of intelligence proposed in this volume. According to the present view, an adequate test would have to measure, at minimum, the aspects of intelligence dealt with by each of the three subtheories of intelligence. The aspects of the theory that are dealt with most inadequately by present tests are, I believe, (a) adaptation to, selection of, and shaping of real-world environments; (b) dealing with novel kinds of tasks and situations; and (c) metacomponential planning and decision making. The present tests measure best (a) the outcomes of knowledge-acquisition components (via crystallized ability tests such as vocabulary and reading) and (b) the current functioning of performance components (via fluid ability tests).

The conceptual orientation underlying current uses of intelligence tests is incomplete. Test constructors and users have long recognized the importance of choosing tasks that tap processes important to intellectual functioning: Even factor theorists, who have tended not to emphasize information processing in their theories (with a few notable exceptions, such as Guilford, 1967), have recognized that individual differences in information processing are at least in part responsible for obtained factorial outcomes. But the kinds of interindividual comparisons test users often want to make – for example, across different sociocultural groups – are often invalid because (a) existing tests measure only products of intellectual functioning, and these products may be obtained by various processes and strategies that have different distributions of usage across sociocultural groups; and (b) even if the processes and strategies are used in comparable proportions by members of the various groups, cross-group comparisons will be unfair if the processes and strategies required are either differentially adaptive, novel, or automatized across groups.

There is, I believe, a pressing need for much more innovation in the testing of intelligence. In recent years, there have been, as far as I can tell, only two well-publicized tests that could be labeled as highly innovative, the Feuerstein (1979) Learning Potential Assessment Device (LPAD) and the Kaufman and Kaufman (1983) Assessment Battery for Children (K-ABC). The former test, based in part upon Vygotsky's theory of the zone of potential development and Feuerstein's own version of this theory, appears to be quite promising, although it is in need of further validation. The latter test, the Kaufman and Kaufman Assessment Battery for Children, is an example of largely misguided innovation. The theory upon which it is based, Luria's (1961) theory of simultaneous versus successive processing, has not held up well in the empirical literature, and the test's overreliance upon associative learning (one of two scores from the intelligence battery is for associative learning!) is most unfortunate: Associative learning has been found again and again to be among the poorest measures of intelligence (see Estes, 1982; Jensen, 1970). To the extent that the K-ABC has reduced racial differences, it is because of this overreliance upon associative learning, which does not show much in the way of group differences but also does not show much correlation with other measures of intelligence. Nevertheless, this test, like Feuerstein's, represents at least an effort toward innovation in testing. There are, of course, other innovations of a different nature. For example, computerized adaptive testing promises to lead to genuine advances in the rapid and efficient assessment of intelligence. However, such testing represents a repackaging of existing test materials rather than the creation of wholly new materials. Our own efforts toward new kinds of tests, described in the last chapter, are guided by the triarchic theory and attempt more directly to measure its three aspects than do current tests.

Training of intelligence

The triarchic theory has some fairly straightforward implications for programs that seek to train intelligent performance. (See Sternberg, 1983b, for more details regarding some of these implications.)

First, training of intellectual performance must be socioculturally relevant to the individuals who are exposed to the training program. It is tempting, to say the least, to put together a training program appropriate for white middle-class North Americans and then to attempt to use the program on any available group of subjects, regardless of the similarity of their backgrounds to those of the majority culture in the United States.

How does one decide what constitutes a culturally appropriate intervention? Obviously, a complex question such as this one could not possibly be fully addressed here. Extensive consultations are needed between experts from the target population of interest and experts creating the training program. I believe that a useful starting point for these consultations, and the training program, is in the investigation of implicit theories of intelligence in experts and laypersons from the target population of interest. Do implicit theories of intelligence differ across cultures? There is at least some evidence, presented in Chapter 2, that such theories do, in fact, differ cross-culturally. It is important to recognize that sociocultural differences may occur within countries (as well as communities!) and not just across countries. Within the United States, for example, someone functioning within a predominantly Hispanic or Afro-American subculture may find behaviors to be adaptive that are quite different from those found to be adaptive within the majority culture. Differences in what is adaptive can be a function of economic and social as well as cultural or ethnic identifications, so that it is necessary to examine carefully whether what seems like a homogeneous population truly is one.

It is important, in considering a socioculturally appropriate intervention, to take into account not only the present state of the culture, but also the state it can be expected to enter during the subsequent decade or so. Developing countries, for example, are in periods of rapid change, and to design an intervention that is highly appropriate for their present conditions may be futile: These conditions will soon change. Thus, it is necessary in planning a program for training intellectual skills to focus on what will be needed as well as what is presently needed. This vision of the future should be that of people who know well and possibly may influence the culture's development, not the vision of the psychologist planning or implementing the training program. In order to plan an appropriate intervention, I believe extensive interviewing and possibly a formal research investigation are called for that give the investigator a reasonably clear sense of what is culturally appropriate to train in a given environment: One needs to match the program to the population.

Second, the program should furnish links between the training it provides and real-world behavior. The success of programs that train intellectual skills is often measured by pretest – retest increases of trained individuals on IQ tests relative to increases of untrained individuals on the same tests. In good evaluations, a more pluralistic assessment of success of the training program is used. But few assessments are pluralistic enough to take into account increased levels of adaptive functioning in real-world performance. Yet ultimately it is such performance that training programs ought to seek to improve.

I believe it is necessary for programs to provide links between the training they provide and the real-world behaviors to which they ultimately seek to generalize because a large body of research indicates how difficult it is to obtain transfer of training even under conditions that would seem on their surface to be optimal for transfer to occur (see Borkowski & Cavanaugh, 1979, for an excellent discussion of conditions conducive to transfer). Thus, if one seeks to obtain transfer to a set of tasks and situations very different from those in which training takes place, a real effort must be made to maximize the probability of its occurring. Otherwise, one may find oneself in the same position as those who study versions of the "Missionaries and Cannibals Problem" (e.g., Reed, Ernst, & Banerji, 1974), where it is exceedingly difficult to obtain transfer even between problem isomorphs!

Third, the program should provide explicit training in strategies and tactics for coping with novel kinds of tasks and situations. I believe that many of the most innovative and successful programs, such as Lipman's Philosophy for Children and Feuerstein's Instrumental Enrichment (IE), are successful in large part because of their training of children in new ways of thinking. The less successful programs often merely rehash presentation of skills that children have already been taught in greater or lesser degree. Such programs tend to train to particular tests rather than to generalizable skills that underlie performance on these tests.

Fourth, the program should provide explicit training in both executive and nonexecutive information processing as well as in interactions between the two kinds of information processing. Feuerstein's program, for example, directly deals with both of these kinds of skills, addressing deficits in performance such as inability to select relevant versus irrelevant cues in defining a problem and lack of spontaneous comparative behavior or limitations in its application. Butterfield and Belmont's program for training of learning and recall skills in retarded performers (e.g., Belmont & Butterfield, 1969, 1971; Butterfield & Belmont, 1971, 1977) draws heavily upon both executive and nonexecutive processing. Underlying their research and training is the theoretical view that "competent cognition requires an active, deliberate, planful search for solutions to the information-processing problem at hand" (Butterfield & Belmont, 1977, p. 279). In recent work, Ann Brown (1978; Brown & DeLoache, 1978) has taken a similar point of view.

Fifth, the program should be sensitive to individual differences. If one observes successful and unsuccessful people in every walk of life, it will become clear that the causes of success and failure are numerous. Individuals adopt a wide variety of ways of dealing with the problems life presents, and there are almost always multiple ways both to succeed and to fail. Programs that train intellectual skills should acknowledge and actively encourage individuals to manifest their differences in strategies and styles. In particular, the programs should help students learn their strengths and weaknesses, and they should help them learn to capitalize upon their strengths at the same time that they compensate in whatever ways are available for their weaknesses (Cronbach & Snow, 1977; Snow, 1979).

Any number of studies have shown interactions between students' ability patterns and their effectiveness in implementing particular strategies for solving intellectual tasks. Consider, for example, effects of individuals' relative levels of verbal and spatial abilities on task performance. MacLeod, Hunt, and Mathews (1978) and Mathews, Hunt, and MacLeod (1980) found that subjects' patterns of verbal and spatial abilities interacted with their strategy choice and efficacy in performing a particular strategy. Sternberg and Weil (1980), in their investigation of linear-syllogistic reasoning, found that the effectiveness with which either a primarily verbal or a primarily spatial strategy was carried out depended upon subjects' patterns of verbal and spatial abilities. As expected, the verbal strategy was relatively more effective for high verbals, whereas the spatial strategy was relatively more effective for high spatials. Programs that train intellectual skills will often present problems that can be solved in multiple ways. The program should take into account that what is optimal for some students may not be optimal for others.

Finally, the program should be responsive to motivational as well as intellectual needs of the students it trains. Commenting upon the behavior of the typical "culturally deprived" examinee who is likely to show reduced performance on standard intelligence tests, Feuerstein (1979) has noted that such examinees enter the ability-testing situation with reduced motivation attributable to a lack of curiosity about the situation, a lack of a need system that would endow the tasks to be performed with a specific personal meaning, and an avoidance reaction to the kinds of tasks that have been associated with repeated experiences of failure in the past. Feuerstein thus attributes intellectually deficient performance at least in part to motivational deficits (or at least differences relative to the motivational sets of typical performers).

A champion of the view that reduced intellectual performance often re-sults from motivational as well as from intellectual deficits has been Zigler (1971), who has claimed that reduced cognitive performance is frequently mediated in part by reduced intrinsic motivation. By effecting quantitative and qualitative changes in the motivational levels of retarded children, Zigler and his colleagues have been able to obtain improvements in these children's performance on traditional intelligence tests. Neither Feuerstein nor Zigler has claimed that intellectual deficits in individuals showing re-tarded performance can be accounted for wholly or even primarily in terms of motivational deficits. Certainly, high levels of motivation (whether intrin-sic or extrinsic) are not sufficient for adequate intellectual performance. But like these two investigators, I believe that a fairly high level of motivation is necessary for adequate intellectual performance. Indeed, for student sam-ples restricted in range with respect to intellectual ability (e.g., graduate students or educable mentally retarded students), differences in motivation may account for large shares of differences in observed performance, regard-less of the level the performance is at. A training program that provides intellectual stimulation, no matter how well it does so, will be inadequate if it does not motivate students to learn from the program, to use what they have learned in situations outside the program, and to adopt an attitude of intel-lectual curiosity in their everyday encounters with both academic and non-academic situations. The point is that it doesn't matter what you know if you don't use it, and a program should motivate students not only to learn but also to use what they learn.

The psychologists who seem most to have recognized the importance of motivation to skills training are not those concerned with intellectual skills, but rather those concerned with behavioral problems, such as those prob-lems that lead to obesity, heavy smoking, and drug addiction. Programs to effect behavioral change in these areas, in order to be more effective, must change an individual's motivational set as well as his or her specific behaviors in the training situation. The same holds for behavioral changes as a result of intellectual skills training.

The field of intelligence

Historically, the field of intelligence has tended to be something of an estab-lishment, with its own set of problems and its own way of doing things. Unfortunately, this establishment often proceeded independently of main-stream psychology, with only minor interaction between the mainstream, on the one hand, and the field of intelligence, on the other. The field was never taken too seriously by respectable psychologists, and indeed, I think it fair to say that there was a sentiment that it tended to attract neither the best scholars nor the best research. At some times in the history of the field, this sentiment was probably wrong; at other times, it may have been right. But for intelligence research to attract the most able scholars in psychology, clearly it would have to become a field linked to and accepted by the mainstream of psychological research.

In the 1970s, with the emergence of vigorous responses to Cronbach's (1957) challenge to the two disciplines of scientific psychology (correlational and experimental psychology), the study of intelligence did indeed seem to be on the road toward a greater acceptance by, and linkage to, mainstream psychology (at least in the United States): Many of the articles published in the field were published in mainline psychological journals and thus could influence the thinking of those outside of, or only peripherally involved with, the field of intelligence, as well as the hard core of intelligence researchers. At the same time, Douglas Detterman founded a journal for the field, called, appropriately enough, *Intelligence.* Thus, investigators had the option of publishing in their own journal or in the more mainline journals of the field of psychology as a whole. I believe that there is a need for research on intelligence to continue in the development of its own establishment, but this time with full contact between it and other psychological establishments. On the one hand, one must avoid the pitfall of the past in which intelligence researchers formed a clique, unexciting to and possibly unknown by researchers in other areas. On the other hand, it is essential that the field continue to develop its own traditions, both old and new. Intelligence research cannot afford to be judged by the standards of any one subfield, whether it be cognitive, developmental, differential, or any other area of psychology. The journal *Intelligence* is referred to in its subtitle as "multidisciplinary," and it is important to recognize that the study of intelligence is and should continue to be multidisciplinary. To conform rigidly to the mores of any one discipline will result and, I believe, has resulted in a constriction of the concept of *intelligence* that simply does not do full justice to it. Intelligence cannot be understood solely in terms of cognitive psychology, for example, and as soon as one decides that it is just cognitive psychologists that one wishes to please, the construct will be investigated not in its own right, but in a restricted form tied to the Procrustean bed of any single way of looking at things. The recent *Handbook of Human Intelligence* (Sternberg, 1982g), for example, contains articles by differential, cognitive, comparative, educational, developmental, behavior – genetic, and other kinds of psychologists. Intelligence is, and will have to continue to be, a construct capable of being understood only in a multidisciplinary fashion.

The approach proposed here is certainly cognitive in its bases, like many other contemporary approaches (see Sternberg, in press-b, for a review of these cognitive approaches). At the same time, it is not restricted to the rationales, principles, or methods of cognitive psychology. Most elements of the triarchic theory have been proposed before, in one form or another. If this book represents a new contribution, I would hope it would be in combining those elements that are needed for a theory of intelligence and in deleting those elements that may be relevant to other constructs but not to the construct of intelligence.

The temptations toward simplification and narrow focusing are many. Certain psychologists would like to understand intelligence solely in terms of the measurement of EEG or other psychophysiological indices, as though such indices have a magical causal status that other forms of dependent variables lack. But what exactly does a high correlation between, say, an EEG measure and a test of intelligence mean? Does the correlation mean that the physiological indicant somehow causes intelligence, or that it measures a cause of it? Certainly not, because correlation does not imply causation. It is just as likely that intelligent behavior generates certain physiological responses, or that both the physiological indicants and the intelligent behavior are dependent upon some other element, which itself might be studied at a different level of analysis. Even if IQ correlated perfectly with some physiological measure, what would this correlation tell us about (a) the cognitive processes that underlie intelligent behavior, (b) what constitutes an intelligent behavior, or (c) why intelligence tests as they now exist are so imperfect as predictors of intelligent behavior in the real world? One might as easily fault the physiological index as praise it, arguing that the measure is incomplete in dealing only with the same subset of intelligence as do existing intelligence tests.

Other psychologists would like to understand intelligence solely in terms of the functioning of genes, as though intelligence is precisely that portion of cognitive abilities that is inherited. But accounts that assign a certain proportion of variance to heredity and a certain proportion to environment still fail to answer the fundamental question of just what intelligence is. There is nothing wrong with these accounts, nor is there anything wrong with physiological accounts. The important thing to recognize is that the various kinds of accounts address different questions at different levels of analysis. All of these kinds of research are needed. A problem arises only when an investigator comes to believe that his or her approach supersedes all others. At present, there just does not exist a single approach that answers or even addresses all of the questions one would want answered about the nature of intelligence. Oversimplifications not only narrow one's interpretation of the construct but also narrow the questions one can ask about the construct. If any field has suffered from a focusing on narrow and sometimes peripheral questions, the field of intelligence has.

To conclude, I view the field of intelligence as experiencing a renaissance that is long overdue but that shows every sign of making up for what some might see as lost time. There are many opposing tugs either to make intelligence a branch of some established area of psychology, such as cognitive psychology, or else to make it a sovereign field isolated from all the rest. These tugs are healthy only so long as they cancel each other out. The field needs to establish itself as an independent discipline at the same time that it needs to draw upon and give to other disciplines. So long as investigators continue to be lured from all areas of psychology, and so long as they remain willing to interact with each other and draw upon each others' expertise, I believe that the present surge of research will flourish, as it did in the decade of the 1970s and continues to do in the decade of the 1980s.

Methodological appendix: Testing componential models via componential analysis

The goal of this appendix is to present the techniques of "componential analysis," a methodology for studying cognitive skills that draws upon psychometric and cognitive methodologies and that was used in testing the componential models described in the main body of the book. The appendix will present a series of steps for executing a componential analysis and illustrate the techniques of componential analysis with examples from my research. I have attempted to make the appendix comprehensible without need to refer back to chapters of the book.

In order to achieve some uniformity and continuity, I will draw especially from my componential theory of analogical reasoning (Sternberg, 1977b), as described in Chapter 5. Consider the analogy, LAWYER : CLIENT :: DOCTOR : (a. PATIENT, b. MEDICINE). According to the theory, a subject must *encode* the terms of the problem, perceiving each item and retrieving relevant attributes from long-term memory; *infer* the relation between LAWYER and CLIENT, recognizing that a lawyer renders professional services to a client; *map* the higher-order relation from the first to the second half of the analogy, in this case, recognizing that both halves of the analogy (those headed by LAWYER and by DOCTOR) deal with professional services rendered; *apply* the relation inferred in the first half of the analogy to the second half of the analogy so as to generate an ideal completion that indicates to whom a DOCTOR renders professional services; *compare* the options, PATIENT and MEDICINE, to the ideal response; optionally, *justify* PATIENT as close enough to an ideal response to be correct; and *respond* with the chosen answer.

Overview of componential analysis: selecting or generating a theory of relevant cognition

The first thing one has to do is to decide what it is one wishes to analyze. Such a decision requires a theory of that aspect of cognition for which one wishes to perform the componential analysis. There are any number of criteria on the basis of which one might evaluate either preexisting theories or one's own new theory. I have proposed five criteria that I believe are particularly useful for this purpose (Sternberg, 1977b):

1. *Completeness*. A complete theory is one that accounts for all processes involved in the area of cognition of interest.

2. *Specificity*. A specific theory describes in detail the workings of each aspect of cognition. A theory can be complete but not specific if it accounts for all processes, representations, structures, and so on but does not describe the workings of the processes in detail. A theory can also be specific but not complete if it describes in detail a proper subset of processes, structures, and representations involved in the relevant area of cognition.

3. *Generality*. A theory is general if it is applicable across a wide range of problems within the relevant domain of cognition.

4. *Parsimony*. A theory is parsimonious if it can account for performance in the relevant domain of cognition with a relatively small number of parameters and working assumptions. Parsimony is difficult to evaluate, in part because many theories that appear parsimonious on their surface have hidden assumptions, whereas other theories that appear less parsimonious can be taken more easily at face value. As might be expected, there tends to be a tradeoff between parsimony, on the one hand, and completeness and specificity, on the other. A difficult problem facing theorists is to strike a reasonable balance between them.

5. *Plausibility*. A theory is plausible if it is able to account for experimental (or other) data that provide a test of the theory. Plausibility also involves intuitive judgments about the reasonableness of the theory. If one theory seems less reasonable on its face than another theory, skeptics may require more compelling evidence to convince them of the former theory than to convince them of the latter theory.

Consider as an example of the application of these criteria the componential theory of analogical reasoning.

The theory does quite well by the completeness criterion: The analogical reasoning process is described from beginning to end. This specification is in terms of rather detailed flowchart models for the six processes described earlier. (Explicit flowcharts for various models under the theory are presented in Sternberg, 1977b.) All necessary processes are explicitly stated in the flowchart and their interrelations shown. Of course, the componential theory does not address all aspects of reasoning by analogy: For example, it does not specify the decision rule by which subjects choose one response over the other(s). This specification requires supplementation of the componential theory with a theory of response choice (which is, in fact, presented in Sternberg & Gardner, 1983, and in Chapter 5).

The theory is quite specific in describing the details of the three attribute-comparison processes (inference, mapping, and application). It is less specific in describing the encoding process.

The theory has been shown to be quite general: It has been shown to apply to items presented in both true – false and forced-choice formats; to apply to items with schematic-picture, verbal, and geometric content; and to apply to subjects of ages ranging from about 7 years of age to adulthood.

The theory achieves a reasonable degree of parsimony by specifying all operations but assigning separate information-processing components only to psychologically significant operations. The theory thus manages to be complete while at the same time retaining parsimony. The major aspects of analogical reasoning are accounted for in the five mandatory components and the one optional one. But the minor aspects are represented in flow-charts and in most cases are absorbed into the response component, which is estimated as a regression constant (which includes within it all operations that are constant across analogies of varying difficulties and kinds).

Finally, the plausibility of the theory has been tested rather extensively through a series of experimental investigations (Sternberg, 1977a, 1977b; Sternberg & Gardner, 1983; Sternberg & Nigro, 1980; Sternberg & Rifkin, 1979). Methods for testing plausibility of the theory will be described later. But to date, the empirical evidence has been very supportive in suggesting that the theory provides a good account of a variety of data with various experimental paradigms and subjects.

Selecting one or more tasks for analysis

Tasks can be selected for componential analysis on the basis of their satisfaction of four criteria originally proposed by Sternberg and Tulving (1977) in a different context: quantifiability, reliability, construct validity, and empirical validity.

1. *Quantifiability*. The first criterion, quantifiability, assures the possibility of the "assignment of numerals to objects or events according to rules" (Stevens, 1951, p. 1). Quantification is rarely a problem in research on intellectual abilities. Occasionally, psychologists are content to use subjects' introspective reports or protocols as their final dependent variable. The protocols, used in and of themselves, fail the test of quantification. If, however, aspects of the protocols are quantified (see, e.g., Newell & Simon, 1972) and thus rendered subject to further analysis, these quantifications can be acceptable dependent variables so long as they meet the other criteria.

2. *Reliability*. The second criterion, reliability, measures true-score variation relative to total-score variation. In other words, it measures the extent to which a given set of data is systematic. Reliability needs to be computed in

two different ways, across item types and across subjects. Because the two indices are independent, a high value of one provides no guarantee or even indication of a high value of the other. Each of these two types of reliability can be measured in two ways, at a given time or over time.

3. *Construct validity*. The third criterion, construct validity, assures that the task has been chosen on the basis of some psychological theory. The theory thus dictates the choice of tasks rather than the other way around. A task that is construct-valid is useful for gaining psychological insights through the lens provided by some theory of cognition.

4. *Empirical validity*. The fourth criterion, empirical validity, assures that the task serves the purpose it is supposed to serve. Thus, whereas construct validity guarantees that the selection of a task is motivated by theory, empirical validity tests the extent to which the theory is empirically supportable. Empirical validation is usually performed by correlating task performance with an external criterion.

These four criteria are related to each other in a number of ways. First, they fall into two natural and orthogonal groupings of two criteria each. The first and second criteria are ones of measurement theory; the third and fourth are ones of substantive psychological theory. The first and third criteria are discrete and dichotomous, being either satisfied or not; the second and fourth criteria are continuous, being satisfied in greater or lesser degree. Second, the criteria fall into a natural ordering. The first two criteria, those of measurement theory, are prerequisite for the second two criteria, those of psychological theory: The tasks must satisfy certain measurement properties before their psychological properties can be assessed. Moreover, the criteria are ordered within these groupings as well as between them. The first criterion within each grouping is prerequisite for the second. Reliability presupposes quantification in that reliability measures the extent to which the measurement obtained by the quantification is consistent. Empirical validity presupposes construct validity in that empirical validity measures the extent to which the measurements dictated by the theory correspond to that theory.

Consider as an example of the application of these criteria performance on the analogical problem type to which my componential theory of analogical reasoning has been applied. Performance on analogies satisfies the four criteria described above. First, performance can be quantified in terms of response latency, error rate, or distribution of responses given among the possible responses that might be given. Second, performance on analogical reasoning tasks can be measured reliably. I have shown reliabilities across items of .97 and .89 for schematic-picture and geometric analogies, respectively (Sternberg, 1977a), and standard psychometric tests including sections measuring analogical reasoning typically report reliabilities across subjects in the .80s and .90s. The construct validity of performance on tests of analogical reasoning is unimpeachable: Analogies have served as a major source of theorizing in psychometric, Piagetian, and information-processing investigations of cognition and intelligence. Finally, the empirical validity of performance on analogy items has been demonstrated in my own research and that of others: Analogies (along with figural matrix problems) have served as a primary basis for measuring g (general intelligence) because performance on these items has been found to correlate about as highly with a variety of criteria as any other single item type that has been tried (see Sternberg, 1977b, for documentation of these claims).

Decomposing task performance

Most tasks, indeed all of the tasks that my collaborators and I have investigated, can be decomposed into subtasks, where a subtask is defined in terms of its involvement of a subset of the information-processing components that are involved in the full task. There are a number of reasons for attempting to isolate information-processing components from subtasks rather than from composite tasks. First, it is often possible to isolate information-processing components from subtasks that cannot be isolated from composite tasks. The smaller the number of information-processing components involved in any single subtask, the greater the likelihood that the individual components will be susceptible to isolation. Second, use of subtasks requires the investigator to specify in which subtask or subtasks each information-processing component is executed and thus requires tighter, more nearly complete specification of the relationship between task structure and the components that act on that structure. Third, use of subtasks increases the number of data points to be accounted for and thus helps to guard against the spurious good fit between model and data that can result when the number of parameters to be estimated becomes large relative to the number of data points to be predicted. Fourth, use of subtasks results in component-free estimates of performance for a series of nested processing intervals. These estimates can be valuable when one wants to test alternative predictions about global stages of information processing. The decomposition of composite tasks into subtasks, then, represents a useful intermediate step in the analysis of the nature of mental abilities. There are a number of different ways of decomposing composite tasks into subtasks. Some of these will be considered below.

The precueing method of task decomposition

In the method of precueing, the first step in a componential analysis is to form interval scores from the decomposition of the global task into a series of nested subtasks, as was done by Johnson (1960) in his pioneering method of serial analysis. The method yields *interval scores* for each of the nested subtasks. Each interval score is a score on one of the series of subtasks and measures performance on a subset of the information-processing components required by the total task. Each subtask in the series of subtasks requires successively less information processing and hence should involve reduced processing time and difficulty. Consider two examples of the use of precueing.

Analogies. An example of the use of precueing can be found in the decomposition of performance in analogical reasoning (Sternberg, 1977a, 1977b; see Chapter 5). Consider the analogy "FOUR SCORE AND SEVEN YEARS AGO" : LINCOLN :: "I'M NOT A CROOK" : (a. NIXON, b. CAPONE). In order to decompose the task, one can eliminate from the subject's information processing successive terms of the analogy. Since the analogy has five terms, up to five subtasks can be formed, although there seems to be no good reason for splitting up the two answer options. Consider, then, four subtasks. In each case, we divided presentation trials into two parts. In the first part, the experimenter presents the subject with some amount of precueing to facilitate solution of the analogy. In the second part, that of primary interest, the experimenter presents the full analogy. Solution of the analogy, however, is assumed to require merely a subset of the full set of components (that is, to involve only a subtask of the full task), because the experimenter assumes that the subject utilized the precueing presented in the first part of the trial to reduce his or her processing load in the second part of the trial. Indeed, subjects are encouraged to use the precueing information in order to help their processing in the second part of the trial. In the description of task decomposition that follows, it will be assumed that the analogies are presented either tachistoscopically or via a computer terminal.

In the first subtask (which is identical to the full task), the subject is presented with a blank field (null precueing) in the first part of the trial. The subject indicates when he or she is ready to proceed, and then the full analogy appears. The subject solves the analogy and then presses a button indicating response a or response b. In the second subtask, the subject still needs to perform most of the task in the second part of the trial. The first part of the trial consists merely of precueing with the first term of the analogy. The subject presses a button to indicate that this term has been processed, and then the whole analogy appears on the screen. The subject solves it and then indicates his or her response. Note that although the full analogy was presented in the second part of the trial, only the last four terms needed to be processed, since the first term had been preprocessed during precueing. The third subtask involves a smaller subset of the task to be performed in the second part of the trial. The first part of the trial consists of presentation of the first two terms of the analogy; the second part consists of full presentation. The fourth subtask involves a very small subset of the full task in the second part of the trial. The first part of the trial consists of presentation of the first three terms of the analogy; the second part consists of full presentation but requires processing of only the last two terms.

The task decomposition described above serves to separate components of information processing that would be confounded if only the full task were presented. Suppose only the full task were presented to subjects. Then, according to certain information-processing models of analogical reasoning (described in detail in Sternberg, 1977b) under the general theory, (a) encoding and response would be confounded, since response is constant across all analogy types (five analogy terms always need to be encoded) and (b) inference and application would be confounded, because the relation between the third term and the correct option is always the same as that between the first two terms. But precueing permits disentanglement of components by selective dropout of components required for processing. By varying the amount of encoding required for various subtasks, the method of precueing permits separation of encoding from the response constant. And by eliminating the inference components from the third and fourth subtasks (while retaining the application component), it becomes possible to distinguish inference from application. Recall that in these two subtasks the first two terms of the analogy were presented during precueing, so that inference could be completed before the full analogy was presented.

The precueing method obviously assumes additivity across subtasks. Two methods of testing additivity have been proposed (Sternberg, 1977b).

The first requires testing of interval scores for simplicial structure. This test enables one to determine whether the assumption is justified that subtask (interval) scores requiring less processing are contained in subtask scores requiring more processing. If the scores are indeed additive, they should form a simplex. One tests for simplicial structure by examining the intercorrelation matrix between the complete set of subtask scores, with the scores arranged in order of increasing amounts of information processing required for item solution. If the scores form a simplex, then the intercorrelation matrix for the subtask scores should show a certain property: Correlations near the principal diagonal of a matrix should be high, and they should taper off monotonically as entries move further away from the principal diagonal. In other words, each successive diagonal of the intercorrelation matrix should show decreasing entries as one moves away from the main diagonal. Because of the overlapping nature of the subtask scores, a second prediction can be made. If each subtask score is predicted from every other subtask score, then only predictor subtask scores immediately adjacent to the predicted score will contribute significant variance to the prediction. The reason for this is that since nonadjacent subtask scores either contain or are contained in adjacent scores, any variance contained in the nonadjacent scores that is not also contained in the adjacent ones should be uncorrelated with the predicted variable. Thus, in predicting one subtask score from all the others, only the adjacent scores (those with one more and one less precue) should have significant regression weights.

The second method involves comparison of parameter estimates for the uncued condition alone with those for all the conditions combined. Ideally, this comparison would be done between subjects (just in case the very use of precueing affects performance even on items receiving only null precueing); in practice, the comparison may end up being within-subject. The parameter estimates should be the same whether or not precueing was used. The data from three experiments on analogical reasoning showed reasonable conformity to the assumption of additivity. More importantly, even when the assumption of additivity was violated to some degree, the method of precueing proved to be robust, yielding sensible and informative data nevertheless. The method was quite successful in its application to analogy problems. The best model under the theory of analogical reasoning accounted for 92%, 86%, and 80% of the variance in the latency data for experiments using People Piece (schematic-picture), verbal, and geometric analogies, respectively.

Linear syllogisms. The method of precueing has also been applied in two experiments on linear syllogisms or three-term series problems (Sternberg, 1980e; see Chapter 6). In the first experiment, subjects were presented with problems such as "John is taller than Pete. Pete is taller than Bill. Who is tallest? John Pete Bill." Order of names was counterbalanced. Trials again occurred in two parts. In the first part, subjects received either a blank field or the two premises of the problem. (A third condition, involving presentation of only the first premise, might have been used, but was not.) In the second part, subjects received the whole problem. In each trial, subjects indicated when they were ready to receive the whole item and then indicated as their response one of the three terms of the problem. A possible limitation of this manner of presentation is that it seems to force serial-ordered processing, whereas when left to their own devices, subjects might process the problems differently – for example, by reading the question first. A second experiment was therefore done.

In the second experiment, the same type of problem was used, except that the question was presented first: "Who is tallest? John is taller than Pete. Pete is taller than Bill. John Pete Bill." Again, order of names was counterbalanced. There were three precueing conditions. In the first, a blank field was presented during the first part of the trial. In the second, only the question was presented during the first part of the trial. In the third, the question and the premises were presented during the first part of the trial, so that in the second part of the trial the subjects needed to discover only the ordering of the answer options. The full problem was always presented in the second part of the trial.

The methodology was again quite successful. The best model, my own mixed model (Sternberg, 1980e), accounted for 98% of the variance in the latency data from the first experiment and for 97% of the variance in the latency data from the second experiment. In these experiments (unlike in the analogy experiments), model fits were substantially lower in the conditions comprising the full problems only: 81% and 74%, respectively. Worth noting, however, is that the respective reliabilities of these subsets of the latency data were only .86 and .82, meaning that even here most of the reliable variance was accounted for. The higher fits of the models to data with precueing were due to disentanglement of encoding from response. When only full problems are presented, it is impossible to separate premise encoding time from response time, as both are constant over problem types: There are always two premises and one response. Separation of the encoding component substantially increased the variance in the latency data and hence the values of R^2.

Other problem types. The method of precueing has also been applied in the presentation of classification and series completion problems (Sternberg & Gardner, 1983). In the classification problems, subjects were presented with two groups of two items each and a target item. The subjects had to indicate in which group the target belonged. For example, one group might be (a) ROBIN, SPARROW, and the other, (b) HADDOCK, FLOUNDER. If the target were BLUEJAY, the correct answer would be response a. Precueing was accomplished by presenting either a blank field in the first part of the trial or just the two groups of items without the answer. Further precueing might have been accomplished by presenting just one group of items in the first part of the trial, although this was not done in this particular experiment.

In the series completion problems, subjects were presented with a linear ordering that they had to complete, for example, INFANT, CHILD, ADOLES-CENT, (a) ADULT, (b) TEENAGER. Precueing was accomplished by presenting either a blank field or just the first three terms of the item in the first part of the trial. Again, finer-grained precueing might have been done, but wasn't.

Precueing in these experiments, as in the analogies and linear-syllogisms experiment, was quite successful. Models provided good fits to the latency data for schematic-picture, verbal, and geometric items. Details can be found in Sternberg and Gardner (1983).

Evaluation of method. The method of precueing has both positive and negative aspects. On the positive side: (a) It permits disentanglement of components that otherwise would be confounded; (b) by doing so, it permits comparison of models that otherwise would be indistinguishable; (c) it increases the number of data points to be modeled, thereby helping to guard against the spurious good fit that can result when relatively large numbers of parameters are estimated for relatively small numbers of observations; (d) it requires the investigator to specify in what interval(s) of processing each mental operation takes place, thereby forcing the investigator to explicate his or her model in considerable detail; and (e) it provides scores for performance in a series of nested processing intervals rather than merely for the total task. On the negative side: (a) The method requires at least a semblance of additivity across subtasks; (b) it requires use of tachistoscopic or computer equipment to present each trial; (c) it requires individual testing; and (d) it is not suitable for young children because of its complexity. In the uses to which the method has been put so far, the advantages of precueing have more than offset its limitations.

Method of partial tasks

In the method of partial tasks, complete items are presented involving either a full set of hypothesized components or just some subset of these components. The method differs from the method of precueing in that trials are not split into two parts. Decomposition is effected with unitary trials. The partial and full tasks, however, are assumed to be additively related, as in the method of precueing. Consider two examples of the use of this method.

Linear syllogisms. The method of partial tasks has been used in four experiments on linear syllogisms (Sternberg, 1980d, 1980e). The full task consisted of the standard linear syllogism (three-term series problem) as described earlier. The partial task consists of two-term series problems – for example, "John is taller than Pete. Who is tallest?" (The ungrammatical superlative was used in the question to preserve uniformity with the three-term series problems.) The mixed model of linear-syllogistic reasoning specified component processes involved in both the two- and three-term series problems, specifying the processes involved in the former as a subset of the processes involved in the latter. The values of R^2 were .97, .97, and .97 with all items considered and .84, .88, and .84 with only three-term series problems considered. Note that these values are quite similar to those obtained under the method of precueing. Values of parameters were also remarkably similar, with two exceptions (predicted by the mixed model).

Categorical syllogisms. The method of partial tasks has also been applied in the investigation of categorical syllogisms (Sternberg & Turner, 1981). The full task was a standard categorical syllogism, with premises like "All B are C. Some A are B." The subject was presented with a conclusion, such as "All A are C," and had to indicate whether this conclusion was definitely true, possibly true, or never true of the premises. The partial task involved presentation of only a single premise, such as "Some A are B." The subject again had to decide whether a conclusion, such as "All A are B," was definitely, possibly, or never true of the (in this case, single) premise.

Whereas the primary dependent variable of interest in the previously decribed experiments was solution latency, the primary dependent variable in this experiment was response choice. The preferred model of syllogistic reasoning, the transitive-chain model, accounted for 96% of the variance in the response-choice data from the full task and for 96% of the variance in the response-choice data from the partial task. Fits were not computed for the combined data, as in this particular experiment we happened to be interested in the full task as an "encoding-plus-combination task" and in the partial task as an "encoding-only" task. These data indicate not only that the method of partial tasks can be applied successfully to categorical syllogisms, but that it can be applied to response-choice as well as to latency data.

Evaluation of method. This method seems to share all of the advantages of the method of precueing but only one of its disadvantages, namely, the assumption of additivity, in this case between the partial and the full task. The method of partial tasks therefore seems to be the preferred method when one has the option of using either of the two methods. Two additional points need to be considered. First, additivity may be obtained across precueing conditions but not from partial to full tasks or vice versa. Thus, some amount of pilot testing may be needed to determine which method is more likely to yield additivity across conditions. Second, some tasks are decomposable by either method, but others may be decomposable only by one or the other method. I have found the method of precueing applicable to more tasks than the method of partial tasks, although the differential applicability may be a function of the particular tasks I have investigated. In any case, the decision of which method to use can be made only after a careful consideration of task demands and decomposability. In some cases, the investigator may choose to use both methods, as in Sternberg (1980e).

Method of stem splitting

The method of stem splitting involves items requiring the same number of information-processing components but different numbers of executions of the various components. It combines features of the method of precueing with those of the method of partial tasks.

Analogies. So far, the method has been applied only to verbal analogies. Using the method of stem splitting, we presented verbal analogies in three different formats (Sternberg & Nigro, 1980):

1. RED : BLOOD :: WHITE : (a) COLOR, (b) SNOW
2. RED : BLOOD :: (a) WHITE : SNOW, (b) BROWN : COLOR
3. RED : (a) BLOOD :: WHITE : SNOW, (b) BRICK :: BROWN : COLOR

The number of answer options was allowed to vary from two to four for individual items. Consider how the different item types involve different numbers of executions of the same components. The first item requires encoding of five terms, inference of one relation, mapping of one relation, application of two relations, and one response. The second item requires encoding of six terms, inference of one relation, mapping of two relations, application of two relations, and one response. The third item requires encoding of seven terms, inference of two relations, mapping of two relations, application of two relations, and one response. (In each case, exhaustive processing of the item is assumed.) Varying the number of answer options also creates further variance in the numbers of operations required.

This method has been used with subjects as young as the third-grade level and as old as the college level. The data from the experiment were quite encouraging, both for the tested theory and the method. Multiple correlations (R) between predicted and observed data points were .85, .88, .89, and .92 for the preferred models in grades 3, 6, 9, and college respectively.

Evaluation of method. This method has barely been tried, and so I am not in a position to evaluate it fully. On the positive side: (a) It could be (although it has not yet been) used for group testing in conjunction with booklets of the kind described in the next section; (b) it requires no special equipment to administer items; (c) it is feasible with young children; and (d) it seems to create a certain added interest to the problems for the subjects. On the negative side: (a) The success of the method has not yet been adequately tested; (b) the generality of the method to problems other than analogies has not yet been shown; and (c) the method seems more likely than the preceding ones to generate special strategies that are inapplicable to standard (complete) tasks.

Method of systematically varied booklets

In previous methods, the unit of presentation was the single item. In this method, the unit of presentation is the booklet. In previous methods, subjects were given as long as they needed to complete each individual item. In this method, subjects are given a fixed amount of time to complete as many items as they can within a given booklet. The number of items in the booklet should exceed the number of items that subjects can reasonably be expected to complete in the given time period. The key to the method is that all items in the booklet should be homogeneous with respect to the theory or theories being tested. Although the same items are not repeated, each item serves as a replication with respect to the sources of difficulty specified by the theory. Although items within a given booklet are homogeneous, items are heterogeneous across booklets. In this method, specifications of the items within a booklet are varied in the same way that specifications of single items are varied in the preceding methods.

Analogies. The method of systematically varied booklets has been employed only with two types of schematic-picture analogies (Sternberg & Rifkin, 1979). In the two experiments done so far, the method has been used successfully with children as young as second grade and as old as college age. Subjects at each grade level were given 64 seconds in which to solve the 16 analogies contained in each booklet. Independent variables were numbers of schematic features changed between the first and second analogy terms, the first and third analogy terms, and the first and second analogy answer options. Items within a given booklet were identical in each of these respects. Three dependent variables were derived from the raw data. The first was latency for correctly answered items, obtained by dividing 64 by the number of items correctly completed. This measure takes into account both quality and quantity of performance. The second dependent variable was latency for all answered items, obtained by dividing 64 by the number of items completed, whether they were completed correctly or incorrectly. This measure takes into account only quantity of performance. The third dependent variable was error rate, obtained by dividing the number of items answered incorrectly by the number of items answered at all. This measure takes into account only quality of performance.

In a first experiment, model fits (R^2) for the best model were .91, .95, .90, and .94 for latencies of correct responses at grades 2, 4, 6, and college, respectively; they were .87, .94, .93, and .94 for latencies of all responses at each grade level; and they were .26, .86, .52, and .65 for error rates at each level. The fits for errors, although lower than for the latencies, were almost at the same levels as the reliabilities of each of the sets of data, indicating that only slightly better fits could possibly have been obtained. Model fits in a second experiment were slightly lower than in the first experiment, but so were the reliabilities of the data.

Evaluation of method. The method of systematically varied booklets has three distinct advantages and two distinct disadvantages. Its advantages are that (a) it is practical even with very young children; (b) it requires no special equipment for test administration; and (c) it is adopted for group testing. Its disadvantages are that (a) it is not possible to obtain a pure measure of time spent only on items answered correctly (or incorrectly), because times are recorded only for booklets, not for individual items; and (b) the method is not particularly well suited to disentangling components. In some of the models tested, for example, encoding and response, and inference and application, were confounded.

Method of complete tasks (standard method of presentation)

The method of complete tasks is simply the standard method of presenting only the composite item. It is suited to items in which no confoundings of components occur. Consider two examples of the use of the method.

Categorical syllogisms. The method of complete tasks was used in the presentation of categorical syllogisms (Guyote & Sternberg, 1981; see Chapter 6). In a first experiment, subjects were presented with syllogistic premises, such as "All B are C. All A are B," plus four conclusions (called A, E, I, and O in the literature on syllogistic reasoning), "All A are C. No A are C. Some A are C. Some A are not C," plus the further conclusion, "None of the above." Subjects had to choose the preferred conclusion from among the five. In a second experiment, concrete rather than abstract terms were used. Premises were either factual ("No cottages are skyscrapers"), counterfactual ("No milk cartons are containers"), or anomalous ("No headphones are planets"). In a third experiment, the quantifiers *most* and *few* were used instead of *some.* In a fourth experiment, premises were presented in the form "All A are B. X is an A," and subjects were asked simply to judge whether a conclusion such as "X is a B" was valid or invalid. Our transitive-chain model outperformed the other models of response choice to which it was compared, yielding values of R^2 of .97 for abstract content, .91 for concrete factual content, .92 for concrete counterfactual content, .89 for concrete anomalous content, .94 when *most* and *few* were substituted for *some,* and .97 for the simpler syllogisms requiring only a valid – invalid judgment. Latency models were also fit to some of the data, with excellent results.

Conditional syllogisms. The method of complete tasks was also used in testing the transitive-chain model on conditional syllogisms of the form "If A then B. A. Therefore, B." The subject's task was to evaluate the conclusion as either valid or invalid. The model accounted for 95% of the variance in the response-choice data.

Evaluation of method. The main advantages of this method are that it is the simplest of the methods described and that it does not require any assumptions about additivity across conditions of decomposition. The main disadvantage of the method is that in many, if not most, tasks, information-processing components will be confounded. These confoundings can lead to serious consequences, as discussed in Sternberg (1977b). The method is the method of choice only when it is possible to disentangle all component processes of interest.

Quantification of componential model

Once scores have been obtained for the various subtasks (if any) involved in task performance across conditions, it is necessary to quantify the information-processing model (i.e., the model expressed as a flowchart or in other information-processing terms). The exact method of quantification will depend upon the task being studied and the method used to decompose the task. I will therefore first state some general principles of quantification and then give a single example of a quantification – analogies. Other examples of quantifications can be found in others of my writings (e.g., Guyote & Sternberg, 1981, for categorical and conditional syllogisms; Schustack & Sternberg, 1981, for causal inferences; Sternberg, 1980e, for linear syllogisms; Tourangeau & Sternberg, 1981, for metaphors).

Generally, quantification is done so as to use multiple regression as a means of predicting a dependent variable from a series of independent variables. The dependent variable will usually be reaction time, error rate, or probability of a given response or response set. Independent variables will usually be the numbers of times each of a given set of information-processing components is performed. Thus, one predicts latency, error rate, or response probability from numbers of times each of the operations in the model is performed.

Latency parameters (raw regression weights) represent the durations of the various components. Response time is usually hypothesized to equal the sum of the amounts of time spent on each component operation. Hence, a simple linear model can predict response time to be the sum across the different component operations of the numbers of times each component operation is performed (as an independent variable) multiplied by the duration of that component operation (as an estimated parameter).

Proportion of response errors is hypothesized to equal the (appropriately) scaled) sum of the difficulties encountered in executing each component operation. A simple linear model predicts proportion of errors to be the sum across the different component operations of the number of times each component operation is performed (as an independent variable) multiplied by the difficulty of that component operation (as an estimated parameter). This additive combination rule is based upon the assumption that each subject has a limit on processing capacity (or space) (see Osherson, 1974). Each execution of an operation uses up capacity. Until the limit is exceeded, performance is flawless except for constant sources of error (such as motor confusion, carelessness, momentary distractions, etc.). Once the limit is exceeded, however, performance is at a chance level. For a discussion of other kinds of error models, see Mulholland, Pellegrino, and Glaser (1980).

In the response-time models (with solution latency as dependent variable), all component operations must contribute significantly to solution latency, since by definition each execution of an operation consumes some amount of time. In the response-error models (error rate as dependent variable), however, all component operations need not contribute significantly to proportion of errors. The reason for this is that some operations may be so easy that no matter how many times they are executed, they contribute only trivially to prediction of errors.

An example of a quantification: analogies. In the analogy experiments of Sternberg (1977a, 1977b), mathematical modeling was done by linear multiple regression. Parameters of the model were estimated as unstandardized regression coefficients.

Consider the basic equations for predicting analogy solution times in the Sternberg (1977a, 1977b) experiments described earlier. In these experiments, subjects received precueing with either zero, one, two, or three cues and were then asked to solve the full item as rapidly as possible. The equations shown here are for the simplest model, the so-called Model I, in which all operations are assumed to be executed exhaustively. Other models introduce further degrees of complication, and other publications should be consulted for details of their quantification (Sternberg, 1977a, 1977b; Sternberg & Gardner, 1983; see also Chapter 5).

$$RT_0 = 4a + fx + gy + fz + c$$
$$RT_1 = 3a + fx + gy + fz + c$$
$$RT_2 = 2a \quad\quad + gy + fz + c$$
$$RT_3 = \quad a \quad\quad\quad\quad + fz + c$$

In these equations, RT_i refers to reaction time for a given number of precues, i. Among the parameters, a refers to exhaustive encoding time, x refers to exhaustive inference time, y refers to exhaustive mapping time, z refers to exhaustive application time, and c refers to constant response time. Among the independent variables, the number of encodings to be done in each condition are given numerically (4, 3, 2, 1); f refers to the number of attributes to be inferred or applied (in the exhaustive model, they are confounded); g refers to the number of attributes to be mapped.

All parameters of each model enter into analogy processing in the 0-cue condition. The subjects must encode all four terms of the analogy as well as perform the inference, mapping, application, and response processes. The 1-cue condition differs only slightly. The first term was presented during precueing and is assumed to have been encoded at that time. Hence, the 1-cue condition requires the encoding of just three analogy terms rather than all four. In the 2-cue condition, the A and B terms of the analogy were precued, and it is assumed that inference occurred during precueing. Hence, the inference parameter (x) drops out, and there is again one less term to encode. In the 3-cue condition, the A and C terms were precued, and hence it is assumed that mapping as well as inference occurred during precueing. The mapping parameter (y) therefore drops out, and there is again one less term to encode. In general, the successive cueing conditions are characterized by the successive dropout of model parameters.

Parameter dropouts also resulted from null transformations in which no changes occurred from A to B and/or from A to C. These dropouts occurred in degenerate analogies (zero A to B and zero A to C attribute changes) and in semidegenerate analogies (zero A to B or zero A to C attribute changes, but not both zero). Indeed, these degenerate and semidegenerate analogies were originally included to provide a zero baseline for parameter estimation. For example, in the 0-cue condition, the inference and application parameters drop out when no changes occur from A to B, and the mapping parameter drops out when no changes occur from A to C. The same type of selective dropout occurs in all four cueing conditions.

The models make separate attribute-comparison time or error "charges" only for nonnull value transformations. This type of "difference parameter" was used throughout these and other experiments and has been used by many others as well (e.g., Clark & Chase, 1972). Value identities are not separately charged. Subjects are assumed to be preset to recognize null transformations ("sames"), and the parameter is assumed to represent amount of time or difficulty involved in alteration of the initial state.

The optional justification parameter was estimated as a function of the product of the distance from the keyed answer option to the ideal option times the number of previous attribute-comparison operations to be checked, both as determined by ratings provided by subjects otherwise uninvolved in the experiments. The idea is that the further the keyed option is from the ideal one, the more likely is checking to be necessary. If the keyed and ideal options are identical, then the value of the justification parameter will be zero, and it will be irrelevant to analogy solution. If, however, not even the best presented option corresponds to the ideal option, then justification is required. This parameter was used only in the forced-choice geometric analogies.

This description does not contain all of the details included in the models, nor is it intended to be used to reproduce the data in the experiments. Instead, it is intended to be illustrative of the kinds of procedures used in quantification of a particular task.

Model testing: internal validation

Once the model is formulated, it is necessary to test it, either by multiple regression or by other means. There are any number of tests that may be used. I have found the following tests useful in internally validating a componential model. I will illustrate the tests with examples from a study I did with Bathsheva Rifkin on the development of analogical reasoning processes (Sternberg & Rifkin, 1979), drawing in the example only on the adult data:

1. R^2 *for model.* This descriptive statistic is the overall squared correlation between predicted and observed data and thus represents the proportion of variance in the data that the model is able to account for. It is a measure of relative goodness of fit. In our analogies experiment, the best model showed an R^2 of .94 in the prediction of solution latencies.

2. *RMSD for model.* The root-mean-square deviation (RMSD) statistic gives the overall root-mean-square deviation of observed from predicted data. It is a measure of absolute badness of fit. Because it is an "absolute" measure, its value will be affected by the variance of the observed and predicted data. In the Sternberg–Rifkin experiment, we calculated standard errors of estimate rather than RMSDs. (The two statistics are closely related for linear models.) The standard error of estimate for the latency data was .32 second.

3. $F_{regression}$ *for model.* This statistic is the basis for deciding whether to reject the null hypothesis of no fit of the model to the data. Higher values are associated with better fits of the model to the data. Because the regression F value takes into account the number of parameters in the model, I have found the statistic useful in deciding among alternative models with differing numbers of parameters. The regression F for the preferred model in the Sternberg–Rifkin data was 159.94, which was highly significant in rejecting the null hypothesis of no fit of the model to the data.

4. $F_{residual}$ *for model.* This statistic is the basis for deciding whether to reject the null hypothesis of no discrepancy between the proposed model and the data. Lower values are associated with better fits of the model to the data. It is important to compute this statistic or an analogue, in that a model may account for a large proportion of variance in the data and yet be capable of

being rejected relative to the "true" model. Unfortunately, the residual F was not calculated in the Sternberg–Rifkin data, although it seems highly likely, given the systematicity of residuals described below, that it would have been statistically significant in rejecting the proposed model relative to the "true" one. Indeed, with enough power in one's test, virtually any model can be rejected!

5. *Relative values of statistics 1–4 for alternative models.* It is highly desirable to compare the fit of a given model to alternative models. The fact that a given model fits a set of data very well may merely reflect the ease with which that data set can be fit. In some cases, even relatively implausible models may result in good fits. Testing plausible alternative models guards against fits that are good but nevertheless trivial. In the Sternberg–Rifkin experiment, we tested three alternative models of information processing (for schematic-picture analogies with separable attributes). The models differed in terms of their specifications regarding which components of information processing (inference and application) are exhaustively executed and which are executed with self-termination. The model that best fit the data, in terms of the combined criteria, was the one that was maximally self-terminating (i.e., both inference and application self-terminating).

6. *$F_{regression}$ for individual parameter estimates.* Significance of the overall regression F does not imply that each parameter contributes significantly to the model. Thus, individual parameters should be tested for significance in order to assure their nontrivial contribution to the model. In the preferred model of analogical reasoning for the Sternberg–Rifkin data, all parameters contributed significantly to the model.

7. *ΔR^2 for individual parameter estimates.* The ΔR^2 statistic indicates the contribution of each parameter when that parameter is added to all others in the model. When independent variables in the model are intercorrelated, this descriptive statistic gives information different from that obtained in the step above. A parameter may be statistically significant and yet contribute only a very small proportion of variance when added to all of the others. These values were not computed in the Sternberg–Rifkin study.

8. *Interpretability of parameter estimates.* Parameters may pass the two tests described above and yet have nonsensical values. The values may be nonsensical because they are negative (for real-time operations!) or because their values, although positive, are wildly implausible. In the Sternberg–Rifkin study, interpretability of parameter estimates was a key basis for distinguishing among models. One model yielded statistically significant *negative* parameter estimates for real-time operations and was disqualified on this basis alone. Such estimates usually arise when one variable in a model serves as a suppressor variable.

9. *Examination of residuals of observed from predicted data points.* Residuals of observed from predicted data points should be assessed in order to determine the specific places in which the model does and does not predict the data adequately. The residuals will usually later be useful in reformulating the model. In the Sternberg–Rifkin data, examination of residuals revealed a systematic discrepancy between predicted and observed data. Subjects tended to be even more self-terminating than the maximally self-terminating model would allow. This discrepancy suggests that for items with very bad answer options, subjects may be able to short-circuit the full amount of normal processing and to disconfirm a false option on the basis of some kind of preliminary scan (see Sternberg, 1977b).

10. *Substantive plausibility of the model.* This criterion is a substantive rather than a statistical one. The model may "fit" statistically and yet make little or no psychological sense. The model should therefore be considered for its substantive plausibility. In the Sternberg–Rifkin data, the model not only made sense psychologically but corresponded well to the model that people indicated they used when they were asked how they solved the problems.

11. *Heuristic value of the model.* This criterion is again substantive rather than statistical. One should ask whether the model is at the right level of analysis for the questions being asked, whether it will be useful for the purposes to which it later will be put, and whether it is likely to generalize to other tasks and task domains. I believe that the model of analogical reasoning proposed by Sternberg and Rifkin has had at least some heuristic value, in that my colleagues and I have been able to elaborate upon it in subsequent research (e.g., Sternberg & Gardner, 1983; Sternberg & Ketron, 1982).

12. *Consideration of model for individual-subject as well as group-average data.* The analyses described above can be applied to both group-average and individual data. It is important to test the proposed model on individual-subject as well as group-average data. There are at least two reasons for this. First, averaging of data can occasionally generate artifacts whereby the fit of the model to the group data does not accurately reflect its fit to individual subjects. Second, there may be individual differences in strategies used by subjects that can be discerned only through individual-subject model fitting. One wishes to know what individual subjects do as well as what subjects do "on the average." I have found in at least several cases that what individual subjects do does not correspond in every case to the strategy indicated by the best group-average model (e.g., Sternberg & Ketron, 1982; Sternberg & Weil, 1980). In the Sternberg–Rifkin experiment, the preferred model fit individual data well: The mean R^2 for individual subjects was .78, a respectable fit when one considers that model fitting was done on the basis of just a single observation per data point.

Model testing: external validation

External validation requires testing the parameters of the proposed model against external criteria. Such validation actually serves at least two distinct purposes.

First, it provides an additional source of verification for the model. Often, one will make differential predictions regarding correlations of individual parameter estimates with external criteria. The external validation can serve to test these predictions and thus the validity of the model. Consider, for example, my research on linear syllogisms. Some of the components in the mixed model were predicted to operate upon a linguistic representation for information and others to operate upon a spatial representation for information (Sternberg, 1980e). It was important to show that the parameters theorized to operate upon a linguistic representation showed higher correlations with verbal than with spatial ability tests; similarly, it was important to show that the parameters theorized to operate upon a spatial representation showed higher correlations with spatial than with verbal ability tests. These predicted patterns were generally confirmed.

Second, it provides a test of generality for the proposed model. If interesting external criteria cannot be found that show significant and substantial correlations with the individual parameter estimates for the proposed model, then it is unclear that the model, or perhaps the task, is of much interest. For example, for parameters of analogical reasoning to be of theoretical interest, they should be shown to correlate with scores on a variety of inductive reasoning tests, but not with scores on perceptual-speed tests. This differential pattern of correlations was in fact shown (Sternberg, 1977b).

The above examples may serve to point out that two kinds of external validation need to be performed. The first, convergent validation, assures that parameters do in fact correlate with external measures with which they are supposed to correlate; the second, discriminant validation, assures that parameters do not in fact correlate with external measures with which they are not supposed to correlate but with which they might be plausibly correlated according to alternative theories. Some investigators have performed only convergent but not discriminant validation (e.g., Shaver, Pierson, & Lang, 1974), with what seem like auspicious results. The problem, though, is that obtained correlations may be due to the general factor in intellectual performance rather than to the particular operations specified as of interest in the theory. Thus, convergent validation without discriminant validation is usually of little use.

Although I have emphasized correlations of parameters with external measures, it is an unfortunate fact of life that oftentimes parameter estimates for individual subjects will not be as reliable as one would like. In these cases, and even in cases where the estimates are fairly reliable, it is desirable to correlate total task scores as well as subtask scores with the external measures. Although such correlations may reflect various mixtures of operations in the tasks and subtasks, they are likely to be more stable than the correlations obtained for the parameter estimates, simply because of the higher reliability of the composite scores and because of the fact that obtaining correlations for these scores is not dependent upon the correctness of one's theory, as it is for component scores.

The value of external validation for theory testing can be seen, in different ways, both in my work on analogical reasoning and in my work on linear-syllogistic reasoning.

In the former work, initial correlations between parameter estimates and standardized tests of inductive reasoning abilities yielded a curious pattern. Although the attribute-comparison components – inference, mapping, and application – showed relationships with the mental test scores, the highest relationship emerged from the response constant component! Thus, the internal validation procedures showed that the proposed quantified model was doing an excellent job in accounting for the latency data; but the external validation procedures showed that some very important ingredient in analogical reasoning, at least in terms of its relationship to intelligence, was being relegated to the least interesting component. It was this finding that led to the development, in my theorizing, of the notion of metacomponents or executive control processes that, although "constant" over standard experimental manipulations of the analogies, nevertheless are key ingredients in intellectual performance. Thus, the external validation served the purpose of showing an aspect of the theory that was in need of review. Internal validation – the kind used exclusively by many cognitive psychologists – was insufficient to show this need.

In the latter work, my theory of linear-syllogistic reasoning made explicit predictions regarding which components of information processing should correlate with verbal ability tests and which should correlate with spatial ability tests. Although internal validation can address the question of whether a given component contributes to real-time latency or to the commission of errors, it cannot really address the question of whether a given component operates upon one kind of representation or another. Latencies and error rates are simply nondefinitive in indicating forms of representation used. But correlating individual-subject component scores with verbal and spatial ability tests revealed essentially the pattern of convergent and discriminant validation predicted by the theory. With one exception, components theorized to operate upon a linguistic representation correlated with verbal but not spatial tests; components theorized to operate upon a spatial representation correlated with spatial but not verbal tests. Thus, additional validation of the theory was possible beyond that which could be obtained merely from internal validation procedures.

Reformulation of componential model

In practice, most first-pass (and even subsequent) models, whether componential or otherwise, are not correctly formulated. It will often be necessary to reformulate one's model on the basis of a given data set and then to cross-validate the revised model on subsequent sets of data. It is worth underscoring that cross-validation is essential. With enough fiddling, almost any data set can be fit by some model. What is hard is showing that the model fits data sets other than the one that was used in its formulation. The steps described above provide a wealth of data to use in revising one's model. The investigator should use the data to best advantage in reformulating the model. Once the reformulation is complete, the model is ready to be tested again on new data.

In the analogies work, for example, my original fits of model to data were only mediocre, with values of R^2 in the .50s. Clearly, something was either wrong or missing from the model. Investigation of residuals revealed that the model was incomplete: Certain kinds of analogies – in particular, those with either identical A and B terms or identical A and C terms (or both), and also those with extremely inadequate incorrect response options – could be processed more quickly than was predicted by the theory. It appeared that subjects were using dual processing, whereby they would process a given analogy both holistically and analytically at the same time. If the holistic processing yielded an answer, then analytical processing was terminated and a response was emitted. Thus, the holistic processing essentially bypassed the detailed attribute-by-attribute comparison needed for the analytical processing. This dual-processing theory (Sternberg, 1977b), when it replaced the uniprocessing theory, raised the value of R^2 by close to .3 and replicated in subsequent experiments beyond the first. In this and other instances (as noted above), the componential procedures proved useful for reformulation of the theory so as better to account for subjects' performance.

Generalization of componential model

Once a given task has been adequately understood in componential terms, it is important to show that the proposed model is not task-specific. If the model is in fact task-specific, then it is unlikely to be of much psychological interest. My own strategy has been to extend componential models from a single task, task format, and task content first to multiple task formats and contents and later to other tasks. For example, the componential model of analogical reasoning was originally tested on true – false People Piece analogies, then extended to true – false verbal analogies, then extended to forced-choice geometric analogies, and finally generalized to other tasks, including classifications and series completions, both of which were theorized to involve the same inductive components as are required for analogical reasoning (and for each other). This process of generalization is needed in order to establish the priority of the information-processing theory rather than of the task analysis per se. Inevitably, one can start only with the analysis of one or a small number of tasks. But eventually, one must extend one's analysis to multiple tasks, with the choice of tasks being guided by the theory that generated the first task that was studied.

In my analogies work, for example, a criticism that was sometimes made after publication of the initial work (Sternberg, 1977a, 1977b) was that the theory was one of analogical reasoning but not clearly one of anything else. Although I claimed in my 1977 book that the theory could be extended to other kinds of induction items, it was not until this extension was made (Sternberg & Gardner, 1983; see Chapter 5) that I could claim that the theory truly showed some generality as an account of how individuals solve the kinds of induction problems most frequently used to measure general intelligence (namely, analogies, series completions, and classifications).

Conclusions

I have described in this appendix a set of procedures – collectively referred to as "componential analysis" – that can be used in the formulation and testing of theories of cognitive processing. A componential analysis generally involves decomposition of a task into subtasks and then the internal and external validation of one or more componential models of task performance.

Several advantages accrue to the decomposition of a global task into subtasks. Scores from subtasks (a) allow separation of components that otherwise would have been confounded, (b) enable comparison of models that otherwise would have been indistinguishable, (c) increase degrees of freedom for the residual in prediction, (d) require precise specification of the temporal ordering and location of components, (e) prevent distortion of results from external validation, and (f) provide component-free estimates of performance for nested processing intervals.

Further advantages accrue from the use of component scores representing subjects' performance on each of the information-processing components used in task performance. Component scores (a) estimate scores by inferentially powerful componential models, (b) interpret performance in terms of mental processes, (c) pinpoint individual sources of particular strength and weakness for diagnosis and training, and (d) can derive estimates of measurement error from data for individual subjects.

Finally, use of reference ability scores that are correlated with subtask and component scores (a) allows identification of correlates of individual differences in performance for each component, (b) prevents overvaluation of task-specific components, and (c) potentially provides for both convergent and discriminant validation of a componential model.

In sum, then, componential procedures have been shown to be applicable to a large number of cognitive domains and have shown themselves to be valuable in understanding human cognitive performance. But I by no means claim that componential analysis is suitable for all kinds of analyses of cognitive skills. The methodology is not appropriate when parallel processing is used to any great extent, and it is also not appropriate where problems are of such great complexity that quantitative modeling simply becomes impractical; in these cases, other kinds of modeling, such as computer modeling, become more appropriate. Moreover, there exist some tasks that, although not apparently highly complex, resist the kinds of methods described here. For example, we have found classical insight problems of the kinds used by Gestalt psychologists resistant to straightforward componential task decomposition. Perhaps if we had a better grasp of what insight is and how it occurs, we would be in a better position to study such problems componentially, but for the time being we have found other methods of study superior for understanding performance on these very ill-structured kinds of problems. Thus, although componential analysis is useful for the analysis of many kinds of cognitive skills, it is clearly not useful for the analysis of all kinds of cognitive skills, and the investigator will have to make a judgment as to whether the methodology can be tailored so as to be suitable for a given use. In the past, many methodologies have been extended beyond the task domains in which they tend to be most successful (e.g., factor analysis, multidimensional scaling, hierarchical clustering, etc.), and I have no desire to see this overextension happen with componential analysis. I believe the methodology has shown itself to be useful in a wide variety of domains and expect that the methodology will continue to be extended (but, I hope, not overextended) to new domains.

References

Achenbach, T. M. (1970). The children's associative responding test: A possible alternative to group IQ tests. *Journal of Educational Psychology, 61*, 340–348.

Ames, W. S. (1966). The development of a classification scheme of contextual aids. *Reading Research Quarterly, 2*, 57–82.

Anderson, J. R. (1976). *Language, memory, and thought.* Hillsdale, NJ: Erlbaum.

Anderson, J. R., Kline, P. J., & Beasley, Jr., C. M. (1980). Complex learning processes. In R. E. Snow, P. A. Federico, & W. Montague (Eds.), *Aptitude, learning, and instruction,* Vol. 2: *Cognitive process analyses of learning and problem solving.* Hillsdale, NJ: Erlbaum.

Anderson, N. H. (1979). Algebraic rules in psychological measurement. *American Scientist, 67*, 555–563.

Anderson, R. C., & Freebody, P. (1979). *Vocabulary knowledge.* (Tech. Rep. No. 136). Champaign: University of Illinois, Center for the Study of Reading.

Archer, D. (1980). *How to expand your social intelligence quotient.* New York: M. Evans.

Archer, D., & Akert, R. M. (1977a). How well do you read body language? *Psychology Today, 11*, 68–72, 119–120.

Archer, D., & Akert, R. M. (1977b). Words and everything else: Verbal and nonverbal cues in social interpretation. *Journal of Personality and Social Psychology, 35*, 443–449.

Archer, D., & Akert, R. M. (1980). The encoding of meaning: A test of three theories of social interaction. *Social Inquiry, 50*, 393–419.

Argyle, M. (1969). *Social interaction.* Chicago: Aldine.

Aristotle (1927). Poetics. In W. Fyfe (Trans.), *Aristotle: The poetics.* Cambridge, MA: Harvard University Press.

Atkinson, R. C., & Shiffrin, R. M. (1968). Human memory: A proposed system and its control processes. In K. Spence & J. Spence (Eds.), *The psychology of learning and motivation* (Vol. 2). New York: Academic Press.

Baron, J. (1981). Reflective thinking as a goal of education. *Intelligence, 5*, 291–309.

Baron, J. (1982). Personality and intelligence. In R. J. Sternberg (Ed.), *Handbook of human intelligence.* Cambridge: Cambridge University Press.

Baron, J., & Strawson, C. (1976). Use of orthographic and word-specific knowledge in reading words. *Journal of Experimental Psychology: Human Perception and Performance, 2*, 386–393.

Belmont, J. M., & Butterfield, E. C. (1969). The relations of short-term memory to development and intelligence. In L. C. Lipsett & H. W. Reese (Eds.), *Advances in child development and behavior*. New York: Academic Press.

Belmont, J. M., & Butterfield, E. C. (1971). Learning strategies as determinants of memory deficiencies. *Cognitive Psychology, 2*, 411–420.

Berger, M. (1982). The "scientific approach" to intelligence: An overview of its history with special reference to mental speed. In H. J. Eysenck (Ed.), *A model for intelligence*. Berlin: Springer-Verlag.

Berry, J. W. (1974). Radical cultural relativism and the concept of intelligence. In J. W. Berry & P. R. Dasen (Eds.), *Culture and cognition: Readings in cross-cultural psychology*. London: Methuen.

Berry, J. W. (1980). Cultural universality of any theory of human intelligence remains an open question. *Behavioral & Brain Sciences, 3*, 584–585.

Berry, J. W. (1981). Cultural systems and cognitive styles. In M. Friedman, J. P. Das, & N. O'Conner (Eds.), *Intelligence and learning*. New York: Plenum.

Billow, R. (1977). Metaphor: A review of the psychological literature. *Psychological Bulletin, 84*, 81–92.

Binet, A., & Simon, T. (1905). Méthodes nouvelles pour le diagnostic du niveau intellectuel des anormaux. *L'Année psychologique, 11*, 245–336.

Binet, A., & Simon, T. (1908). Le développement de l'intelligence chez les enfants. *L'Année psychologique, 14*, 1–90. (Reprinted in A. Binet and T. S. Simon, *The development of intelligence in children*. Baltimore: Williams & Wilkins, 1916, pp. 182–273.)

Binet, A. & Simon, T. (1973). *Classics in psychology: The development of intelligence in children*. New York: Arno Press.

Bisanz, G. L., & Voss, J. F. (1981). Sources of knowledge in reading comprehension. In A. Lesgold & C. A. Perfetti (Eds.), *Interactive process in reading*. Hillsdale, NJ: Erlbaum.

Black, M. (1962). *Models and metaphors*. Ithaca, NY: Cornell University Press.

Blum, N. L., & Naylor, J. C. (1956). *Industrial psychology: Its theoretical and social foundations*. New York: Harper & Row.

Boring, E. G. (1923). Intelligence as the tests test it. *New Republic*, June 6, pp. 35–37.

Borkowski, J. G., & Cavanaugh, J. C. (1979). Maintenance and generalization of skills and strategies by the retarded. In N. R. Ellis (Ed.), *Handbook of mental deficiency* (2nd ed.). Hillsdale, NJ: Erlbaum.

Brand, C. R., & Deary, I. J. (1982). Intelligence and "inspection time." In H. J. Eysenck (Ed.), *A model for intelligence*. Berlin: Springer-Verlag.

Bransford, J. D., Barclay, J. R., & Franks, J. J. (1972). Sentence memory: A constructive versus interpretive approach. *Cognitive Psychology, 3*, 193–209.

Brody, E. B., & Brody, N. (1976). *Intelligence: nature, determinants, and consequences*. New York: Academic Press.

Brown, A. L. (1974). The role of strategic behavior in retardate memory. In N. R. Ellis (Ed.), *International review of research in mental retardation* (Vol. 1). New York: Academic Press.

Brown, A. L. (1978). Knowing when, where, and how to remember: A problem of metacognition. In R. Glaser (Ed.), *Advances in instructional psychology* (Vol. 1). Hillsdale, NJ: Erlbaum.

Brown, A. L., Campione, J. C., & Murphy, M. D. (1977). Maintenance and generalization of trained metamnemonic awareness by educable retarded children: Span estimation. *Journal of Experimental Child Psychology, 24,* 191–211.

Brown, A. L., & DeLoache, J. S. (1978). Skills, plans, and self-regulation. In R. Siegler (Ed.), *Children's thinking: What develops?* Hillsdale, NJ: Erlbaum.

Brown, W., & Thomson, G. H. (1921). *The essentials of mental measurement.* Cambridge: Cambridge University Press.

Bruner, J. S., Goodnow, J. J., & Austin, G. A. (1956). *A study of thinking.* New York: Wiley.

Bruner, J. S., Shapiro, D., & Tagiuri, R. (1958). The meaning of traits in isolation and in combination. In R. Tagiuri & L. Petrollo (Eds.), *Person perception and interpersonal behavior.* Stanford, CA: Stanford University Press.

Bryant, P. E., & Trabasso, T. (1971). Transitive inferences and memory in young children. *Nature, 232,* 456–458.

Burt, C. (1919). The development of reasoning in school children. *Journal of Experimental Psychology, 5,* 68–77.

Burt, C. (1940). *The factors of the mind.* London: University of London Press.

Butcher, H. J. (1970). *Human intelligence: Its nature and assessment.* London: Methuen.

Butterfield, E. C., & Belmont, J. M. (1971). Relations of storage and retrieval strategies as short-term memory processes. *Journal of Experimental Psychology, 89,* 319–328.

Butterfield, E. C., & Belmont, J. M. (1977). Assessing and improving the cognition of mentally retarded people. In I. Bialer & M. Sternlicht (Eds.), *Psychology of mental retardation: Issues and approaches.* New York: Psychological Dimensions.

Butterfield, E. C., Wambold, C., & Belmont, J. M. (1973). On the theory and practice of improving short-term memory. *American Journal of Mental Deficiency, 77,* 654–669.

Campione, J. C., & Brown, A. L. (1977). Memory and metamemory development in educable retarded children. In R. V. Kail, Jr., & J. W. Hagen (Eds.), *The development of memory and cognition.* Hillsdale, NJ: Erlbaum.

Campione, J. C., & Brown, A. L. (1979). Toward a theory of intelligence: Contributions from research with retarded children. In R. J. Sternberg & D. K. Detterman (Eds.), *Human intelligence: Perspectives on its theory and measurement.* Norwood, NJ: Ablex.

Campione, J. C., Brown, A. L., & Ferrara, R. A. (1982). Mental retardation and intelligence. In R. J. Sternberg (Ed.), *Handbook of human intelligence.* Cambridge: Cambridge University Press.

Cantor, N. (1978). Prototypicality and personality judgments. Doctoral dissertation. Department of Psychology, Stanford University.

Carpenter, P. A., & Just, M. A. (1975). Sentence comprehension: A psycholinguistic model of verification. *Psychological Review, 82,* 45–73.

Carroll, J. B. (1976). Psychometric tests as cognitive tasks: A new "structure of intellect." In L. B. Resnick (Ed.), *The nature of intelligence.* Hillsdale, NJ: Erlbaum.

Carroll, J. B. (1980). *Individual difference relations in psychometric and experimental cognitive tasks.* (NR 150-406 ONR Final Report). Chapel Hill, NC: L. L. Thurstone Psychometric Laboratory, University of North Carolina.

Carroll, J. B. (1981). Ability and task difficulty in cognitive psychology. *Educational Researcher, 10,* 11–21.

Carroll, J. B. (in press). Second-language abilities. In R. J. Sternberg (Ed.), *Human abilities: An information-processing approach.* San Francisco: Freeman.

Case, R. (1974a). Mental strategies, mental capacity, and instruction: A neo-Piagetian investigation. *Journal of Experimental Child Psychology, 18,* 372–397.

Case, R. (1974b). Structures and strictures: Some functional limitations on the course of cognitive growth. *Cognitive Psychology, 6,* 544–573.

Case, R. (1978). Intellectual development from birth to adolescence: A neo-Piagetian interpretation. In R. Siegler (Ed.), *Children's thinking: What develops?* Hillsdale, NJ: Erlbaum.

Cattell, J. M. (1890). Mental tests and measurements. *Mind, 15,* 373–380.

Cattell, R. B. (1971). *Abilities: Their structure, growth, and action.* Boston: Houghton Mifflin.

Cattell, R. B., & Cattell, A. K. (1963). *Test of g: Culture fair, Scale 3.* Champaign, IL: Institute for Personality and Ability Testing.

Ceraso, J., & Provitera, A. (1971). Sources of error in syllogistic reasoning. *Cognitive Psychology, 2,* 400–410.

Chapin, F. S. (1967). *The social insight test.* Palo Alto, CA: Consulting Psychologists Press.

Chapman, L. J., & Chapman, J. P. (1959). Atmosphere effect re-examined. *Journal of Experimental Psychology, 58,* 220–226.

Charlesworth, W. R. A. (1976). Human intelligence as adaption: An ethological approach. In L. B. Resnick (Ed.), *The nature of intelligence.* Hillsdale, NJ: Erlbaum.

Charlesworth, W. R. (1979a). An ethological approach to studying intelligence. *Human Development, 22,* 212–216.

Charlesworth, W. R. (1979b). Ethology: Understanding the other half of intelligence. In M. von Cranach, K. Koppa, W. Lepenies, & D. Ploog (Eds.), *Human ethology: Claims and limits of a new discipline.* Cambridge: Cambridge University Press.

Charness, N. (1981). Aging and skilled problem solving. *Journal of Experimental Psychology: General, 110,* 21–38.

Chase, W. G., & Simon, H. A. (1973). The mind's eye in chess. In W. G. Chase (Ed.), *Visual information processing.* New York: Academic Press.

Chi, M. T. H. (1978). Knowledge structures and memory development. In R. S. Siegler (Ed.), *Children's thinking: What develops?* Hillsdale, NJ: Erlbaum.

Chi, M. T. H., Glaser, R., & Rees, E. (1982). Expertise in problem solving. In R. J. Sternberg (Ed.), *Advances in the psychology of human intelligence* (Vol. 1). Hillsdale, NJ: Erlbaum.

Clark, H. H. (1969a). The influence of language in solving three-term series problems. *Journal of Experimental Psychology, 82,* 205–215.

Clark, H. H. (1969b). Linguistic processes in deductive reasoning. *Psychological Review, 76*, 387–404.

Clark, H. H. (1971). More about "adjectives, comparatives, and syllogisms": A reply to Huttenlocher and Higgins. *Psychological Review, 78*, 505–514.

Clark, H. H. (1972a). Difficulties people have answering the question "where is it?" *Journal of Verbal Learning and Verbal Behavior, 11,* 265–277.

Clark, H. H. (1972b). On the evidence concerning J. Huttenlocher and E. T. Higgins' theory of reasoning: A second reply. *Psychological Review, 79*, 428–432.

Clark, H. H. (1973). Semantics and comprehension. In T. A. Sebeok (Ed.), *Current trends in linguistics,* Vol. 12: *Linguistics and adjacent arts and sciences.* The Hague: Mouton.

Clark, H. H., & Chase, W. G. (1972). On the process of comparing sentences against pictures. *Cognitive Psychology, 3*, 472–517.

Clark, H. H., & Clark, E. V. (1977). *Psychology and language.* New York: Harcourt Brace Jovanovich.

Cole, M. (1979–1980). Mind as a cultural achievement: Implications for IQ testing. In *Annual report of the research and clinical center for child development.* Sapporo, Japan: Hokkaido University, Faculty of Education.

Cole, M., Gay, J., Glick, J., & Sharp, D. W. (1971). *The cultural context of learning and thinking.* New York: Basic Books.

Cole, M., & Means, B. (1981). *Comparative studies of how people think.* Cambridge, MA: Harvard University Press.

Collins, A. M., & Loftus, E. F. (1975). A spreading-activation theory of semantic processing. *Psychological Review, 82*, 407–428.

Collins, A., & Smith, E. E. (1982). Teaching the process of reading comprehension. In D. K. Detterman & R. J. Sternberg (Eds.), *How and how much can intelligence be increased?* Norwood, NJ: Ablex.

Collins, A., Warnock, E. H., Aiello, N., & Miller, M. L. (1975). Reasoning from incomplete knowledge. In D. Bobrow & A. Collins (Eds.), *Representation and understanding: Studies in cognitive science.* New York: Academic Press.

Cook, M. (1971). *Interpersonal perception.* Baltimore: Penguin Books.

Cooper, L. A., & Shepard, R. N. (1973). Chronometric studies of the rotation of mental images. In W. G. Chase (Ed.), *Visual information processing.* New York: Academic Press.

Cornelius, S. W., Willis, S. L., Blow, S., & Baltes, P. B. (1983). Training research in aging: Attention processes. *Journal of Educational Psychology, 75*, 257–270.

Craik, F. I., & Lockhart, R. S. (1972). Levels of processing: A framework for memory research. *Journal of Verbal Learning and Verbal Behavior, 11*, 671–684.

Cronbach, L. J. (1957). The two disciplines of scientific psychology. *American Psychologist, 12*, 671–684.

Cronbach, L. J. (1970). *Essentials of psychological testing* (3rd ed.). New York: Harper & Row.

Cronbach, L. J., & Snow, R. E. (1977). *Aptitudes and instructional methods.* New York: Irvington.

Crowder, R. G. (1982). *The psychology of reading: An introduction.* Oxford: Oxford University Press.

Daalen-Kapteijns, Van, M. M., & Elshout-Mohr, M. (1981). The acquisition of word meanings as a cognitive learning process. *Journal of Verbal Learning and Verbal Behavior, 20,* 386–399.

Davidson, J. E., & Sternberg, R. J. (1982, November). "Insights about insight." Paper presented at the annual meeting of the Psychonomic Society, Minneapolis.

Davidson, J. E., & Sternberg, R. J. (1984). The role of insight in intellectual giftedness. *Gifted Child Quarterly, 28,* 58–64.

DeSoto, C. B., London, M. & Handel, S. (1965). Social reasoning and spatial paralogic. *Journal of Personality and Social Psychology, 2,* 513–521.

Dewey, J. (1957). *Human nature and conduct.* New York: Modern Library.

Diller, K. C. (1978). *The language teaching controversy.* Rowley, MA: Newbury House.

Dockrell, W. B. (1970). *On intelligence.* Toronto: Ontario Institute for Studies in Education.

Downing, C. J., Sternberg, R. J., & Ross, B. (1983). Multicausal inference: Evaluation of evidence in causally complex situations. Typescript.

Egan, D. E., & Greeno, J. G. (1973). Acquiring cognitive structure by discovery and rule learning. *Journal of Educational Psychology, 64,* 85–97.

Egan, D. E., & Grimes-Farrow, D. D. (1982). Differences in mental representations spontaneously adopted for reasoning. *Memory and Cognition, 10,* 297–307.

Ekman, P. (1964). Body position, facial expression, and verbal behavior during interviews. *Journal of Abnormal and Social Psychology, 68,* 295–301.

Ellis, N. R. (1963). The stimulus trace and behavioral inadequacy. In N. R. Ellis (Ed.), *Handbook of mental deficiency.* New York: McGraw-Hill.

Ellis, N. R. (1970). Memory processes in retardates and normals. In N. R. Ellis (Ed.), *International review of research in mental retardation.* New York: Academic Press.

Ellsworth, P. C., & Carlsmith, J. M. (1968). Effects of eye contact and verbal content on affective response to a dyadic interaction. *Journal of Personality and Social Psychology, 10,* 15–20.

Erickson, J. R. (1974). A set analysis theory of behavior in formal syllogistic reasoning tasks. In R. Solso (Ed.), *Loyola symposium on cognition* (Vol. 2). Hillsdale, NJ: Erlbaum.

Erickson, J. R. (1978). Research on syllogistic reasoning. In R. Revlin & R. E. Mayer (Eds.), *Human reasoning.* Washington, D.C.: Winston.

Estes, W. K. (1982). Learning, memory, and intelligence. In R. J. Sternberg (Ed.), *Handbook of human intelligence.* Cambridge: Cambridge University Press.

Evans, T. G. (1968). A program for the solution of geometric-analogy intelligence test questions. In M. Minsky (Ed.), *Semantic information processing.* Cambridge: MIT Press.

Eysenck, H. J. (1953). *Uses and abuses of psychology.* Harmondsworth, England: Penguin.

Eysenck, H. J. (1967). Intelligence assessment: A theoretical and experimental approach. *British Journal of Educational Psychology, 37,* 81–98.

Eysenck, H. J. (Ed.). (1982). *A model for intelligence.* Berlin: Springer-Verlag.

Feldman, R. D. (1982). *Whatever happened to the quiz kids?* Chicago: Chicago Review Press.

Feuerstein, R. (1979). *The dynamic assessment of retarded performers: The learning potential assessment device, theory, instruments, and techniques.* Baltimore: University Park Press.

Feuerstein, R. (1980). *Instrumental enrichment: An intervention program for cognitive modifiability.* Baltimore: University Park Press.

Flavell, J. H. (1977). *Cognitive development.* Englewood Cliffs, NJ: Prentice-Hall.

Flavell, J. H. (1981). *Cognitive monitoring.* In W. P. Dickson (Ed.), *Children's oral communication skills.* New York: Academic Press.

Flavell, J. H., Botkin, P. T., Fry, C. L., Jr., Wright, J. W., & Jarvis, P. E. (1968). *The development of role-taking and communication skills in children.* New York: Wiley.

Flavell, J. H., & Wohlwill, J. F. (1969). Formal and functional aspects of cognitive development. In D. Elkind & J. H. Flavell (Eds.), *Studies in cognitive development: Essays in honor of Jean Piaget.* New York: Oxford University Press.

Fleishman, E. A. (1965). The prediction of total task performance from prior practice on task components. *Human Factors, 7,* 18–27.

Fleishman, E. A., & Hempel, Jr., W. E. (1955). The relation between abilities and improvement with practice in a visual discrimination reaction task. *Journal of Experimental Psychology, 49,* 301–312.

Ford, M. E. (1982). Social cognition and social competence in adolescence. *Developmental Psychology, 18,* 323–340.

Ford, M. E., & Miura, I. (1983). Children's and adult's conception of social competence. Manuscript in preparation.

Ford, M. E., & Tisak, M. S. (1983). A further search for social intelligence. *Journal of Educational Psychology, 75,* 197–206.

Frandsen, A. N., & Holder, J. R. (1969). Spatial visualization in solving complex problems. *Journal of Psychology, 73,* 229–233.

Frederiksen, J. R. (1980). Component skills in reading: Measurement of individual differences through chronometric analysis. In R. E. Snow, P. A. Federico, & W. E. Montague (Eds.), *Aptitude, learning, and instruction: Cognitive process analyses of aptitude* (Vol. 1). Hillsdale, NJ: Erlbaum.

Frederiksen, J. R. (1982). A componential theory of reading skills and their interactions. In R. J. Sternberg (Ed.), *Advances in the psychology of human intelligence* (Vol. 1). Hillsdale, NJ: Erlbaum.

Frederiksen, N. (1962). Factors in in-basket performance. *Psychological Monographs: General and Applied, 76* (22, Whole No. 541).

Frederiksen, N., Saunders, D. R., & Ward, B. (1957). The in-basket test. *Psychological Monographs, 71* (9, Whole No. 438).

Frege, G. (1952). On sense and reference. In P. Geach & M. Black (Eds.), *Translations from the philosophical writings of Gottolb Frege.* Oxford: Basil Blackwell & Mott.

French, J., Ekstrom, R., & Price, I. (1963). Kit of reference tests for cognitive factors. Princeton, NJ: Educational Testing Service.

Galton, F. (1883). *Inquiry into human faculty and its development.* London: Macmillan.

Gardner, H. (1983). *Frames of mind: The theory of multiple intelligences.* New York: Basic Books.

Garner, W. R. (1974). *The processing of information and structure.* New York: Wiley.

Geiselman, R. E., Woodward, J. A., & Beatty, J. (1982). Individual differences in verbal memory performance: A test of alternative information-processing models. *Journal of Experimental Psychology: General, 111,* 109–134.

Gelman, R., & Gallistel, C. R. (1978). *The child's understanding of number.* Cambridge MA: Harvard University Press.

Gentner, D. (1977). Children's performance on a spatial analogies task. *Child Development, 48,* 1034–1039.

Gentner, D. (1983). Structure-mapping: A theoretical framework for analogy. *Cognitive Science, 7,* 155–170.

Ghiselli, E. E. (1966). *The validity of occupational aptitude tests.* New York: Wiley.

Gladwin, T. (1970). *East is a big bird.* Cambridge: Harvard University Press.

Glaser, R. (1967). Some implications of previous work on learning and individual differences. In R. M. Gagne (Ed.), *Learning and individual differences.* Columbus, OH: Merrill.

Glaser, R., & Chi, M. (1979). Progress report presented at Office of Naval Research contractor's meeting, New Orleans.

Goldberg, R. A., Schwartz, S., & Stewart, M. (1977). Individual differences in cognitive processes. *Journal of Educational Psychology, 69,* 9–14.

Goodman, N. (1955). *Fact, fiction, and forecast.* Cambridge, MA: Harvard University Press.

Goodnow, J. J. (1976). The nature of intelligent behavior: Questions raised by cross-cultural studies. In L. B. Resnick (Ed.), *The nature of intelligence.* Hillsdale, NJ: Erlbaum.

Gordon, E. W., & Terrell, M. D. (1981). The changed social context of testing. *American Psychologist, 36,* 1167–1171.

Gough, H. G. (1966). Appraisal of social maturity by means of the CPI. *Journal of Abnormal Psychology, 71,* 189–195.

Greeno, J. G. (1978). Natures of problem-solving abilities. In W. K. Estes (Ed.), *Handbook of learning and cognitive processes,* Vol. 5: *Human information processing.* Hillsdale, NJ: Erlbaum.

Gresham, F. M. (1981). Validity of social skills measures for assessing social competence in low-status children. *Developmental Psychology, 17,* 390–398.

Guilford, J. P. (1952). When not to factor analyze. *Psychological Bulletin, 49,* 26–37.

Guilford, J. P. (1967). *The nature of human intelligence.* New York: McGraw-Hill.

Guilford, J. P. (1980). Components versus factors. *Behavioral and Brain Sciences, 3,* 591–592.

Guilford, J. P. (1982). Cognitive psychology's ambiguities: Some suggested remedies. *Psychological Review, 89,* 48–59.

Guilford, J. P., & Hoepfner, R. (1971). *The analysis of intelligence.* New York: McGraw-Hill.

Guthrie, E. R. (1935). *The psychology of learning.* New York: Harper & Row.

Guttman, L. (1954). A new approach to factor analysis: The radex. In P. E. Lazarsfeld, (Ed.), *Mathematical thinking in the social sciences,* Glencoe, IL: Free Press.

Guttman, L. (1965). A faceted definition of intelligence. In R. R. Eiferman (Ed.), *Scripta Hierosolymitana* (Vol. 14). Jerusalem: Magnes Press.

Guyote, M. J. & Sternberg, R. J. (1981). A transitive-chain theory of syllogistic reasoning. *Cognitive psychology, 13,* 461–525.

Halberstadt, A. G., & Hall, J. A. (1980). Who's getting the message? Children's nonverbal skills and their evaluation by teachers. *Developmental Psychology, 16,* 564–573.

Hampton, J. A. (1979). Polymorphous concepts in semantic memory. *Journal of Verbal Learning and Verbal Behavior, 18,* 441–461.

Handel, S., DeSoto, C. B., & London, M. (1968). Reasoning and spatial representations. *Journal of Verbal Learning and Verbal Behavior, 7,* 351–357.

Hebb, D. O. (1949). *The organization of behavior.* New York: Wiley.

Hendrickson, A. E. (1982). The biological basis of intelligence. Part 1: Theory. In H. J. Eysenck (Ed.), *A model for intelligence.* Berlin: Springer-Verlag.

Henley, N. M. (1969). A psychological study of the semantics of animal terms. *Journal of Verbal Learning and Verbal Behavior, 8,* 176–184.

Hogaboam, T. W., & Pellegrino, J. W. (1978). Hunting for individual differences: Verbal ability and semantic processing of pictures and words. *Memory and Cognition, 6,* 189–193.

Holzinger, K. J. (1938). Relationships between three multiple orthogonal factors and four bifactors. *Journal of Educational Psychology, 29,* 513–519.

Holzman, T. G., Glaser, R., & Pellegrino, J. W. (1976). Process training derived from a computer simulation theory. *Memory and Cognition, 4,* 349–356.

Horn, J. L. (1968). Organization of abilities and the development of intelligence. *Psychological Review, 75,* 242–259.

Horn, J. L. (1979). Trends in the measurement of intelligence. In R. J. Sternberg & D. K. Detterman (Ed.), *Human intelligence: Perspectives on its theory and measurement.* Norwood, NJ: Ablex.

Horn, J. L., & Cattell, R. B. (1966). Refinement and test of the theory of fluid and crystallized ability intelligences. *Journal of Educational Psychology, 57,* 253–270.

Horn, J. L., & Knapp, J. R. (1973). On the subjective character of the empirical base of Guilford's structure-of-intellect model. *Psychological Bulletin, 80,* 33–43.

Humphreys, L. G. (1962). The organization of human abilities. *American Psychologist, 17,* 475–483.

Humphreys, L. G. (1979). The construct of general intelligence. *Intelligence, 3,* 105–120.

Hunt, E. (1971). What kind of computer is man? *Cognitive Psychology, 2,* 57–98.

Hunt, E. B. (1978). Mechanics of verbal ability. *Psychological Review, 85,* 109–130.

Hunt, E. B. (1980). Intelligence as an information-processing concept. *British Journal of Psychology, 71,* 449–474.

Hunt, E. B., Frost, N., & Lunneborg, C. (1973). Individual differences in cognition: A new approach to intelligence. In G. Bower (Ed.), *The psychology of learning and motivation* (Vol. 7). New York: Academic Press.

Hunt, E., Lunneborg, C., & Lewis, J. (1975). What does it mean to be high verbal? *Cognitive Psychology, 7,* 194–227.

Hunt, E. B., & Poltrock, S. (1974). Mechanics of thought. In B. Kantowitz (Ed.), *Human information processing: Tutorials in performance and cognition*. Hillsdale, NJ: Erlbaum.

Hunt, T. (1928). The measurement of social intelligence. *Journal of Applied Psychology, 12*, 317–334.

Hunter, I. M. L. (1957). The solving of three term series problems. *British Journal of Psychology, 48*, 286–298.

Huttenlocher, J. (1968). Constructing spatial images: A strategy in reasoning. *Psychological Review, 75*, 550–560.

Huttenlocher, J., & Higgins, E. T. (1971). Adjectives, comparatives, and syllogisms. *Psychological Review, 78*, 487–504.

Huttenlocher, J., & Higgins, E. T. (1972). On reasoning, congruence, and other matters. *Psychological Review, 79*, 420–427.

Huttenlocher, J., Higgins, E. T., Milligan, C., & Kauffman, B. (1970). The mystery of the "negative equative" construction. *Journal of Verbal Learning and Verbal Behavior, 9*, 334–341.

Inhelder, B., & Piaget, J. (1958). *The growth of logical thinking from childhood to adolescence*. New York: Basic Books.

Intelligence and its measurement: A symposium (1921). *Journal of Educational Psychology, 12*, 123–147, 195–216, 271–275.

Jackson, M. D., & McClelland, J. L. (1979). Processing determinants of reading speed. *Journal of Experimental Psychology: General, 108*, 151–181.

Jencks, C. (1972). *Inequality*. New York: Harper & Row.

Jensen, A. R. (1969). How much can we boost IQ and scholastic achievement? *Harvard Educational Review, 39*, 1–123.

Jensen, A. R. (1970). Hierarchical theories of mental ability. In W. B. Dockrell (Ed.), *On intelligence*. Toronto: Ontario Institute for Studies in Education.

Jensen, A. R. (1979). *g*: Outmoded theory or unconquered frontier? *Creative Science and Technology, 2*, 16–29.

Jensen, A. R. (1980). *Bias in mental testing*. New York: Free Press.

Jensen, A. R. (1982). Reaction time and psychometric *g*. In H. J. Eysenck (Ed.), *A model for intelligence*. Berlin: Springer-Verlag.

Johnson, D. D., & Pearson, P. D. (1978). *Teaching and reading vocabulary*. New York: Holt, Rinehart and Winston.

Johnson, D. M. (1960). Serial analysis of thinking. In *Annals of the New York Academy of Sciences* (Vol. 91). New York: New York Academy of Sciences.

Johnson-Laird, P. N. (1972). The three-term series problem. *Cognition, 1*, 57–82.

Johnson-Laird, P. N., & Steedman, M. (1978). The psychology of syllogisms. *Cognitive Psychology, 10*, 64–99.

Just, M. A., & Carpenter, P. A. (1980). A theory of reading: From eye fixations to comprehension. *Psychological Review, 87*, 329–354.

Kail, R., Pellegrino, J., & Carter, P. (1980). Developmental changes in mental rotation. *Journal of Experimental Child Psychology, 29*, 102–116.

Kaufman, A. S., & Kaufman, N. L. (1983). *Kaufman assessment battery for children (K-ABC)*. Circle Pines, MN: American Guidance Service.

Kaye, D. B., & Sternberg, R. J. (1983). Development of lexical decomposition ability. Typescript.

Keating, D. P. (1978). A search for social intelligence. *Journal of Educational Psychology, 70,* 218–223.

Keating, D. P. (1980). Thinking processes in adolescence. In J. Adelson (Ed.), *Handbook of adolescent psychology.* New York: Wiley.

Keating, D. (1984). The emperor's new clothes: The "new look" in intelligence research. In R. J. Sternberg (Ed.), *Advances in the psychology of human intelligence* (Vol. 2). Hillsdale, NJ: Erlbaum.

Keating, D. P., & Bobbitt, B. L. (1978). Individual and developmental differences in cognitive processing components of mental ability. *Child Development, 49,* 155–167.

Keil, F. C. (1979). *Semantic and conceptual development.* Cambridge: Harvard University Press.

Keil, F. C. (1981). Constraints on knowledge and cognitive development. *Psychological Review, 88,* 197–227.

Keil, F. C. (1984). Mechanisms of cognitive development and the structure of knowledge. In R. J. Sternberg (Ed.), *Mechanisms of cognitive development.* San Francisco: Freeman.

Kessen, W. (1968). The construction and selection of environments. In *Biology and behavior: Environmental influences.* New York: Russell Sage.

Kintsch, W., & van Dijk, T. A. (1978). Toward a model of text comprehension and production. *Psychological Review, 85,* 363–394.

Klahr, D. (1979). Self-modifying production systems as models of cognitive development. Typescript. Carnegie–Mellon University.

Klahr, D. (1984). Transition processes in quantitative development. In R. J. Sternberg (Ed.), *Mechanisms of cognitive development.* San Francisco: Freeman.

Klahr, D., & Wallace, J. G. (1976). *Cognitive development: An information processing view.* Hillsdale, NJ: Erlbaum.

Koffka, K. (1935). *Principles of Gestalt psychology.* New York: Harcourt, Brace.

Köhler, W. (1927). *The mentality of apes.* New York: Harcourt, Brace.

Köhler, W. (1947). *An introduction to the new concepts in modern psychology.* New York: Liveright.

Kosslyn, S. M. (1975). Information representation in visual images. *Cognitive Psychology, 7,* 341–370.

Kotovsky, K., & Simon, H. A. (1973). Empirical tests of a theory of human acquisition of concepts for sequential events. *Cognitive Psychology, 4,* 399–424.

Kounin, J. (1941a). Experimental studies of rigidity. I: The measurement of rigidity in normal and feebleminded persons. *Character and Personality, 9,* 251–272.

Kounin, J. S. (1941b). Experimental studies of rigidity. II: The explanatory power of the concept of rigidity as applied to feeblemindedness. *Character and Personality, 9,* 273–282.

Kuhn, T. S. (1970). *The structure of scientific revolutions* (2nd ed.). Chicago: University of Chicago Press.

Kurtines, W., & Grief, E. (1974). The development of moral thought: A review and evaluation of Kohlberg's approach. *Psychological Bulletin, 81,* 453–470.

LaBerge, D., & Samuels, J. (1974). Toward a theory of automatic information processing in reading. *Cognitive Psychology, 6*, 293–323.

Laboratory of Comparative Human Cognition (1982). Culture and intelligence. In R. J. Sternberg (Ed.), *Handbook of human intelligence.* Cambridge: Cambridge University Press.

Laboratory of Comparative Human Cognition (1983). Culture and cognitive development. In P. Mussen (Series Ed.) & W. Kessen (Vol. Ed.), *Handbook of child psychology* (Vol. 1). New York: Wiley.

Lally, M., & Nettelbeck, T. (1977). Intelligence, reaction time, and inspection time. *American Journal of Mental Deficiency, 82*, 273–281.

Lansman, M., Donaldson, G., Hunt, E., & Yantis, S. (1982). Ability factors and cognitive processes. *Intelligence, 6*, 347–386.

Larkin, J., McDermott, J., Simon, D. P., & Simon, H. A. (1980). Expert and novice performance in solving physics problems. *Science, 208*, 1335–1342.

Lawson, R. (1977). Representation of individual sentences and holistic ideas. *Journal of Experimental Psychology: Human Learning and Memory. 3*, 1–9.

Lemmon, V. W. (1927). The relation of reaction time to measures of intelligence, memory, and learning. *Archives of Psychology, 15*, 5–38.

Lipman, M., Sharp, A. M., & Oscanyan, F. S. (1980). *Philosophy in the classroom* (2nd ed.). Philadelphia: Temple University Press.

Luce, R. D. (1959). *Individual choice behavior.* New York: Wiley.

Lunneborg, C. E. (1977). Choice reaction time: What role in ability measurement? *Applied Psychological Measurement, 1*, 309–330.

Lunzer, E. A. (1965). Problems of formal reasoning in test situations. In P. H. Mussen (Ed.), *European research in cognitive development.* Monographs of the Society for Research in Child Development, Vol. 30, (2, Serial No. 100), 19–46.

Luria, A. R. (1961). An objective approach to the study of the abnormal child. *American Journal of Orthopsychiatry, 31*, 1–16.

McClelland, D. C. (1953). *The achievement motive.* New York: Appleton-Century-Crofts.

McClelland, D. C. (1961). *The achieving society.* Princeton, NJ: Van Nostrand.

McClelland, D. C. (1973). Testing for competence rather than for "intelligence." *American Psychologist, 28*, 1–14.

McCullough, C. M. (1958). Context aids in reading. *Reading Teacher, 11*, 225–229.

MacLeod, C. M., Hunt, E. B., & Matthews, N. N. (1978). Individual differences in the verification of sentence–picture relationships. *Journal of Verbal Learning and Verbal Behavior, 17*, 493–507.

McNamara, T. P., & Sternberg, R. J. (1983). Mental models of word meaning. *Journal of Verbal Learning and Verbal Behavior, 22*, 449–474.

McNemar, Q. (1951). The factors in factoring behavior. *Psychometrika, 16*, 353–359.

McNemar, Q. (1964). Lost our intelligence? Why? *American Psychologist, 19*, 871–882.

Maier, N. R. F. (1930). Reasoning in humans. I: on direction. *Journal of Comparative Psychology, 12*, 115–143.

Malgady, R., & Johnson, M. (1976). Modifiers in metaphors: Effects of constituent phrase similarity on the interpretation of figurative sentences. *Journal of Psycholinguistic Research, 5*, 43–52.

Markman, E. M. (1977). Realizing that you don't understand: A preliminary investigation. *Child Development, 48*, 986–992.

Markman, E. M. (1979). Realizing that you don't understand: Elementary school children's awareness of inconsistencies. *Child Development, 50*, 643–655.

Markman, E. M. (1981). Comprehension monitoring. In W. P. Dickson (Ed.), *Children's oral communication skills*. New York: Academic Press.

Marshalek, B. (1981). *Trait and process aspects of vocabulary knowledge and verbal ability* (NR154-376 ONR Tech. Rep. No. 15). Stanford, CA: School of Education, Stanford University.

Matarazzo, J. D. (1972). *Wechsler's measurement and appraisal of adult intelligence* (5th ed.). Baltimore: Williams & Wilkins.

Mathews, N. N., Hunt, E. B., & MacLeod, C. M. (1980). Strategy choice and strategy training in sentence–picture verification. *Journal of Verbal Learning and Verbal Behavior, 19*, 531–548.

Mayer, R., & Greeno, J. G. (1972). Structural differences between learning outcomes produced by different instructional methods. *Journal of Educational Psychology, 63*, 165–173.

Mehrabian, A. (1972). *Nonverbal communication*. Chicago: Aldine.

Miles, T. R. (1957). On defining intelligence. *British Journal of Educational Psychology, 27*, 153–165.

Miller, G. A. (1956). The magical number seven plus or minus two: Some limits on our capacity for processing information. *Psychological Review, 63*, 81–97.

Miller, G. A. (1979). Images and models, similes and metaphors. In A. Ortony (Ed.), *Metaphor and thought*. Cambridge: Cambridge University Press.

Miller, G., Galanter, E., & Pribram, K. (1960). *Plans and the structure of behavior*. New York: Holt.

Miller, G. A., & Johnson-Laird, P. N. (1976). *Language and perception*. Cambridge: Harvard University Press.

Mischel, W. (1968). *Personality and assessment*. New York: Wiley.

Moss, F. A., & Hunt, T. (1927). Are you socially intelligent? *Scientific American, 137*, 108–110.

Moss, F. A., Hunt, T., Omwake, K. T., & Woodward, L. G. (1949). *Social intelligence test, George Washington University series*. Washington, D.C.: Center for Psychological Service.

Mulholland, T. M., Pellegrino, J. W., & Glaser, R. (1980). Components of geometric analogy solution. *Cognitive Psychology, 12*, 252–284.

Neisser, U. (1976). *Cognition and reality: Principles and implications of cognitive psychology*. San Francisco: Freeman.

Neisser, U. (1979). The concept of intelligence. *Intelligence, 3*, 217–227.

Newell, A. (1973). Production systems: Models of control structures. In W. G. Chase (Ed.), *Visual information processing*. New York: Academic Press.

Newell, A., Shaw, J. C., & Simon, H. A. (1958). Elements of a theory of human problem solving. *Psychological Review, 65*, 151–166.

Newell, A., & Simon, H. (1972). *Human problem solving.* Englewood Cliffs, NJ: Prentice-Hall.

Nisbett, R., & Ross, L. (1980). *Human inference: Strategies and shortcomings of social judgment.* Englewood Cliffs, NJ: Prentice-Hall.

Noble, C. E., Noble, J. L., & Alcock, W. T. (1958). Prediction of individual differences in human trial-and-error learning. *Perceptual and Motor Skills, 8,* 151–172.

O'Rourke, J. P. (1974). *Toward a science of vocabulary development.* The Hague: Mouton.

Osgood, C., Suci, G., & Tannenbaum, P. (1957). *The measurement of meaning.* Urbana: University of Illinois Press.

Osherson, D. N. (1974). *Logical abilities in children,* Vol. 2: *Logical inference: Underlying operations.* Hillsdale, NJ: Erlbaum.

Osherson, D. N. (1975). *Logical abilities in children,* Vol. 3: *Reasoning in adolescence: Deductive inference.* Hillsdale, NJ: Erlbaum.

Pachella, R. G. (1974). The interpretation of reaction time in information-processing research. In B. H. Kantowitz (Ed.), *Human information processing: Tutorials in performance and cognition.* Hillsdale, NJ: Erlbaum.

Paivio, A. (1971). *Imagery and verbal processes.* New York: Holt, Rinehart and Winston.

Parseghian, P. E., & Pellegrino, J. W. (1980). *Components of individual differences in verbal classification performance.* Paper presented at the Annual Meeting of the American Educational Research Association, Boston, April.

Pascual-Leone, J. (1970). A mathematical model for the transition rule in Piaget's developmental stages. *Acta Psychologica, 63,* 301–345.

Pellegrino, J. W., & Glaser, R. (1979). Cognitive correlates and components in the analysis of individual differences. In R. J. Sternberg & D. K. Detterman (Eds.), *Human intelligence: Perspectives on its theory and measurement.* Norwood, NJ: Ablex.

Pellegrino, J. W., & Glaser, R. (1980). Components of inductive reasoning. In R. Snow, P. A. Federico, & W. Montague (Eds.), *Aptitude, learning, and instruction: Cognitive process analyses of aptitude* (Vol. 1). Hillsdale, NJ: Erlbaum.

Pellegrino, J. W., & Glaser, R. (1982). Analyzing aptitudes for learning: Inductive reasoning. In R. Glaser (Ed.), *Advances in instructional psychology* (Vol. 2). Hillsdale, NJ: Erlbaum.

Pellegrino, J. W., & Lyon, D. R. (1979). The components of a componential analysis. *Intelligence, 3,* 169–186.

Perfetti, C. A., & Lesgold, A. M. (1977). Discourse comprehension and individual differences. In P. Carpenter & M. Just (Eds.), *Cognitive processes in comprehension: The Twelfth Annual Carnegie Symposium on Cognition.* Hillsdale, NJ: Erlbaum.

Perkins, D. (1981). *The mind's best work.* Cambridge: Harvard University Press.

Piaget, J. (1921). Une forme verbale de la comparaison chez l'enfant. *Archives de Psychologie,* 141–142.

Piaget, J. (1928). *Judgment and reasoning in the child.* London: Routledge & Kegan Paul.

Piaget, J. (1955). *The language and thought of the child.* New York: New York American Library.

Piaget, J. (1970). Piaget's theory. In P. H. Mussen (Ed.), *Carmichael's manual of child psychology* (Vol. 1, 3rd ed.). New York: Wiley.

Piaget, J. (1972). *The psychology of intelligence.* Totowa, NJ: Littlefield Adams.

Pintner, R. (1921). Contribution to "Intelligence and its measurement: A symposium." *Journal of Educational Psychology, 12,* 139–142.

Posner, M. I., & Mitchell, R. F. (1967). Chronometric analysis of classification. *Psychological Review, 74,* 392–409.

Potts, G. R., & Scholz, K. W. (1975). The internal representation of a three-term series problem. *Journal of Verbal Learning and Verbal Behavior, 14,* 439–452.

Quinton, G., & Fellows, B. (1975). "Perceptual" strategies in the solving of three-term series problems. *British Journal of Psychology, 66,* 69–78.

Raaheim, K. (1974). *Problem solving and intelligence.* Oslo: Universitetsforlaget.

Reed, S. K., Ernst, G. W., & Banerji, R. (1974). The role of analogy in transfer between similar problem states. *Cognitive Psychology, 6,* 436–450.

Reitman, W. (1965). *Cognition and thought.* New York: Wiley.

Renzulli, J. S. (1976). The enrichment trial model: A guide for developing defensible programs for the gifted and talented. *Gifted Child Quarterly, 20,* 303–326.

Resnick, L. B. (Ed.) (1976). *The nature of intelligence.* Hillsdale, NJ: Erlbaum.

Resnick, L. B., & Glaser, R. (1976). Problem solving and intelligence. In L. B. Resnick (Ed.), *The nature of intelligence.* Hillsdale, NJ: Erlbaum.

Revlin, R., & Leirer, V. (1978). The effect of personal biases on syllogistic reasoning: Rational decisions from personalized representations. In R. Revlin & R. E. Mayer (Eds.), *Human reasoning.* Washington, D.C.: Winston.

Revlis, R. (1975). Two models of syllogistic reasoning: Feature selection and conversion. *Journal of Verbal Learning and Verbal Behavior, 14,* 180–195.

Richards, I. (1936). *The philosophy of rhetoric.* Oxford: Oxford University Press.

Rieger, C. (1975). Conceptual memory. In P. C. Schank (Ed.), *Conceptual information processing.* Amsterdam: North-Holland.

Riley, C. A., & Trabasso, T. (1974). Comparatives, logical structures, and encoding in a transitive inference task. *Journal of Experimental Child Psychology, 17,* 187–203.

Rogoff, B. (1982). Integrating context and cognitive development. In M. E. Lamb & A. L. Brown (Eds.), *Advances in developmental psychology* (Vol. 2). Hillsdale, NJ: Erlbaum.

Rosch, E. (1978). Principles of categorization. In E. Rosch & B. B. Lloyd (Eds.), *Cognition and categorization.* Hillsdale, NJ: Erlbaum.

Rosenthal, R. (Ed.) (1979). *Skill in nonverbal communication: Individual differences.* Cambridge, MA: Oelgeschlager, Gunn & Hain.

Rosenthal, R., Hall, J. A., DiMatteo, M. R., Rogers, P. L., & Archer, D. (1979). *Sensitivity to nonverbal communication: The PONS test.* Baltimore: Johns Hopkins Press.

Royce, J. R. (1963). Factors as theoretical constructs. *American Psychologist, 18,* 522–27.

Royce, J. R. (1973). The conceptual framework for a multi-factor theory of individuality. In J. R. Royce (Ed.), *Multivariate analysis and psychological theory*. New York: Academic Press.

Royce, J. R. (1979). The factor-gene basis of individuality. In J. R. Royce & L. P. Mos (Eds.), *Theoretical advances in behavior genetics*. Alphen aan der Rijn, Netherlands: Sijthoof & Noordhoff.

Royce, J. R. (1980). Factor analysis is alive and well. *American Psychologist, 35,* 390–392.

Rubin, D. C. (1976). The effectiveness of context before, after, and around a missing word. *Perception and Psychophysics 19,* 214–216.

Rumelhart, D. E. (1980). Schemata: The building blocks of cognition. In R. J. Spiro, B. C. Bruce, & W. F. Brewer (Eds.), *Theoretical issues in reading comprehension: Perspectives from cognitive psychology, linguistics, artificial intelligence, and education*. Hillsdale, NJ: Erlbaum.

Rumelhart, D. E., & Abrahamson, A. A. (1973). A model for analogical reasoning. *Cognitive Psychology, 5,* 1–28.

Rumelhart, D. E., & Norman, D. A. (1975). The problem of reference. In D. A. Norman & D. E. Rumelhart, *Explorations in cognition*. San Francisco: Freeman.

Russell, B. (1956). On denoting. In R. C. Marsh (Ed.), *Logic and knowledge*. London: George Allen & Unwin.

Scarr, S. (1981). Testing for children: Assessment and the many determinants of intellectual competence. *American Psychologist, 36,* 1159–1166.

Schank R. (1980). How much intelligence is there in artificial intelligence? *Intelligence, 4,* 1–14.

Schank, R. C., & Abelson, R. P. (1977). *Scripts, plans, goals, and understanding*. Hillsdale, NJ: Erlbaum.

Schmidt, F. L., & Hunter, J. E. (1981). Development of a general solution to the problem of validity generalization. *Journal of Applied Psychology, 62,* 529–540.

Schneider, W., & Shiffrin, R. (1977). Controlled and automated human information processing. I: Detection, search, and attention. *Psychological Review, 84,* 1–66.

Schustack, M. W., & Sternberg, R. J. (1981). Evaluation of evidence in casual inference. *Journal of Experimental Psychology: General, 110,* 101–120.

Schwartz, S. P. (1977). *Naming, necessity, and natural kinds*. London: Cornell University Press.

Serpell, R. (1976a). Estimates of intelligence in a rural community of Eastern Zambia. Human Development Research Unit Reports, No. 25. Mimeo. Lusaka: University of Zambia.

Serpell, R. (1976b). Strategies for investigating intelligence in its cultural context. *Quarterly Newsletter of the Institute for Comparative Human Development,* 11–15.

Shaver, P., Pierson, L., & Lang, S. (1974). Converging evidence for the functional significance of imagery in problem solving. *Cognition, 3,* 359–375.

Shepard, R. N., & Metzler, J. (1971). Mental rotation of three-dimensional objects. *Science, 171,* 701–703.

Shiffrin, R. M., & Schneider, W. (1977). Controlled and automatic human information processing. II: Perceptual learning, automatic attending, and a general theory. *Psychological Review, 84,* 127–190.

Siegler, R. S (1978). The origins of scientific reasoning. In R. S. Siegler (Ed.), *Children's thinking: What develops?* Hillsdale, NJ: Erlbaum.

Siegler, R. S. (1981). Developmental sequences within and between concepts. *Monographs of the Society for Research in Child Development, 46* (Serial No. 189).

Siegler, R. S. (1984). Mechanisms of cognitive growth: Variation and selection. In R. J. Sternberg (Ed.), *Mechanisms of cognitive development.* San Francisco: Freeman.

Siegler, R. S., & Richards, D. D. (1982). The development of intelligence. In R. J. Sternberg (Ed.), *Handbook of human intelligence.* Cambridge: Cambridge University Press.

Simon, H. A. (1976). Identifying basic abilities underlying intelligent performance of complex tasks. In L. B. Resnick (Ed.), *The nature of intelligence.* Hillsdale, NJ: Erlbaum.

Simon, H. A., & Kotovsky, K. (1963). Human acquisition of concepts for sequential patterns. *Psychological Review, 70,* 534–546.

Smith, E. E., Shoben, E. J., & Rips, L. J. (1974). Structure and process in semantic memory: A featural model for semantic decisions. *Psychological Review, 81,* 214–241.

Snow, R. E. (1979). Theory and method for research on aptitude process. In R. J. Sternberg & D. K. Detterman (Eds.), *Human intelligence: Perspectives on its theory and measurement.* Norwood, NJ: Ablex.

Snow, R. E. (1980). Aptitude processes. In R. E. Snow, P. A. Federico, & W. E. Montague (Eds.), *Aptitude, learning, and instruction: Cognitive process analyses of aptitude* (Vol. 1). Hillsdale, NJ: Erlbaum.

Snow, R. E. (1981). Toward a theory of aptitude for learning. I: Fluid and crystallized abilities and their correlates. In M. Friedman, J. P. Das, & N. O'Conner (Eds.), *Intelligence and learning.* New York: Plenum Press.

Spache, G. D., & Spache, E. B. (1973). *Reading in the elementary school* (3rd ed.). Boston: Allyn & Bacon.

Spear, L. C., & Sternberg, R. J. (in press). An information-processing framework for understanding reading disabilities. In S. Ceci (Ed.), *Handbook of cognitive, social, and neuropsychological aspects of learning disabilities* (Vol. 2). Hillsdale, NJ: Erlbaum.

Spearman, C. (1904). General intelligence, objectively determined and measured. *American Journal of Psychology, 15,* 201–293.

Spearman, C. (1923). *The nature of "intelligence" and the principles of cognition.* London: Macmillan.

Spearman, C. (1927). *The abilities of man.* New York: Macmillan.

Spitz, H. H., Borys, S. V., & Webster, N. A. (1982). Mentally retarded individuals outperform college graduates in judging the nonconservation of space and perimeter. *Intelligence, 6,* 331–345.

Stenhouse, D. (1973). *The evolution of intelligence: A general theory and some of its implications.* New York: Harper & Row.

Sternberg, R. J. (1974). *How to prepare for the Miller Analogies Test.* Woodbury, NY: Baron's Educational Series.

Sternberg, R. J. (1977a). Component processes in analogical reasoning. *Psychological Review, 84,* 353–378.

Sternberg, R. J. (1977b). *Intelligence, information processing, and analogical reasoning: The componential analysis of human abilities.* Hillsdale, NJ: Erlbaum.

Sternberg, R. J. (1978a). Isolating the components of intelligence. *Intelligence, 2,* 117–128.

Sternberg, R. J. (1978b). Intelligence research at the interface between differential and cognitive psychology. *Intelligence, 2,* 195–222.

Sternberg, R. J. (1979a). Developmental patterns in the encoding and combination of logical connectives. *Journal of Experimental Child Psychology, 28,* 469–498.

Sternberg, R. J. (1979b). The nature of mental abilities. *American Psychologist, 34,* 214–230.

Sternberg, R. J. (1980a). The construct validity of aptitude tests: An information-processing assessment. In *Construct validity in psychological measurement.* Princeton: Educational Testing Service.

Sternberg, R. J. (1980b). The development of linear syllogistic reasoning. *Journal of Experimental Child Psychology, 29,* 340–356.

Sternberg, R. J. (1980c). Factor theories of intelligence are all right almost. *Educational Researcher, 9,* 6–13, 18.

Sternberg, R. J. (1980d). A proposed resolution of curious conflicts in the literature on linear syllogisms. In R. Nickerson (Ed.), *Attention and performance VIII.* Hillsdale, NJ: Erlbaum.

Sternberg, R. J. (1980e). Representation and process in linear syllogistic reasoning. *Journal of Experimental Psychology: General, 109,* 119–159.

Sternberg, R. J. (1980f). Sketch of a componential subtheory of human intelligence. *Behavioral and Brain Sciences, 3,* 573–584.

Sternberg, R. J. (1981a). Cognitive–behavioral approaches to the training of intelligence in the retarded. *Journal of Special Education, 15,* 165–183.

Sternberg, R. J. (1981b). A componential theory of intellectual giftedness. *Gifted Child Quarterly, 25,* 86–93.

Sternberg, R. J. (1981c). The evolution of theories of intelligence. *Intelligence, 5,* 209–229.

Sternberg, R. J. (1981d). Intelligence and nonentrenchment. *Journal of Educational Psychology, 73,* 1–16.

Sternberg, R. J. (1981e). Intelligence as thinking and learning skills. *Educational Leadership, 39,* 18–20.

Sternberg, R. J. (1981f). The nature of intelligence. *New York University Education Quarterly, 12,* 3, 10–17.

Sternberg, R. J. (1981g). Nothing fails like success: The search for an intelligent paradigm for studying intelligence. *Journal of Educational Psychology, 73,* 142–155.

Sternberg, R. J. (1981h). Novelty-seeking, novelty-finding, and the developmental continuity of intelligence. *Intelligence, 5,* 149–155.

Sternberg, R. J. (1981i). Reasoning with determinate and indeterminate linear syllogisms. *British Journal of Psychology, 72,* 407–420.

Sternberg, R. J. (1981j). Testing and cognitive psychology. *American Psychologist, 36,* 1181–1189.

Sternberg, R. J. (1981k). Toward a unified componential theory of human intelligence. I: Fluid abilities. In M. Friedman, J. Das, & N. O'Conner (Eds.), *Intelligence and learning.* New York: Plenum.

Sternberg, R. J. (Ed.) (1982a). *Advances in the psychology of human intelligence* (Vol. 1). Hillsdale, NJ: Erlbaum.

Sternberg, R. J. (1982b). A componential approach to intellectual development. In R. J. Sternberg (Ed.), *Advances in the psychology of human intelligence* (Vol. 1). Hillsdale, NJ: Erlbaum.

Sternberg, R. J. (Ed.) (1982c). *Handbook of human intelligence.* Cambridge: Cambridge University Press.

Sternberg, R. J. (1982d). Lies we live by: Misapplication of tests in identifying the gifted. *Gifted Child Quarterly, 26,* 157–161.

Sternberg, R. J. (1982e). Natural, unnatural, and supernatural concepts. *Cognitive Psychology, 14,* 451–488.

Sternberg, R. J. (1982f). Nonentrenchment in the assessment of intellectual giftedness. *Gifted Child Quarterly, 26,* 63–67.

Sternberg, R. J. (1982g). Reasoning, problem solving, and intelligence. In R. J. Sternberg (Ed.), *Handbook of human intelligence.* Cambridge: Cambridge University Press.

Sternberg, R. J. (1982h). Who's intelligent? *Psychology Today, 16,* April, 30–39.

Sternberg, R. J. (1983a). Components of human intelligence. *Cognition, 15,* 1–48.

Sternberg, R. J. (1983b). Criteria for intellectual skills training. *Educational Researcher, 12,* 6–12, 26.

Sternberg, R. J. (1984a). Facets of intelligence. In J. R. Anderson & S. M. Kosslyn (Eds.), *Tutorials in learning and memory: Essays in honor of Gordon Bower.* San Francisco: Freeman.

Sternberg, R. J. (1984b). Higher-order reasoning in post-formal-operational thought. In M. Commons & C. Armon (Eds.), *Beyond formal operations: Late adolescent and adult cognitive development.* New York: Praeger.

Sternberg, R. J. (Ed.). (1984c). *Mechanisms of cognitive development.* San Francisco: Freeman.

Sternberg, R. J. (1984d). Mechanisms of cognitive development: A componential approach. In R. J. Sternberg (Ed.), *Mechanisms of cognitive development.* San Francisco, Freeman.

Sternberg, R. J. (1984e). A theory of knowledge acquisition in the development of verbal concepts. *Developmental Review, 4,* 113–138.

Sternberg, R. J. (1984f). What cognitive psychology can (and cannot) do for test development. In B. S. Plake (Ed.), *Social and technical issues in testing: Implications for test construction and usage.* Hillsdale, NJ: Erlbaum.

Sternberg, R. J. (in press-a). A contextual view of the nature of intelligence. *International Journal of Psychology.*

Sternberg, R. J. (Ed.). (in press-b). *Human abilities: An information-processing approach.* San Francisco: Freeman.

Sternberg, R. J. (in press-c). Instrumental and componential approaches to the training of intelligence. In S. Chipman, J. Segal, & R. Glaser (Eds.), *Thinking and learning skills: Current research and open questions* (Vol. 2). Hillsdale, NJ: Erlbaum.

Sternberg, R. J. (in press-d). Macrocomponents and microcomponents of human intelligence: Some proposed loci of mental retardation. In P. H. Brooks, R. Sperber, & C. McCauley (Eds.), *Learning and cognition in the mentally retarded.* Hillsdale, NJ: Erlbaum.

Sternberg, R. J., & Bower, G. H. (1974). Transfer in part – whole and whole – part free recall: A comparative evaluation of theories. *Journal of Verbal Learning and Verbal Behavior, 13,* 1 – 26.

Sternberg, R. J., Conway, B. E., Ketron, J. L., & Bernstein, M. (1981). People's conceptions of intelligence. *Journal of Personality and Social Psychology, 41,* 37 – 55.

Sternberg, R. J., & Davidson, J. E. (1982). The mind of the puzzler. *Psychology Today, 16,* June, 37 – 44.

Sternberg, R. J., & Davidson, J. E. (1983). Insight in the gifted. *Educational Psychologist, 18,* 51 – 57.

Sternberg, R. J., & Detterman, D. K. (Eds.) (1979). *Human intelligence: Perspectives on its theory and measurement.* Norwood, NJ: Ablex.

Sternberg, R. J., & Downing, C. J. (1982). The development of higher-order reasoning in adolescence. *Child Development, 53,* 209 – 221.

Sternberg, R. J., & Gardner, M. K. (1982). A componential interpretation of the general factor in human intelligence. In H. J. Eysenck (Ed.), *A model for intelligence.* Berlin: Springer-Verlag.

Sternberg, R. J., & Gardner, M. K. (1983). Unities in inductive reasoning. *Journal of Experimental Psychology: General, 112,* 80 – 116.

Sternberg, R. J., Guyote, M. J., & Turner, M. E. (1980). Deductive reasoning. In R. E. Snow, P. A. Federico, & W. Montague (Eds.), *Aptitude, learning, and instruction: Cognitive process analyses of aptitude* (Vol. 1). Hillsdale, NJ: Erlbaum.

Sternberg, R. J., & Ketron, J. L. (1982). Selection and implementation of strategies in reasoning by analogy. *Journal of Educational Psychology, 74,* 399 – 413.

Sternberg, R. J., Ketron, J. L., & Powell, J. S. (1982). Componential approaches to the training of intelligent performance. In D. K. Detterman & R. J. Sternberg (Eds.), *How and how much can intelligence be increased?* Norwood, NJ: Ablex.

Sternberg, R. J., & McNamara, T. P. (in press). The representation and processing of information in real-time verbal comprehension. In S. E. Embretson (Ed.), *Test design: Contributions from psychology, education, and psychometrics.* New York: Academic Press.

Sternberg, R. J., & Neuse, E. (1983). Utilization of context in verbal comprehension. Manuscript submitted for publication.

Sternberg, R. J., & Nigro, G. (1980). Developmental patterns in the solution of verbal analogies. *Child Development, 51,* 27 – 38.

Sternberg, R. J., & Nigro, G. (1983). Interaction and analogy in the comprehension and appreciation of metaphors. *Quarterly Journal of Experimental Psychology*, *35A*, 17–38.

Sternberg, R. J., & Powell, J. S. (1982). Theories of intelligence. In R. J. Sternberg (Ed.), *Handbook of human intelligence*. Cambridge: Cambridge University Press.

Sternberg, R. J., & Powell, J. S. (1983). Comprehending verbal comprehension. *American Psychologist*, *38*, 878–893.

Sternberg, R. J., Powell, J. S., & Kaye, D. B. (1983). Teaching vocabulary-building skills: A contextual approach. In A. C. Wilkson (Ed.), *Classroom computers and cognitive science*. New York: Academic Press.

Sternberg, R. J., & Rifkin, B. (1979). The development of analogical reasoning processes. *Journal of Experimental Child Psychology*, *27*, 195–232.

Sternberg, R. J., & Salter, W. (1982). Conceptions of intelligence. In R. J. Sternberg (Ed.), *Handbook of human intelligence*. Cambridge: Cambridge University Press.

Sternberg, R. J., & Schustack, M. W. (1980). Components of casual inference. *Naval Research Reviews*, *33*, 48–62.

Sternberg, R. J., & Smith, C. (in press). Components of social intelligence *Social Cognition.*

Sternberg, R. J., & Spear, L. C. (in press). A triarchic theory of mental retardation. In N. Ellis & N. Bray (Eds.), *International review of research in mental retardation*, vol. 13. New York: Academic Press.

Sternberg, R. J., Tourangeau, R., & Nigro, G. (1979). Metaphor, induction, and social policy: The convergence of macroscopic and microscopic views. In A. Ortony (Ed.), *Metaphor and thought*. Cambridge: Cambridge University Press.

Sternberg, R. J., & Tulving, E. (1977). The measurement of subjective organization in free recall. *Psychological Bulletin*, *84*, 353–378.

Sternberg, R. J., & Turner, M. E. (1981). Components of syllogistic reasoning. *Acta Psychologica*, *41*, 37–55.

Sternberg, R. J., & Wagner, R. K. (1982). Automatization failure in learning disabilities. *Topics in learning and learning disabilities*, *2*, July, 1–11.

Sternberg, R. J., & Weil, E. M. (1980). An aptitude–strategy interaction in linear syllogistic reasoning. *Journal of Educational Psychology*, *72*, 226–234.

Sternberg, S. (1969). High-speed scanning in human memory. *Science*, *153*, 652–654.

Stevens, S. S. (1951). Mathematics, measurement, and psychophysics. In S. S. Stevens (Ed.), *Handbook of experimental psychology*. New York: Wiley.

Strang, R. (1930). Measures of social intelligence. *American Journal of Sociology*, *36*, 263–269.

Super, C. M. (1982). Application of multi-dimensional scaling techniques to the estimation of children's ages in field research. Manuscript in preparation.

Test of Basic Skills (1977). Princeton, NJ: Educational Testing Service.

Thomson, G. H. (1939). *The factorial analysis of human ability*. London: University of London Press.

Thorndike, E. L. (1920). Intelligence and its uses. *Harper's Magazine*, *140*, 227–235.

Thorndike, E. L. (1924). The measurement of intelligence: Present status. *Psychological Review, 31*, 219–252.

Thorndike, E. L. (1931). *Human learning.* New York: Century.

Thorndike, E. L., Bregman, E. O., Cobb, M. V., & Woodyard, E. I. (1926). *The measurement of intelligence.* New York: Teachers College.

Thurstone, L. L. (1924). *The nature of intelligence.* New York: Harcourt, Brace.

Thurstone, L. L. (1938). *Primary mental abilities.* Chicago: University of Chicago Press.

Thurstone, L. L. (1947). *Multiple factor analysis.* Chicago: University of Chicago Press.

Thurstone, L. L., & Thurstone, T. G. (1962). *Tests of Primary Mental Abilities* (rev. ed.). Chicago: Science Research Associates.

Tourangeau, R., & Sternberg, R. J. (1981). Aptness in metaphor. *Cognitive Psychology, 13*, 27–55.

Tourangeau, R., & Sternberg, R. J. (1982). Understanding and appreciating metaphors. *Cognition, 11*, 203–244.

Trabasso, T. (1972). Mental operations in language comprehension. In J. B. Carroll & R. O. Freedle (Eds.), *Language comprehension and the acquisition of knowledge.* Washington, D.C.: Winston.

Verbrugge, R., & McCarrell, N. (1977). Metaphoric comprehension: Studies in reminding and resembling. *Cognitive Psychology, 9*, 494–533.

Vernon, P. E. (1933). Some characteristics of the good judge of personality. *Journal of Social Psychology, 4*, 42–51.

Vernon, P. E. (1971). *The structure of human abilities.* London: Methuen.

Vernon, P. E. (1979). *Intelligence: Heredity and environment.* San Francisco: Freeman.

Vurpillot, E. (1968). The development of scanning strategies and their relation to visual differentiation. *Journal of Experimental Child Psychology, 6*, 632–650.

Vygotsky, L. S. (1978). *Mind in society: The development of higher psychological processes.* Cambridge: Harvard University Press.

Wagner, R. K., & Sternberg, R. J. (1983). Executive control of reading. Manuscript submitted for publication.

Wagner, R. K., & Sternberg, R. J. (in press). Practical intelligence in real-world pursuits: The role of tacit knowledge. *Journal of Personality and Social Psychology.*

Walker, R. E., & Foley, J. M. (1973). Social intelligence: Its history and measurement. *Psychological Reports, 33*, 839–864.

Wason, P. C. (1960). On the failure to eliminate hypotheses in a conceptual task. *Quarterly Journal of Experimental Psychology, 12*, 129–140.

Watson, J. B. (1930). *Behaviorism* (rev. ed.). New York: Norton.

Webster's New Collegiate Dictionary. (1976). Springfield, MA: G. & C. Merriam.

Wechsler, D. (1950). *The measurement and appraisal of adult intelligence* (4th ed.). Baltimore: Williams & Wilkins.

Wechsler, D. (1958). *The measurement and appraisal of adult intelligence* (5th ed.). Baltimore: Williams & Wilkins.

Wedeck, J. (1947). The relationship between personality and "psychological ability." *British Journal of Psychology, 37*, 133–151.

Weisz, J. R., Yeates, K. O., & Zigler, E. (1982). Piagetian evidence and the developmental-difference controversy. In E. Zigler & D. Balla (Eds.), *Mental retardation: The developmental-difference controversy.* Hillsdale, NJ: Erlbaum.

Werner, H., & Kaplan, E. (1952). *The acquisition of word meanings: A developmental study.* Monographs of the Society for Research in Child Development, No. 51.

Wertheimer, M. (1959). *Productive thinking* (rev. ed). New York: Harper & Row.

Whitely, S. E. (1980). Latent trait models in the study of intelligence. *Intelligence, 4*, 97–132.

Whitely, S. E., & Barnes, G. M. (1979). The implications of processing event sequences for theories of analogical reasoning. *Memory and Cognition, 7*, 323–331.

Wilkins, M. C. (1928). The effect of changed material on ability to do formal syllogistic reasoning. *Archives of Psychology* (No. 102).

Williams, D. S. (1972). Computer program organization induced from problem examples. In H. A. Simon & L. Siklossy (Eds.), *Representation and meaning: Experiments with information processing systems.* Englewood Cliffs, NJ: Prentice-Hall.

Willis, S. L., Schaie, K. W., & Lueers, N. (1982). Fluid-crystallized ability correlates of real-life tasks. Typescript. Pennsylvania State University.

Winston, P. H. (1974). Learning structural descriptions from examples. In P. H. Winston (Ed.), *The psychology of computer vision.* New York: McGraw-Hill.

Wissler, C. (1901). The correlation of mental and physical tests. *Psychological Review, Monograph Supplement, 3* (6).

Wittgenstein, L. (1953). *Philosophical investigations.* Oxford: Basil Blackwell & Mott.

Wober, M. (1974). Towards an understanding of the Kiganda concept of intelligence. In J. W. Berry & P. R. Dasen (Eds.), *Culture and cognition: Readings in cross-cultural psychology.* London: Methuen.

Wolford, G., & Fowler, C. A. (1982). Differential use of partial information by good and poor readers. In T. Tighe & B. Shepp (Eds.), *Interactions: Perception, cognition, and development: A second Dartmouth multidisciplinary conference.* Hillsdale, NJ: Erlbaum.

Wood, D., Shotter, J., & Godden, D. (1974). An investigation of the relationships between problem solving strategies, representation, and memory. *Quarterly Journal of Experimental Psychology, 26*, 252–257.

Woodworth, R. S., & Sells, S. B. (1935). An atmosphere effect in formal syllogistic reasoning. *Journal of Experimental Psychology, 18*, 451–460.

Yussen, S. R., & Kane, P. (in press). Children's concept of intelligence. In S. R. Yussen (Ed.), *The growth of reflection in children.* New York: Academic Press.

Zeaman, D., & House, B. J. (1963). The role of attention in retardate discrimination learning. In N. R. Ellis (Ed.), *Handbook of mental deficiency.* New York: McGraw-Hill.

Zeaman, D., & House, B. J. (1979). A review of attention theory. In N. R. Ellis (Ed.),

Handbook of mental deficiency, psychological theory, and research (2nd ed.). Hillsdale, NJ: Erlbaum.

Zigler, E. (1971). The retarded child as a whole person. In H. E. Adams & W. K. Boardman (Eds.), *Advances in experimental clinical psychology* (Vol. 1). New York: Pergamon Press.

Zigler, E. (1982). Developmental versus difference theories of mental retardation and the problem of motivation. In E. Zigler & D. Balla (Eds.), *Mental retardation: The developmental-difference controversy*. Hillsdale, NJ: Erlbaum.

Zigler, E., & Balla, D. (Eds.) (1982). *Mental retardation: The developmental-difference controversy*. Hillsdale, NJ: Erlbaum.

Author index

Subject index

abilities, 4, 12, 33, 77–8
  see also crystallized abilities; fluid abilities
ability tests, 190–1, 193, 251
abstract concepts, 224–5
abstract reasoning test, 124–5
academic intelligence, 59, 60, 61, 62, 63
academic psychology, 271–5
accommodation, 69
accuracy, 126–7
achievement, 269
  intelligence tests as predictors of, 124–5,
    306–8
adaptation (adaptive behavior), 41, 45–6,
  49–50, 58, 70, 326, 338
  and change, 54
  culture-specific, 53
  definition of, in triarchic theory, 329
  difference across groups, situations, 55–6,
    336, 338
  difficulty in, in retarded, 294
  see also environment, adaptation to,
    selection of, shaping of
adjunct information, 254–7
analogical reasoning, 108, 141–2, 164–5
  in testing models for componential
    analysis, 345, 346–7, 350–2, 368
  tests of componential theory of, 142–5,
    153–6
analogies, 6, 78, 131, 132, 332
  as basis of metaphor, 165, 166, 170–1, 172
  componential model of, 135–6, 356, 357,
    359–62
  inductive reasoning, 138–9
  as measure of intelligence, 5, 75, 108
  precueing in, 350–2
analogies task, 12–13, 126
  for children, 99–100, 101
  metacomponents in, 102–4
animal-name analysis, 156–7

anxiety (test-taking), 311, 312
application(s), 5, 12, 13, 305, 306
  componential analysis, 345, 347
  inductive reasoning, 134, 135, 138, 144,
    165, 332
  second-order relatedness of correspond-
    ing, 159–60, 161
application components, 106
aptitude–treatment interaction, 72
assessment, 38–9
  see also psychometric measurement of
    intelligence
Assessment Battery for Children (K-ABC),
  337
assimilation, 69
associative learning, 337
associative relatedness, 160–1, 162–3
atmosphere theory of categorical-syllogistic
  reasoning, 204
attention allocation, 94, 104–5, 111
attribute–value representation, 142–3, 150
attributes of words
  encoding and comparison, 242–57
  importance of, 245, 246
automatization of information processing,
  41–2, 71–3, 125, 318, 322, 326–7, 331
  components in, 128
  by gifted, 291
  inadequate, in retarded, 281, 292, 293, 298
  measurement of, 74, 75, 76, 77, 78, 93–6,
    304, 308–9
  production system use in, 116
  relation of ability to deal with novelty
    and, 73–4

Baganda (tribe), 34
Batoro (tribe), 34
behavior, 6, 120
  intelligent, 59, 60, 61–2, 63, 128, 322

task comprehension, 69–70, 71–2, 78,
  99–100
  model of, 92–93
task hierarchy, 111–14
task latencies, 74
task performance, 69–70, 71–2, 78, 79–83,
  268
  in automatic information processing, 93
  decomposing, in componential analysis,
    349–59, 368–9
  novelty in, 78, 79–83
  real-time verbal comprehension, 253–4,
    255–7
  typical, 36
task selection, 75–6, 337
  componential analysis, 347–50
  failure of explicit theories to provide basis
    for, 30–1
  giftedness research, 290
  in implicit theories, 68–70
  past use basis for, 67
task–situation–person interactions, 70,
  72–3
temporal cues (context), 221, 223, 234
test scores, 4, 313–14
tests, 5, 6, 8
  see also intelligence tests
Thematic Aperception Test, 269
theory construction, 39
third-order analogies, 157–8, 160–1, 162–4
time allocation, 332
  global/local planning, 302, 304, 332
  problem solution, 300, 301, 302–4, 305
  real-time verbal comprehension, 242,
    252–4, 257
top–down approach, 215, 217–19
  in triarchic theory, 319–22
TOTE (Test–Operate–Test–Exit), 97,
  114–15, 116
training of intelligence, 28, 38, 127, 338–41
  strategy, 153–6, 193–5
  transfer of, 339
  validation of theory of external decontex-
    tualization, 234–5
  vocabulary-acquisition skills, 219, 223
trait and behavioral checklists, 268–9
transformations (product), 6, 118
transitive inferences, 181–2
  linguistic–spatial mixture theory, 182–98
transitive-chain theory, 198–204, 205–7,
  208–13, 333
triarchic theory, 342–4
  giftedness in, 292
  goal of, 317–18
  implications of, 279, 315, 317–35

implications of, for intelligence testing,
  299–314
retardation in, 292–8
status of, 328–35
structure of, 318–28
subtheories, 41–2
tests of, 129–30
see also componential subtheory;
  contextual subtheory; experiential
  subtheory
"trick" problems, 81, 82, 83

unicausal inference, 175–6
unintelligence (behavior), 59, 61
United States
  intelligence in sociocultural milieu of, 58
  subcultures, 338
units (product), 6
units of analysis, 21, 24, 29, 37, 335
  componential subtheory, 97–114
  components' interrelations with, 114–18
unordered arrangement of factors, 6–7

vagueness
  of contextual views, 54, 57
validation
  criteria for, 344–5
  explicit theories of intelligence, 15–17
  implicit theories of intelligence, 34–5
  test items, 75
  triarchic theory, 328–35
  see also convergent validation; discrimi-
    nant validation; external validation;
    internal validation
value cues (context), 221
verbal ability(ies), 35, 73, 78, 101, 330
  in contextually based implicit theory, 58,
    60, 65–6, 68
  individual differences in, 340
verbal comprehension, 130
  acquisition of, 214–40
  defined, 214
  measurement of, 5, 214
  performance components in, 333–4
  real-time, 130, 241–57
  theories of acquisition of, 215–19
verbal concepts, 220
  acquisition of, 226–32
verbal intelligence, see abilities
verbal mediation (theory), 296
visual content, 6
visual scanning, 183, 187, 198
visualizability, 166, 207
vocabulary, 130
  achievement loading of, 306, 307